TREATMENT OF SHOCK
Principles and Practice

TREATMENT OF SHOCK

Principles and Practice

JOHN BARRETT, M.D.

Assistant Professor of Surgery
University of Illinois College of Medicine at Chicago;
Director, Trauma Unit
Cook County Hospital
Chicago, Illinois

LLOYD M. NYHUS, M.D.

Warren H. Cole Professor and Head of the Department of Surgery
University of Illinois College of Medicine at Chicago;
Surgeon-in-Chief
University of Illinois Hospital
Chicago, Illinois

Second Edition

Lea & Febiger   1986   Philadelphia

Lea & Febiger
600 Washington Square
Philadelphia, PA 19106-4198
U.S.A.
(215)922-1330

Library of Congress Cataloging-in-Publication Data
Main entry under title:

Treatment of shock.

Bibliography: p.
Includes index.
1. Shock. I. Barrett, John, 1945–   . II. Nyhus,
Lloyd M., 1923.
RB150.S5T73   1986   617'.21   85–18170
ISBN 0–8121–1008–0

First Edition, 1974

PRINTED IN THE UNITED STATES OF AMERICA

Print No.   4   3   2   1

Preface

In the 12 years that have elapsed since the first edition of this book was published, we have seen enormous strides in our understanding of the pathophysiology of the shock state. This new edition has been extensively rewritten to reflect this new understanding of shock and the methods necessary for its treatment. Part I of the book consists of an update of the effects of shock on the microcirculation and reflects our current understanding of the pathophysiology and treatment of these lesions. Part II is a much expanded view of the effects of shock on the vital organs and includes completely new sections on the brain and the liver as well as expanded concepts of the effects of shock on the lungs, heart, and kidney. The treatment of the underlying cause of shock is found in Part III, which includes a new section on the initial management of the patient in traumatic shock as well as new sections on the pharmacologic treatment of shock and the management of shock in infants and children.

Throughout the work, we have attempted to maintain a practical orientation for the physician who is called on to manage patients in shock. We have attempted to provide an understanding of the pathophysiology of shock as a background for the modern concepts of therapy.

With the increasing sophistication of modern medicine, and the rapid and rational delivery of patients in shock to medical facilities, the shock patient is now a more common sight in the emergency department, operating room, and intensive care sections of our hospitals. Many patients who formerly would have died are now surviving to present the clinician with the challenge of management of the shock state.

In 1872, Gross defined the shock state as "the rude unhinging of the machinery of life." Although modern understanding of shock now permits a more precise definition, shock continues to exert profound effects on the entire organism and on all organ systems. It is only by constantly updating our understanding of what shock is and what it does that we can plan a rational treatment approach. We have provided in this volume a current view of the state of the art of shock management by renowned national and international experts. We wish to thank each of them individually for their contribution to this work, as well as Ms. Catherine Judge in the publications office of the Department of Surgery at the University of Illinois, and the many people at Lea & Febiger, especially Raymond Kersey, without whose help this work would not have been possible.

Chicago

John Barrett, M.D.
Lloyd M. Nyhus, M.D.

Contributors

MICHAEL F. ADINOLFI, M.D.
Clinical Assistant Professor of Surgery,
Tulane University School of Medicine,
New Orleans, Louisiana

JOHN BARRETT, M.D.
Assistant Professor of Surgery,
University of Illinois College of Medicine at Chicago;
Director, Trauma Unit,
Cook County Hospital,
Chicago, Illinois

ARNOLD G. CORAN, M.D.
Professor of Surgery,
Head, Section of Pediatric Surgery,
Surgeon-in-Chief,
Mott Children's Hospital,
University of Michigan Medical School,
Ann Arbor, Michigan

ROBERT M. ELENBAAS, Pharm. D.
Associate Professor of Clinical Pharmacy,
Schools of Pharmacy and Medicine,
University of Missouri, Kansas City;
Clinical Pharmacist,
Department of Emergency Health Services,
Truman Medical Center,
Kansas City, Missouri

GLENN C. HAMILTON, M.D.
Associate Professor of Emergency Medicine and Internal Medicine,
Chairman and Program Director,
Department of Emergency Medicine,
Wright State University School of Medicine,
Dayton, Ohio

TAKASHI KAWASAKI, M.D., Ph.D.
Professor of Biochemistry,
Hiroshima University School of Medicine,
Hiroshima, Japan

WILLIAM ST. JOHN LACORTE, M.D.
Chief of Staff of Primary Care,
Tulane Medical Center,
New Orleans, Louisiana

ALLAN M. LEFER, Ph.D.
Ciba-Geigy Distinguished Scholar,
Professor and Chairman,
Department of Physiology,
Jefferson Medical College,
Philadelphia, Pennsylvania

SUSAN J. MARKOWSKY, Pharm. D.
Assistant Professor of Clinical Pharmacy,
College of Pharmacy,
University of Minnesota;
Clinical Pharmacist,
Department of Clinical Pharmacology,
St. Paul Ramsey Medical Center;
St. Paul, Minnesota

SEIJI MARUBAYASHI, M.D.
Research Associate,
Department of Biochemistry, and Department of Surgery,
Hiroshima University School of Medicine
Hiroshima, Japan

LOUIS MARZELLA, M.D., Ph.D.
Assistant Professor,
Department of Pathology,
University of Maryland, School of Medicine;
Research Programs,
Maryland Institute for Emergency Medical Services Systems,
Baltimore, Maryland

WOLFGANG J. MERGNER, M.D., Ph.D.
Professor, Department of Pathology,
University of Maryland;
University of Maryland Medical Systems,
University Hospital,
Baltimore, Maryland

LOREN D. NELSON, M.D.
Assistant Professor of Surgery and Anesthesiology,
University of Miami School of Medicine;
Associate Director, Surgical Intensive Care Unit,
Jackson Memorial Medical Center,
Miami, Florida

RONALD LEE NICHOLS, M.D.
Henderson Professor and Vice-Chairman, Department of Surgery;
Professor of Microbiology and Immunology,
Tulane University School of Medicine,
New Orleans, Louisiana

LLOYD M. NYHUS, M.D.
Warren H. Cole Professor and Head of the Department of Surgery,
University of Illinois College of Medicine at Chicago;
Surgeon-in-Chief,
University of Illinois Hospital,
Chicago, Illinois

MARC D. PALTER, M.D.
Research Fellow,
Section on Critical Care Medicine, Division of Surgery,
Boston University Medical Center,
Boston, Massachusetts

MATTI SALO, M.D.
Assistant Professor of Anesthesiology,
University of Turku;
Assistant Chief Anesthetist,
Turku University Central Hospital,
Turku, Finland

WILLIAM M. STAHL, M.D.
Professor and Vice-Chairman, Department of Surgery,
New York Medical College, New York;
Director of Surgery,
Lincoln Medical and Mental Health Center,
Bronx, New York

JOHN R. WESLEY, M.D.
Associate Professor of Surgery,
Attending Surgeon,
Section of Pediatric Surgery,
Mott Children's Hospital,
University of Michigan Medical School,
Ann Arbor, Michigan

BLAINE C. WHITE, M.D.
Associate Professor of Emergency Medicine and Research Coordinator,
Section of Emergency Medicine,
Michigan State University,
East Lansing, Michigan

STUART K. WILLIAMS, Ph.D.,
Searle Scholar,
Associate Professor,
Department of Physiology,
Jefferson Medical College,
Philadelphia, Pennsylvania

NEIL S. YESTON, M.D.
Associate Professor of Surgery; Chief, Section on Critical Care Medicine,
Division of Surgery,
Boston University Medical Center,
Boston, Massachusetts

Contents

PART III. TREATING THE UNDERLYING CAUSE

Part I
TREATING THE MICROCIRCULATORY LESIONS

Chapter 1
MICROCIRCULATION IN SHOCK

Allan M. Lefer • Stuart K. Williams

Shock is a multifaceted disorder that has a number of causes and a variety of pathophysiologic mechanisms. Our discussion is concerned with "circulatory shock" to differentiate it from other types of shock including anaphylactic shock, neurogenic shock, and electric shock, all of which are quite different from circulatory shock and involve primary disturbances in organ systems other than the circulatory system, e.g., respiratory, nervous, etc.

Circulatory shock can be defined as a sustained reduction in blood flow perfusing the vital tissues and cells of the body to an extent that results in significant tissue damage, and if uncorrected, can lead to death. There are a variety of types of circulatory shock including hemorrhagic (oligemic, hypovolemic), septic (endotoxic, bacteremic), cardiogenic (cardiac), traumatic, intestinal ischemic (splanchnic ischemic), acute pancreatitis (pancreatic), and burn (thermal) shock. Although these types of shock all have characteristic hemodynamic features and somewhat different time courses,[1] all have several common features. Nevertheless, all types of circulatory shock result in a severe hypotensive state at some stage in their development, and virtually all involve an early splanchnic vascular hypoperfusion and a later impairment of cardiac function. One important and consistent feature of circulatory shock is a fundamental insufficiency of microcirculatory flow leading to inadequate perfusion of the somatic cells of many of the important organs of the body. These alterations in the microcirculation, the effects of the resultant ischemia of the cells, and the modification of the components of the microcirculation are the major themes of this chapter.

FLUID AND ELECTROLYTE SHIFTS IN SHOCK

The sequelae of microvascular complications can be described simply as an insufficiency of blood perfusion to peripheral tissues resulting in cellular hypoxia and death. Concurrent with this insufficiency of flow is microcirculatory failure resulting from a chain of metabolic events. In the past, investigations into the effects of shock have focused on the macrocirculation since it was assumed that the microvascular bed suffers little damage until the shock process has become irreversible. However, a new understanding of the importance of the microcirculation in disease states has led to the belief that early in the shock state, damage occurs in the intrinsic regulatory processes that influence microvascular blood flow and exchange.

After a fall in mean arterial blood pressure, at least four major changes occur in the microcirculation. These include 1. disturbed diffusional transport, 2. loss of

Supported in part by the W.W. Smith Charitable Trust

3

myogenic adjustments, 3. nutritional shunting, and 4. rheological changes. All of these conditions can be summarized as the inability of the terminal vascular bed to regulate the orderly distribution of blood flow.

Severe circulatory shock can be considered the net result of several contributing factors. All of these factors can be linked directly to the deterioration of microcirculatory function and can be considered as altered performance of either blood flow, vascular exchange, or both. Alterations in blood flow are thus related to the suppression of autoregulation,[2] the occurrence of spontaneous vasomotion,[2] and diminished smooth muscle cell reactivity.[3] Changes in microcirculatory exchange function are related to an imbalance of hydraulic pressure and osmotic forces, a change from net fluid filtration to absorption resulting in hemodilution followed secondarily by the loss of fluid, the occurrence of plasma protein leakage, and later to impaired lymphatic drainage.

Elements of the Microcirculation

The major components of the microcirculation are arterioles, capillaries, and venules. The afferent vessels, the arterioles, as they approach the capillaries, are a single endothelial cell lining surrounded by layers of circular smooth muscle cells.[4] The smooth muscle layer becomes a single discontinuous layer at the level of the arteriolar-capillary junction. The arterioles are innervated primarily with adrenergic and a limited number of cholinergic fibers.[5] Capillaries consist of single endothelial cell tubes with no smooth muscle cell investment. The morphology of capillaries differs between tissues and generally relates to the permeability function in each tissue.[6] In the liver, spleen, and bone marrow, the capillaries are described as discontinuous, exhibiting gaps at interendothelial junctions.[7] Capillaries in the brain, heart, lungs, and muscle are characterized as continuous since the interendothelial junctions exhibit tight associations.[8] Venules are characterized by increasing diameter and increasing investment of smooth muscle cells.[6] There is sparse innervation of the small venules.

Changes in Microvascular Flow

During the initial stages of shock, as a direct result of lowered mean arterial blood pressure, the larger arterioles of the microvascular tree constrict.[9] This initial constriction can be terminated by treatment with sympatholytic drugs or α-adrenergic blockers indicating that this constriction is a result of compensatory neurogenic feedback.[10] The constriction of precapillary sphincters will subsequently lead to ischemia and a progression toward irreversibility. Further responses are the suppression of vasomotion,[9] a blunted response to constrictor stimuli,[3] and the inability to maintain intracapillary pressure.[11] In addition, because of the sustained arteriolar vasoconstriction, changes in precapillary sphincter activity have little effect on capillary blood flow. This results in the buildup of metabolic byproducts, and after several hours of oligemia, the terminal vascular bed becomes a passive structure incapable of compensatory adjustment.[10]

Microvascular Exchange in Shock

The maintenance of microcirculatory homeostasis exists as a balance between flow and capillary surface area, against hydraulic and osmotic pressure. The major determinant of fluid flux is capillary pressure (Pc) which is determined by 1. volume flow, 2. fluid exchange, and 3. autoregulation. The Starling equation permits the quantitative interpretation of the relationship between the major factors that influence fluid exchange in the microcirculation:

$$Q = k(Pc + \Pi i) - (Pi + \Pi p)$$

In this equation, Q represents net fluid flux (ml/min/100 g tissue), Pc is net capillary hydraulic pressure (mm Hg), Πi is interstitial or tissue pressure (mm Hg), Pi is interstitial hydraulic pressure (mm Hg), Πp is the capillary osmotic pressure (mm Hg), and k is the filtration constant of the endothelial cell membrane. Shock has an effect on all of these hemodynamic forces. The net effect of these forces on fluid flux is shown in Figure 1–1A. The major force of filtration is capillary hydraulic pressure (Pc) and the major force of absorption is the plasma oncotic pressure (Πp) whose major determinant is the concentration of plasma proteins.

Capillary pressure, Pc, is assumed to fall dramatically during initial shock, although this fall is somewhat offset by local regulation.[12] After prolonged hypotension and the onset of erratic microvascular flow, Pc drops precipitously and becomes variable throughout the microcirculation. Finally, with the drop of systemic pressure below 40 mm Hg, the observed Pc may be close to venous levels. This change is shown in Figure 1–1B. The final low Pc is mostly a result of the complete closure of terminal arterioles.[10] The net fluid movement during these stages can be seen as initial fluid absorption resulting in hemodilution, followed by a gradual changeover to a final small but persistent net filtration.[10]

With the fall in capillary pressure and subsequent hemodilution, the plasma colloid osmotic pressure (Πp) falls steadily from a level of approximately 25 mm Hg to values as low as 12 mm Hg. During the initial stages of shock, Πp remains low followed by a slow gradual increase. This reversal is most probably related to a rise in hematocrit.[10] Finally, the terminal phase of shock is characterized by an increase in hematocrit with concomitantly decreased Πp. The latter effect is exacerbated by the increased loss of plasma proteins during this stage because of increased permeability of the capillary endothelium.

To summarize, the shock state results in dramatic changes in both capillary pressure and plasma oncotic pressure. These changes result in marked shifts in the forces regulating fluid flux and in increased fluid levels in the extravascular space. Since many organs are relatively unaffected by changes in fluid permeability, it is unusual for peripheral edema to affect tissue survival. The lung, however, is extremely sensitive to increased extravasation of fluid resulting in the observed deleterious effects of pulmonary edema and other complications, i.e., adult respiratory distress syndrome (ARDS).

Blood Rheology and Shock

One problem often overlooked in discussions of hemodynamic changes observed during cardiovascular disease is the commonly observed changes in the rheologic properties of blood. Factors that govern rheologic properties are the concentration, shape, size, and deformability of suspended particles, the extent of cellular adhesion and aggregation, and finally the composition of the plasma.[13] With the occurrence of shock and associated changes in the plasma and blood components, we must pay closer attention to subsequent abnormalities in blood rheology. New interest has focused toward optimization of blood viscosity

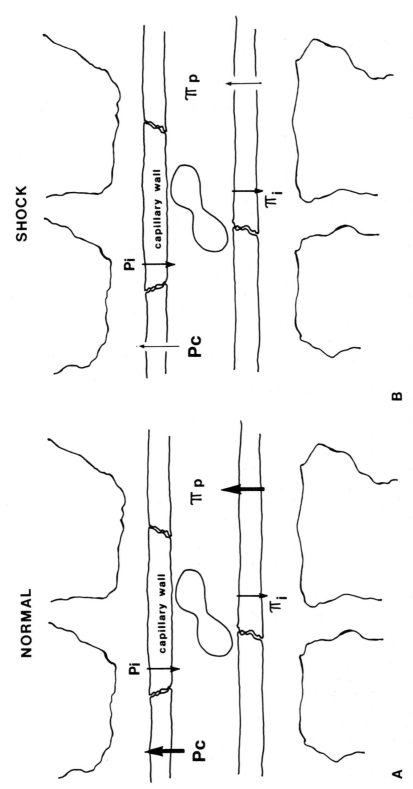

Fig. 1–1. Schematic diagram of pressure and osmotic forces that regulate fluid flux across the capillary wall. Normally (A) a near balance exists among Pc (capillary hydraulic pressure), Pi (interstitial hydraulic pressure), π_i (interstitial osmotic pressure), and π_p (plasma osmotic pressure). During shock (B) Pc falls dramatically, resulting in reduced fluid filtration. The osmotic effects of π also change as a result of hemodilution and increased permeability of the capillary wall to proteins.

through regulation of proper hematocrit, enabling blood flow to increase during ischemic states.[14] Furthermore, hematocrit-dependent blood flow is more sensitive in specific organs; specifically, blood flow to the heart and brain is extremely susceptible to changes in hematocrit.[14] As described earlier, shock leads to dramatic shifts in the forces governing the flow of fluid to and from the microcirculation resulting in associated changes in hematocrit. With shifts in hematocrit, the microcirculation would be expected to be severely compromised because of changes in blood viscosity. Moreover, the autoregulatory capacity of the vasculature is severely compromised at high hematocrit readings.[15] The complex interaction between shock-induced blood rheologic changes and compromised microcirculatory function is not fully understood. Future studies are essential to focus on these relationships.

SUBCELLULAR ALTERATIONS IN CIRCULATORY SHOCK

To understand the basic pathophysiologic mechanism of shock, we must analyze abnormal cellular processes as a consequence of the shock state. In general, investigations have clarified certain aspects of cellular biology during circulatory shock.

General Cell Changes

One of the basic cellular responses to a variety of types of shock is cell swelling. In general, most cells swell in response to ischemia, presumably because of inhibition of cell-membrane ion pumps, and the subsequent accumulation of cellular water. Hemorrhage has been shown to induce nuclear swelling in certain cells of the cerebral cortex but usually not in the cerebellar cortex.[1] Although swelling may be an early response to ischemia, several other types of ultrastructural alterations occur. Mitochondria have been shown to swell and to undergo degenerative changes such as invagination and breakup of internal cristae[1] in response to hemorrhage, endotoxin, or hypoxia. These changes occur in such diverse organs as liver, posterior pituitary gland, kidney, and skeletal muscle.

In addition to these mitochondrial changes, important alterations occur in other subcellular organelles. Thus, the endoplasmic reticulum is frequently splayed and scattered about the cytoplasm, alterations in the cell membrane can be readily observed, large invaginations in the sarcoplasmic reticulum can be seen, nuclear envelope damage often results, zymogen granules and other secretory granules are often broken or lysed (sometimes only remnants of their membrane are present), and there is an enlargement of the lysosomal vacuolar apparatus. Lysosomes may be increased or decreased in number depending on the metabolic and functional status of the cell. However, lysosomes usually appear as distended structures with large prominent vacuoles in shock. These vacuoles may be filled with cell debris or with a relatively clear fluid.

Mitochondria

In addition to ultrastructural evidence, physiologic and biochemical studies also show mitochondrial damage in shock. In general, there appears to be a significant degree of uncoupling of oxidative phosphorylation as reflected in a decreased mitochondrial P/O ratio, i.e., ratio of high-energy phosphate bonds generated per mole of oxygen consumed.[16] Perhaps even more significant is the well-documented decrease in state 3 respiratory activity (i.e., O_2 consumption occurring during phosphorylation in the presence of ADP and Pi) and in respiratory control ratios (RCR) indicative of uncoupling of oxidative phosphorylation.[17] These changes are much more prominent in hepatic rather than cardiac mitochondria, perhaps related to the degree of cellular acidosis present. In this regard, hepatocyte pH drops from about 7.1 to 5.9 in hemorrhagic shock, whereas myocardial cell pH appears to increase from 6.6 to 7.2 under the same conditions. Recently, efforts have been made to determine the subcellular basis for the impairment of mitochondrial function. One factor that is known to be crucial to mitochondrial function is the permeability and transport characteristics of the mitochondrial membrane. Thus, as mitochondrial function deteriorates, enhanced Na^+ entry[18] and greater K^+ loss from cells occur. Whether these ionic changes induce mitochondrial failure or whether they are a consequence of mitochondrial damage is not clear at present. Moreover, Ca^{++} transport across rat liver mitochondrial membranes is seriously impaired early in endotoxemia. This may be a critical step in mitochondrial damage, although more direct data are needed to interpret these findings.[19]

Another phenomenon that has received attention is the release of large amounts of acid hydrolases by lysosomes early in shock, which effectively attack and destroy the mitochondria during shock. This hypothesis has been verified in vitro, where lysosomal extracts were added to mitochondrial fractions in vitro and significant damage to the mitochondria resulted. The major lysosomal factor apparently responsible for mitochondrial swelling and uncoupling was a phospholipase. Lysosomal enzymes also inhibit mitochondrial calcium transport.[20]

Cell Membranes

Cell membrane function is another area of cell integrity that appears to be altered during shock. Although ultrastructural damage can occasionally be observed in the cell membrane, no quantitative morphometric data of cell membrane integrity during shock are presently available. Studies of this type would be extremely difficult to perform, and interpretation would be subject to a variety of problems such as sampling population size or fixation artifacts. Nevertheless, significant alterations in cell membrane function occur during circulatory shock. As an example, transport of Na^+ and K^+ across liver cell membranes is impaired in hemorrhagic shock. This membrane defect can be corrected by early treatment with fluid therapy. More recently, investigators have measured the resting transmembrane potential (E_m) of muscle cells as an index of active transport mechanisms of the cell membrane. These studies indicate that a decrease in E_m on the order of 20 mV occurs in skeletal muscle cells during hemorrhagic shock.[21] This change in membrane potential is associated with a decrease in extracellular water and an increase in intracellular Na^+. Once E_m decreases, the rate of rise and amplitude of the muscle action potential also decreases, which can result in impaired excitation of muscle. Although these changes themselves probably are not responsible for cell death, they undoubtedly contribute to conditions that result in cell damage during shock.

Lysosomes

Lysosomes are subcellular organelles that play a key role in the economy and life cycle of most mammalian cells. Lysosomes take many forms, shapes, and sizes, and may contain differing amounts of a variety of acid hydrolases. Despite the heterogeneity of form and function, lysosomes appear to play a relatively similar role in many organs during circulatory shock. In general, during hemorrhagic, endotoxic, intestinal ischemic, cardiogenic, and acute pancreatitic shock, lysosomes undergo marked degenerative changes. These changes occur principally in the organs that become ischemic or hypoxic during the shock state. Usually these tissues are the soft splanchnic organs, i.e., liver, pancreas, spleen, intestine, and sometimes other areas are involved such as kidney and skeletal muscle. In cardiogenic shock there is a direct myocardial lysosomal involvement as well. Janoff and co-workers[22] were the first investigators to recognize the importance of lysosomal changes in the pathophysiology of endotoxic and traumatic shock. Since then, many groups have substantiated and extended these findings in hemorrhagic, endotoxic, cardiogenic, intestinal ischemic, traumatic, and acute pancreatitic shock.[23] Thus, lysosomal involvement is well documented in circulatory shock.

Changes in lysosomes during shock appear to be related to the permeability of the lysosomal membrane, the configuration of the vacuolar apparatus of lysosomes, and the amount and type of acid hydrolase within the lysosome. Since lysosomes contain proteases, lipases, phospholipases, sulfatases, glucuronidases, glucosidases, and other acid hydrolases, their disruption and subsequent release of enzymes into the surrounding cytoplasm can be quite damaging to the structural integrity and metabolic functions of the cell.

Lysosomes are important intracellular organelles that normally play an important role in the economy and metabolism of somatic cells. Nevertheless, when shock develops, lysosomal membranes become leakier, largely in response to the localized hypoxia and ischemia.[24] Evidence of this tendency toward leakage is the finding of high activities of lysosomal hydrolases in the circulation, decreased activity of these enzymes in certain tissues, e.g., liver and pancreas, increased free-to-bound ratios of these enzymes in tissues, and enlarged lysosomes containing large vacuoles.[24] Lysosomal disruption also occurs early in myocardial ischemia.[24,25]

Lysosomal enzymes and products of lysosomal hydrolases, when injected or infused into normal animals, induce a variety of pathologic events including increased vascular permeability, pulmonary and cardiac damage, and production of a myocardial depressant factor (MDF), which is also produced in circulatory shock.[24]

Lysosomes therefore play an important role in the pathogenesis of shock. These organelles contribute to the proteolysis and lipolysis occurring in shock, as well as potentiate a variety of pathophysiologic events. Early use of lysosomal stabilizing agents such as cytoprotective prostaglandins or high doses of glucocorticoids prevents or minimizes lysosomal disruption and its consequences. Indeed, lysosomal membrane-stabilizing agents are among the most successful class of pharmacologic substances currently used in the treatment of circulatory shock.

NEW DIRECTIONS OF MICROCIRCULATORY PATHOPHYSIOLOGY IN SHOCK

Endothelium in Shock

The vascular endothelium has recently become the center of interest in biomedical research dealing with vascular related diseases. For years the endothelium was considered a quiescent cell with little metabolic, albeit some functional, importance in the maintenance of normal physiology. The current surge of interest is in part attributable to new techniques that have permitted the isolation of capillary and large vessel endothelial cells.[26-28] Recently developed techniques now permit the long-term culture of adult human endothelial cells.[29] With intense interest in the function of endothelial cells and the availability of new approaches for the in vivo and in vitro study of these cells, the importance of this cell in pathologic states is becoming defined.

ENDOTHELIAL CELL-MEDIATED EXCHANGE

The basic function that the exchange vessels of the microvasculature perform, namely exchange, is the most critical function of the cardiovascular system. This exchange function is most highly developed in humans and, as is so often the case, has the least inherent margin of safety. With the arrest of blood flow as experienced in shock, exchange is compromised rapidly, often leading to cell death. Our understanding of how exchange, or more precisely, vascular permeability, is compromised during shock is limited in part by our limited understanding of the mechanism of transendothelial solute and fluid transport. The endothelial cell is extremely permeable to water and thus does not restrict the passage of fluid. Fluid transport is determined by the Starling forces previously described. On the other hand, solute transport, most notably plasma protein transport, is highly restricted by the endothelial cell.[30] As shown in Figure 1-2, the continuous capillary, in this instance a coronary capillary, exhibits a continuous membrane barrier to solute transport. The major morphologic features that take part in transport are the numerous micropinocytic vesicles and the interendothelial junctions. The transport vesicles are highly selective in their capacity to transport proteins and may not play a significant role in the transport of bulk quantities of protein.[31] Junctional complexes vary between elements of the microvasculature differing in their degree of tightness.[8] Capillary junctions are characterized as tight, mostly because of their inability to transport even small molecules.[32] The junctions of the postcapillary venule, on the other hand, are less complex[33], and it is this area of the microvasculature that appears susceptible to dramatic increases in permeability during pathologic conditions.[34] Ischemic events result in the extravasation of protein and a permeability edema as a result of junctional opening at the postcapillary venules or in the case of the coronary microcirculation, a smaller focal leakage throughout all elements of the microcirculation.[35] The mechanisms that may explain this change in endothelial permeability include cell swelling, rheologic properties and effects of arachidonic acid metabolites, oxygen radicals, inflammation responses, and endothelial metabolic products.

ARACHIDONIC ACID METABOLISM

Arachidonic acid, a normal membrane constituent, can be metabolized to a number of biologically active cyclooxygenase and lipoxygenase products including prostacyclin (PGI_2), thromboxane A_2, bisenoic prostaglandins (e.g., PGD_2, PGE_2, and $PGF_{2\alpha}$), the hydroxy acids, and leukotrienes. The importance of these products in normal cardiovascular function is seen through their reported effects on platelet aggregation, contraction, and vascular tone and their effects on cellular metabolic function.

Under normal conditions, the endothelial cell acts as a physical barrier to solute

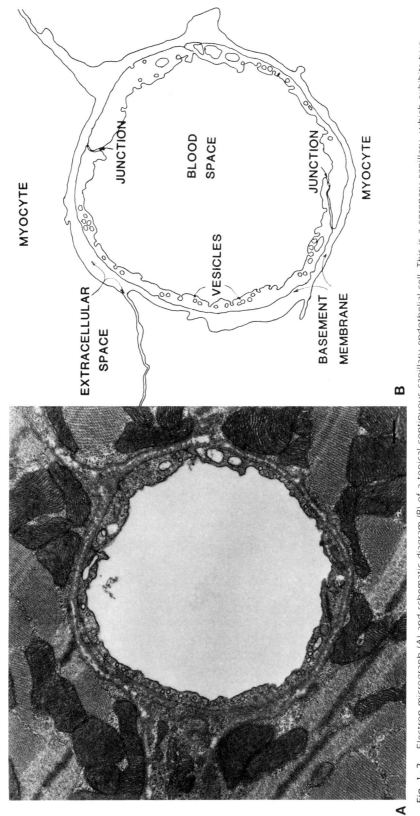

Fig. 1–2. Electron micrograph (A) and schematic diagram (B) of a topical continuous capillary endothelial cell. This is a coronary capillary, which exhibits two possible routes for transcapillary solute exchange, specifically intraendothelial junctional complexes and micropinocytic vesicles. The myocytes are closely associated with capillary endothelium resulting in a limited interstitial space.

11

and cellular exchange. For example, circulating platelets do not interact with undamaged endothelial cells lining blood vessel walls. The exact mechanism of this nonadherent factor is unknown; it is established, however, that the endothelial cell exhibits the capacity to produce prostacyclin (PGI$_2$), a known inhibitor of platelet aggregation. PGI$_2$ inhibits the actions of thromboxane A$_2$, which induces platelet aggregation.[36] Thus, a balance between PGI$_2$ and thromboxane A$_2$ production exists in the endothelial cell, which favors reduced platelet aggregation. Following injury, the endothelial cell exhibits increased adhesion of platelets, suggesting this balance has been altered.[37] Evidence also suggests that endothelial cells and platelets exhibit the ability to share substrates.[38] Endoperoxide precursors synthesized by platelets can be transferred to proximal endothelial cells resulting in the accumulation of metabolites. Thus, a great deal of cell-to-cell interaction occurs as would occur at the site of a growing thrombus. Finally, fatty acids themselves can damage the endothelial cell lining, resulting in either metabolic derangement or microvascular leakage.[39]

HEMOSTATIC ASPECTS OF SHOCK

A major function of the endothelial cell lining of both the macrocirculation and the microcirculation is the maintenance of a nonthrombogenic surface. The endothelial cell exhibits the ability to retard both the coagulation cascade and the adherence of circulating blood cells. However, following injury to the endothelial cell lining of the vascular system, metabolic activities are stimulated, resulting in the formation of microthrombi.

A major factor observed during shock that results in the alteration of normal hemostatic mechanisms is the occurrence of either reduced flow or cessation of blood flow. Under conditions of reduced flow, coagulation and cell aggregation begin, resulting in thrombus formation. The endothelial cell acts as a nidus for this reaction. At the same time, however, the fibrinolytic system is activated, leading to the dissolution of clots and the re-establishment of unobstructed blood flow. Recent evidence suggests that the endothelial cell plays an integral role in the production of plasmin, the major fibrinolytic enzyme in the blood.[40] Plasmin is derived from circulating plasminogen, a zymogen cleaved upon the action of plasminogen activator (PA). In vitro experiments have established that the endothelial cell has the capacity to synthesize and release plasminogen activator, suggesting that endothelium is actively involved in the regulation of clot dissolution.[40] Further progress must be made in establishing the ability of endothelium to secrete PA under the pathologic conditions observed during shock. The susceptibility of microvascular beds to "no-reflow" phenomena,[35] possibly as a direct result of the compromised ability of the microcirculation to reverse the clotting process through fibrinolysis, is an important unresolved question in shock.

LEUKOCYTE INTERACTION WITH THE ENDOTHELIAL CELL

Under normal conditions, both platelets and leukocytes exhibit minimal affinity for the endothelial cell lining of the vascular wall. Injury to the endothelial cell results in the synthesis or release of a number of active metabolites. The initial event in this cascade is the adherence of cells to the vascular wall stimulated by the appearance of chemo-attractant substances. For leukocytes, the major attractants known are complement intermediates (C5a), formyl peptide analogues, bacterial exudates, activated serum (zymosan), and leukotrienes formed by arachidonic acid metabolism, e.g., LTB$_4$.[41] The increased adhesion of leukocytes to the endothelial cell surface results from not only increased stickiness of leukocytes but also to the apparent activation of the endothelial cell surface. Thus, the leukocyte and the endothelial cell both appear to be activated following injury leading to increased cell-to-cell interaction. Although many metabolites and mediators have been reported to stimulate leukocyte-endothelial cell interaction, recent results with arachidonic acid derivatives are particularly exciting. The relatively low concentration necessary to stimulate this interaction suggests the importance of the pathophysiologic role of these metabolites in vivo.[41]

PLATELET-ENDOTHELIAL CELL INTERACTIONS

While major damage to the microvascular wall will lead to platelet adhesion to exposed interstitial collagen, simple injury of the endothelial cell lining without denudation is sufficient to stimulate a platelet response.[37] The nonadhesive nature of the normal endothelial cell has been attributed, in part, to the production of PGI$_2$, an extremely potent inhibitor of platelet aggregation.[42] However, results of pharmacologic studies suggest that other properties of the endothelial cell may be altered, resulting in platelet adhesion and aggregation. One proposed explanation is altered collagen synthesis of damaged endothelial cells.[43] Normal endothelium synthesizes predominantly basement membrane collagens (Types IV and V); following damage, however, the endothelium secretes interstitial collagens (Types I/III).[43] The expression of Types I/III collagens, rather than the more typical Types IV/V collagens on the surface of damaged endothelium, may provide one explanation for the increased platelet reactivity in injured endothelial cells. The belief that increased vascular reactivity to platelets and leukocytes requires extensive damage to the endothelium must be revised because minimal damage to the endothelial lining may be sufficient to alter metabolic function leading to increased cellular adhesiveness.

The elements of shock, including hypoxia, stagnated flow, buildup of endothelial cell metabolites, and the appearance of toxic agents provide the circumstances necessary for the occurrence of a dysfunctional endothelium. We must now consider that the endothelium actively maintains a normal nonthrombogenic surface through metabolic processes, and after injury these processes are disrupted. This metabolic shift, which may be caused by a number of factors, leads to altered adhesion of cells, loss of microvascular patency, insufficient perfusion, and cellular death.

ANGIOTENSIN CONVERTING ENZYME

As the importance of the endothelial cell in normal physiology has gained prominence, newer functional and metabolic properties of this cell have been identified and studied intensively. One enzymatic property identified as an exclusive function of endothelial cells is angiotensin-converting enzyme (ACE) activity.[44] This enzyme cleaves the relatively inactive decapeptide angiotensin I to the extremely potent vasopressor octapeptide angiotensin II. Immunocytochemical studies have localized this enzyme to the plasma membrane of the endothelial cell, and thus circulating angiotensin can rapidly be metabolized to active substrate without the requirement of cellular uptake.[44] Less is known concerning the regulation of this enzyme; however, both in vivo and in vitro data suggest that the activity may be altered in part by the availability of oxygen.[45] In this regard, hypoxia appears to cause a reduction in ACE activity.[46] This reduction results not only in the reduction in plasma angiotensin II concentration but in the appearance of elevated levels of precursors of the renin-angiotensin cascade, most notably renin. In addition, the reduction of ACE activity as a result of reduced PO_2 leads to increased bradykinin concentration. The buildup of bradykinin, as would be expected in shock-induced hypoxia, has profound effects on capillary permeability—most strikingly, increased permeability of plasma proteins. This leakage would result in increased fluid flow and in certain organs, a permeability edema. The cellular effects of bradykinin are focused on the opening of postcapillary venular junctions resulting in the rapid extravasation of protein. Intravital microscopic examinations indicate that bradykinin is one of the most potent agonists of venular protein leakage.[47] In addition, these substances may also have effects on the vesicular pathway of macromolecular leakage.

ENDOTHELIAL CELL CONTRACTILITY

Cytoplasmic proteins such as actin and myosin, and cytoskeletal proteins participate in the maintenance of cellular architecture during motility as well as the maintenance of shape in response to shear stress.[48] The endothelial cell exhibits the ability to reorganize cytoskeletal and contractile elements during changes in shear stress.[49] In addition, endothelial cells localized in the postcapillary venule respond to numerous agents by creating leaky sites, presumably by some form of cellular contraction. In vitro and in vivo experiments have indicated that endothelial cells possess bundles of contractile proteins that resemble stress fibers of cultured cells.[50] The appearance of these stress fibers can be changed by altered velocity and turbulence of blood flow. During hemodynamic stress, as is experienced during shock, the maintenance of normal intimal as well as cell-to-cell integrity may be compromised. This stress may be the direct result of changes in rheologic factors such as blood viscosity or reduced flow, or may be the result of action of metabolites on contractile proteins.

ENDOTHELIUM IN SHOCK

We have just begun to appreciate the role of the endothelial cell in maintaining not only normal cardiovascular function but the integral role the endothelial cell plays in pathophysiologic processes such as shock. The functional importance of endothelial cells to these conditions spans membrane processes such as vesicular transport and cell-to-cell interaction, metabolic functions such as arachidonic acid metabolism and generation of vasoactive substances, to new studies on the contractile nature of the endothelium. An endothelial cell relaxing factor has been discovered in the endothelium of large arteries.[51] This unknown substance, thought to be a lipid, has the remarkable ability to produce vasodilation when activated or released by a variety of vasoactive substances. The derangement of endothelial cell function in shock, and the resultant complications observed in the microcirculation amplify our need to understand more fully the functional importance of this cell.

New Pharmacologic Approaches to Shock Relating to the Microcirculation

The pharmacologic treatment of shock has evolved over the past thirty years from vasopressors to α-adrenergic blockers to glucocorticoids to a variety of newer agents including eicosanoids, cardiotonics, and membrane-stabilizing agents. Among the newer, more successful pharmacologic agents employed in shock are a number of classes of compounds that involve the regulation of transport of key substances across the cell membrane (e.g., calcium entry blockers) to substances that either enhance or modulate the role of the endothelium. In this connection, angiotensin-converting enzyme inhibitors, which block the conversion of angiotensin I to angiotensin II (a process that occurs almost exclusively in the endothelium), as well as prostacyclin, an eicosanoid produced largely by the vascular endothelium, have proved to be valuable therapeutic agents in the treatment of circulatory shock. Figure 1–3 illustrates the actions of these three classes of therapeutic agents and their interaction with the microcirculation and the cells it perfuses.

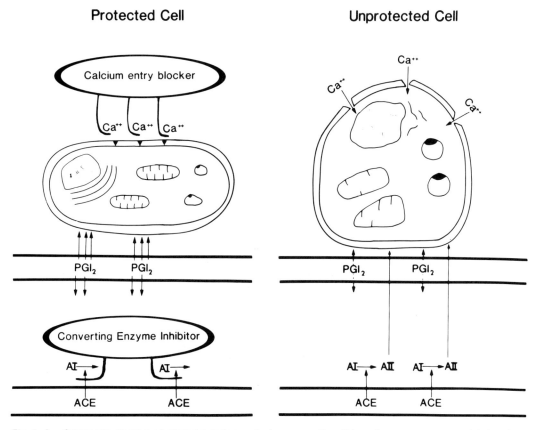

Fig. 1–3. Schematic diagram of microcirculation perfusing a somatic cell (e.g., liver, pancreas, muscle) showing a nucleus, endoplasmic reticulum, mitochondria, and lysosomes. Prostacyclin (PGI$_2$) and angiotensin-converting enzyme (ACE) are generated in the endothelium. Extracellular calcium (Ca^{++}) enters by specific calcium channels. Protection against cell damage is achieved by angiotensin-converting enzyme preventing the formation of angiotensin II (AII), calcium entry blockers preventing calcium flooding of the cell, or by enhancing PGI$_2$ production.

CALCIUM ENTRY BLOCKERS IN SHOCK

Calcium is known to play a vital role in a broad range of biological functions. Flooding of the cell with calcium is generally thought to mediate many of the damaging processes occurring in ischemia and shock (Fig. 1–3). Agents that prevent the accumulation of calcium in the cytosol markedly alter a variety of intracellular processes and protect the cell from damage. Calcium entry blockers are classified as vasodilators primarily because of their ability to block the inward transsarcolemmal Ca^{++} flux in the smooth muscle of peripheral arterioles.[52] However, additional vasodilator mechanisms have also been hypothesized for these agents. Calcium entry blockers reduce myocardial contractility, thereby reducing myocardial oxygen demand, and produce coronary dilation, which increases myocardial oxygen supply.[53] In addition, calcium entry blockers have been reported to inhibit thromboxane-induced vasoconstriction,[54] protect against arachidonate-induced sudden death in rabbits,[55] and preserve the integrity of hepatocytes in hypoxic, perfused liver preparations.[56]

The efficacy of calcium entry blockers as therapeutic agents in circulatory shock has not been widely investigated. Hackel et al.[57] reported increased survival rates in dogs in hemorrhagic shock given verapamil when compared with untreated dogs in hemorrhagic shock; they also reported a decreased occurrence of myocardial lesions. Others report a reduction in portal hypertension and a less severe small intestinal hemorrhage.[58] Hess et al.[59] also reported that verapamil protects in hemorrhagic shock. Beneficial actions of nimodipine have also been reported in traumatic shock in rats,[60] including increased survival rates and reduced accumulation of plasma MDF. Nitrendipine, a new dihydroperidine analog, has been found to improve circulatory function and prolong survival in hemorrhagic[61] and traumatic[62] shock. Thus, the consensus is that calcium entry blockers, if given carefully so as not to reduce myocardial function or blood pressure too precipitously, can protect in shock states.

ANGIOTENSIN CONVERTING ENZYME INHIBITORS IN SHOCK

Angiotensin II is a naturally occurring peptide that exerts prominent vasoconstriction as well as producing cardiac lesions resulting from damage to the coronary endothelium. The discovery of angiotensin-converting enzyme inhibitors (CEI) by Ferriera[63] has led to the advent of converting enzyme inhibitors as specific means of examining the role of the renin-angiotensin system. Since converting enzyme is localized to a large extent in the pulmonary endothelium, this enzyme is ultimately related to the microcirculation (see Fig. 1–3). The first use of converting enzyme inhibitors in shock was conducted in dogs subjected to hemorrhage and anesthetized with pentobarbital sodium.[64] These investigators noted enhanced cardiac output and decreased total peripheral resistance in shocked dogs treated with a nonapeptide inhibitor of converting enzyme (teprotide). This effect was observed immediately upon administration of the converting enzyme inhibitors even during oligemia while mean arterial blood pressure (MABP) was maintained at 40 mm Hg. No effect on mean bleedout volume was observed. Morton et al.[65] later also found increased survival rates in dogs subjected to hemorrhage and treated with teprotide.

Trachte and Lefer[66] in a more comprehensive study showed that captopril exerted a marked protective effect in cats subjected to hemorrhagic shock. Moreover, these workers measured plasma angiotensin II concentrations by a specific radioimmunoassay and showed a 70 to 80% inhibition of angiotensin II formation during hemorrhage. Later, these workers showed that infusion of angiotensin II to animals given captopril reversed the protective effect of the drug,[67] suggesting that the prevention of angiotensin II formation was the key action of captopril. More recently, a nonsulfhydryl-converting enzyme inhibitor, enalapril, has been shown to also protect during hemorrhagic shock.[68] Enalapril and its parent compound enalaprilat also have the added beneficial effects of antagonizing the coronary constrictor effect of angiotension II and not exerting some of the side effects of sulfhydryl group containing agents.[69]

Thus, angiotensin-converting enzyme inhibitors, by preventing the endothelium from forming the potent vasoconstrictor and cardiac-lesion producing substance, angiotensin II, can exert a marked protective effect in circulatory shock, particularly during hemorrhagic shock.

PROSTACYCLIN IN CIRCULATORY SHOCK

Prostacyclin (PGI$_2$) is a prostanoid generated by the vascular endothelium, and was discovered by Vane and Moncada in 1976.[70] PGI$_2$ is thought to protect the endothelium from the potentially damaging effects of platelets or chemotactic stimuli (see Fig. 1–3). Prostacyclin is the most potent inhibitor of platelet aggregation and the most potent vasodilator and membrane-stabilizing agent of all the prostaglandins thus far studied.[71] Despite these and other desirable properties, prostacyclin has not been widely studied as a therapeutic agent in shock. This is partially a result of its recent discovery and its general unavailability until a few years ago. Also, early usage of prostacyclin suggested that its vasodepressor effects were so strong that PGI$_2$ might not be useful in shock.[70]

Recently, lower doses of prostacyclin were found to exert important protective effects in traumatic shock in rats[72,73] and endotoxic shock in cats and dogs.[74,75] The results of these studies indicate that prostacyclin dilates the splanchnic[76] and systemic[71] vascular beds, prevents platelet aggregation,[71] stabilizes lysosomal membranes, and prevents formation of the cardiotoxic peptide MDF,[75,76] and improves survival. These results were achieved at low to moderate doses of PGI$_2$ (20 to 200 ng/kg/min).

Similar doses of prostacyclin were also shown to preserve the integrity of the ischemic heart,[77] liver,[78] and limb.[79] Prostacyclin exerts a cytoprotective action both in the intact blood-perfused animal[77] or patient as well as in physiologic salt solutions given to constant flow-perfused organs.[78] Therefore, inhibition of platelet aggregation and increasing perfusion to the ischemic organ do not appear to be primary mechanisms in the protection against ischemic damage. Rather, cytoprotection may prove to be the decisive action of prostacyclin in these settings. Cytoprotection may take the form of membrane stabilization, prevention of proteolysis, increases in cyclic AMP levels in cells, and prevention of toxic factor formation, as well as other actions. Certainly, vasodilation and prevention of platelet aggregation may contribute to these cytoprotective effects of prostacyclin in the intact animal. Further investigations on prostacyclin in shock and in ischemic states will undoubtedly reveal complex mechanisms of action of this interesting prostaglandin.

One drawback in the use of prostacyclin is its lack of biological stability. Recently, some derivatives of prostacyclin, including 6,9-thiaprostacyclin[76] and carbocyclic prostacyclin[80,81] have been shown to have many of the important effects of prostacyclin but are much more chemically stable. A metabolically stable prostacyclin derivative would be of great importance in the treatment of shock. Nevertheless, prostacyclin, a product of the endothelium, appears to be a useful agent in circulatory shock and in related ischemic disorders. For a review of all the prostaglandins in circulatory shock, the reader is referred to a recent review.[82]

In summary, all three modes of therapy have in common the preservation of cellular integrity and the protection of subcellular organelles from the consequences of ischemia, hypoxia, and acidosis. Calcium entry blockers prevent the entry of calcium into the cell and modulate the deleterious effect of calcium flooding of the cell; prostacyclin stabilizes cell membranes and increases cyclic 3'5'-AMP levels inside many cell types; and converting enzyme inhibitors prevent the severe vasoconstrictor and ischemia-producing effects of angiotensin II. Moreover, all three agents prevent the formation of toxic factors in shock as exemplified by myocardial depressant factor (MDF). It is therefore of considerable interest that agents closely related to microcirculatory function are also of primary importance in therapy for shock states.

REFERENCES

1. Lefer, A.M., and Spath, J.A., Jr.: Pharmacologic basis for the treatment of circulatory shock. *In* Cardiovascular Pharmacology, 2nd Ed. Edited by M. Antonaccio. New York, Raven Press, 1984.
2. Hinshaw, L.B.: Autoregulation in normal and pathological states including shock and ischemia. Circ. Res., *28*:46, 1971.
3. Zweifach, B.W.: Etiology of the shock syndrome. Heart Bull., *14*:21, 1965.
4. Jeffords, J.G.,and Knisely, M.H.: Concerning the geometric shapes of arteries and arterioles. A contribution to the biophysics of health disease and death. Angiology, *7*:105, 1956.
5. Bloch, E.H.: Principles of the microvascular system. Invest. Ophthal., *5*:250, 1966.
6. Wolff, J.R.: Ultrastructure of the terminal vascular bed as related to function. *In* Microcirculation. Vol. 1. Edited by G. Kaley and B.M. Altura. Baltimore, University Park Press, 1977.
7. Weiss, L.: Bone marrow. *In* Histology, 4th Ed. Edited by L. Weiss and R.O. Greep. New York, McGraw-Hill, 1977.
8. Simionescu, N., Simionescu, M., and Palade, G.E.: Structural basis of permeability in sequential segments of the microvasculature. II. Pathways followed by microperoxidase across endothelium. Microvasc. Res., *15*:17, 1978.
9. Zweifach, B.W.: Microcirculatory derangements as a basis for the lethal manifestations of experimental shock. Br. J. Anaesthesiol., *30*:466, 1958.
10. Zweifach, B.W., and Fronek, A.: The interplay of central and peripheral factors in irreversible hemorrhagic shock. Prog. Cardiovasc. Dis., *18*:147, 1975.
11. Zweifach, B.W., and Intaglietta, M.: Fluid exchange across capillaries during hemorrhagic hypotension. Fed. Proc., *27*:512, 1968.
12. Zweifach, B.W.: Local regulation of capillary pressure. Circ. Res., *28*:129, 1971.
13. Nordt, F.J.: Hemorheology in cerebrovascular diseases: approaches to drug development. Ann. N.Y. Acad. Sci., *416*:651, 1983.
14. Fan, F., Chen, R.Y.Z., Schuessler, G.B., and Chien, S. Effects of hematocrit variations on regional hemodynamics and oxygen transport in the dog. Am. J. Physiol., *238*:H545, 1980.
15. Crowell, J.W., and Smith, E.E. Determinant of optimal hematocrit. J. Appl. Physiol., *22*:501, 1967.
16. White, R.R., Mela, L., Bacalzo, L.V. Jr., Olofsson, K., and Miller, L.: Hepatic ultrastructure in endotoxemia, hemorrhage, and hypoxia: Emphasis on mitochondrial changes. Surgery, *73*:525, 1973.
17. Schumer, W., Das Gupta, T.K., Moss, G.S., and Nyhus, L.M.: Effect of endotoxemia on liver cell mitochondria in man. Ann. Surg., *71*:875, 1970.
18. Baue, A.E., Wurth, M.A., and Sayeed, M.: Alterations in hepatic cell function during hemorrhagic shock. Bull. Soc. Int. Chir., *5*:387, 1972.

19. Chaudry, I.H.: Cellular mechanisms in shock and ischemia and their correction. Am. J. Physiol., *245*:R117, 1983.
20. Mellors, A., Tappel, A.L., Sawant, P.L., and Desai, I.D.: Mitochondrial swelling and uncoupling of oxidative phosphorylation by lysosomes. Biochem. Biophys. Acta, *143*:299, 1967.
21. Trunkey, D.D., Illner, H., Wagner, I.Y., and Shires, G.T.: The effect of hemorrhagic shock on intracellular muscle action potentials in the primate. Surgery, *74*:241, 1973.
22. Janoff, A., Weissmann, G., Zweifach, B.W., and Thomas, L.: Pathogenesis of experimental shock: IV. Studies on lysosomes in normal and tolerant animals subjected to lethal trauma and endotoxemia. J. Exp. Med., *116*:451, 1962.
23. Lefer, A.M.: The role of lysosomes in circulatory shock. A minireview. Life Sci., *19*:1803, 1976.
24. Lefer, A.M.: Lysosomes in the pathogenesis of circulatory shock. *In* Handbook of Shock and Trauma. Vol. 1. Edited by B.M. Altura, A.M. Lefer, and W. Schumer. New York, Raven Press, 1983.
25. Spath, J.A., Jr., Lane, D.L., and Lefer, A.M.: Protective action of methylprednisolone on the myocardium during experimental myocardial ischemia in the cat. Circ. Res., *35*:44, 1974.
26. Jaffe, E.A., Nachman, R.L., Becker, C.G., and Minick, C.R. Culture of human endothelial cells derived from umbilical veins. J. Clin. Invest., *52*:2745, 1973.
27. Wagner, R.C., and Matthews, M.A.: The isolation and culture of capillary endothelium from epididymal fat. Microvasc. Res., *10*:286, 1975.
28. Williams, S.K., Gillis, J.F., Matthews, M.A., Wagner, R.C., and Bitensky, M.W.: Isolation and culture of brain endothelial cells: morphology and enzyme activity. J. Neurochem., *35*:374, 1980.
29. Jarrell, B.W., Shapiro, S.S., Williams, S.K., Carabasi, R.A., Levine, E., Mueller, S., and Thornton, S.: Human adult endothelial cell growth in culture. J. Vasc. Res., *1*:757, 1984.
30. Renkin, E.M.: Transport of proteins by diffusion, bulk flow and vesicular mechanisms. Physiologist, *23*:57, 1980.
31. Williams, S.K.: Vesicular transport of proteins by capillary endothelium. Ann. N.Y. Acad. Sci., *416*:457, 1983.
32. Wissig, S.L.: Identification of the small pore in muscle capillaries. Acta Physiol. Scand., *463*:33, 1979.
33. Simionescu, N., Simionescu, M., and Palade, G.E.: Open junctions in the endothelium of the post capillary venules of the diaphragm. J. Cell Biol., *79*:27, 1978.
34. Arfors, K.E., Rutili, G., and Svensjo, E.: Microvascular transport of macromolecules in normal and inflammatory conditions. Acta Physiol. Scand., *463*:93, 1979.
35. McDonagh, P.F.: The role of the coronary microcirculation in myocardial recovery from ischemia. Yale J. Biol. Med., *56*:303, 1983.
36. Marcus, A.J., Weksler, B.B., and Jaffe, E.A.: Enzymatic conversion of prostaglandin endoperoxide (PGH_2) and arachidonic acid to prostacyclin by cultured human endothelial cells. J. Biol. Chem., *253*:7138, 1978.
37. Curwen, K., Gimbrone, M.A., Jr., and Handin, R.I.: In vitro studies of thromboresistance: the role of prostacyclin (PGI_2) in platelet adhesion to cultured normal and virally transformed human vascular endothelial cells. Lab. Invest., *42*:366, 1980.
38. Marcus, A.J., Weksler, B.B., Jaffe, E.A., and Broekman, M.J.: Synthesis of prostacyclin from platelet-derived endoperoxides by cultured human endothelial cells. J. Clin. Invest., *66*:979, 1980.
39. Sedar, A.W., Silver, M.J., Kocsis, J.J., and Smith, J.B.: Fatty acids and the initial events of endothelial damage seen by scanning and transmission electron microscopy. Atherosclerosis, *30*:273, 1978.
40. Luskutoff, D.J., Levin, E.G., and Mussoni, L.: Fibrinolytic components of cultured endothelial cells. *In* Pathobiology of the Endothelial Cell. Edited by H. Nossel and H.J. Vogel. New York, Academic Press, 1982.
41. Hoover, R.L., Folger, W.A., Haering, B.R., Ware, B.R., and Karnovsky, M.J.: Adhesion of leukocytes to endothelium: roles of divalent cations, surface charge, chemotactic agents and substrate. J. Cell Sci., *45*:73, 1980.
42. Moncada, S., Gryglewski, S., Bunting, S., and Vane, J.R.: An enzyme isolated from arteries transforms prostaglandin endoperoxides to an unstable substance that inhibits platelet aggregation. Nature, *263*:663, 1976.
43. Gimbrone, M.A., and Buchanan, M.R.: Interactions of platelets and leukocytes with vascular endothelium: in vitro studies. Ann. N.Y. Acad. Sci., *401*:171, 1982.
44. Ryan, U.S., Ryan, J.W., Whitacker, C., and Chiu, A.: Localization of angiotensin converting enzyme (Kininase II). Immunocytochemical and immunofluorescence. Tissue Cell, *8*:125, 1976.
45. Milledge, J.S., and Catley, D.M.: Renin, aldosterone, and converting enzyme during exercise and acute hypoxia in humans. J. Appl. Physiol., *52*:320, 1982.
46. Stalcup, S.A., Lipset, J.S., Woan, J.M., Leunberger, P.J., and Mellins, R.B.: Inhibition of angiotensin converting enzyme activity in culture endothelial cells by hypoxia. J. Clin. Invest., *63*:966, 1979.
47. Delmaestro, R.F., Bjork, J., and Arfors, K.E.: Increase in microvascular permeability induced by

enzymatically generated free radicals. II. Role of superoxide anion radical, hydrogen peroxide, and hydroxyl radical. Microvasc. Res., *22*:255, 1981.

48. Herman, I.M., Crisona, N., and Pollard, T.D.: Relation between cell activity and the distribution of cytoplasmic actin and myosin. J. Cell Biol., *90*:84, 1981.

49. Wong, A., Pollard, T.D., and Herman, I.M.: Endothelial cells contain stress fibers in vivo. J. Cell Biol., *91*:299a, 1981.

50. Herman, I.M., Pollard, T.D., and Wong, A.J.: Contractile proteins in endothelial cells. Ann. N.Y. Acad. Sci., *401*:50, 1982.

51. Furchgott, R.F.: The role of the endothelium in the responses of vascular smooth muscle to drugs. Annu. Rev. Pharmacol. Toxicol., *24*:175, 1984.

52. Henry, P.D.: Comparative pharmacology of Ca^{2+}-antagonists: nifedipine, verapamil, diltiazem. Am. J. Cardiol., *46*:1047, 1980.

53. Stoepel, K., Heise, A., and Kazda, S.: Pharmacological studies of the antihypertensive effect of nitrendipine. Arzneim. Forsch., *31*:2056, 1981.

54. Smith, E.F., III, Lefer, A.M., and Nicolaou, K.C.: Mechanism of coronary vasoconstriction induced by carbocyclic thromboxane A_2. Am. J. Physiol., *240*:H493, 1981.

55. Okamatsu, S., Peck, R.C., and Lefer, A.M.: Effects of calcium channel blockers on arachidonate-induced sudden death in rabbits. Proc. Soc. Exp. Biol. Med., *166*:551, 1981.

56. Lefer, A.M.; Hepatoprotective actions of calcium channel blockers. *In* Falk Symposium #38: Mechanisms of Hepatocyte Injury and Death. Edited by D. Keppler, H. Popper, L. Bianchi, and D. Reutter. Lancaster, England, M.T.P. Press, 1985, p. 361.

57. Hackel, D.B., Mikat, E.M., Whalen, G., Reimer, K., and Rochlani, S.P.: Treatment of hemorrhagic shock in dogs with verapamil: effects on survival and on cardiovascular lesions. Lab. Invest., *41*:356, 1979.

58. Whalen, G.F., Hackel, D.B., and Mikat, E.: Prevention of portal hypertension and small bowel hemorrhage in dogs treated with verapamil during hemorrhagic shock. Circ. Shock, *7*:399, 1980.

59. Hess, M.L., Mahany, T.M., and Greenfield, L.J.: Calcium channel blockers in shock. *In* Molecular and Cellular Aspects of Shock and Trauma. Vol. 3. Edited by A.M. Lefer and W. Schumer. New York, Alan R. Liss, Inc., 1983.

60. Lefer, A.M., and Carrow, B.A.: Salutary actions of nimodipine in traumatic shock. Life Sci., *29*:1347, 1981.

61. Hock, C.E., Su, J.-Y., and Lefer, A.M.: Salutary effects of nitrendipine, A new calcium entry blocker in hemorrhagic shock. Eur. J. Pharmacol., *97*:37, 1984.

62. Lefer, A.M., Hock, C.E., and Su, J.-Y.: Beneficial actions of nitrendipine during traumatic shock in rats. *In* Nitrendipine: A Ca^{2+} Antagonist. Edited by A. Scriabine, S. Vanov, and K. Deck. Baltimore, Urban & Schwarzenberg, 1984.

63. Ferriera, S.H.: A bradykinin potentiating factor (BPF) present in the venom of Bothrops jararaca. Br. J. Pharmacol. Chemother., *24*:163, 1965.

64. Errington, M.L., and Rocha e Silva, M.: On the role of vasopressin and angiotensin in the development of irreversible haemorrhagic shock. J. Physiol. (London), *242*:119, 1974.

65. Morton, J.J., Semple, P.F., Ledingham, I.M., Stuart, B., Tehrani, M.A., Garcia, A.R., and McGarrity, G.: Effect of angiotensin-converting enzyme inhibitor (SQ 20,881) on the plasma concentration of angiotensin I, angiotensin II and arginine vasopressin in the dog during hemorrhagic shock. Circ. Res., *41*:301, 1977.

66. Trachte, G.J., and Lefer, A.M.: Beneficial action of a new converting enzyme inhibitor (SQ 14,225) in hemorrhagic shock in cats. Circ. Res., *43*:576, 1978.

67. Trachte, G.J., and Lefer, A.M.: Mechanism of the protective effect of angiotensin converting enzyme inhibition in hemorrhagic shock. Proc. Soc. Exp. Biol. Med., *162*:54, 1979.

68. Freeman, J.G., Hock, C.E., Edmonds, J.S., and Lefer, A.M.: Anti-shock actions of a new converting enzyme inhibitor, enalaprilic acid, in hemorrhagic shock in cats. J. Pharmacol. Exp. Ther., *231*:610, 1984.

69. Lefer, D.J., and Lefer, A.M.: Coronary vascular actions of the converting enzyme inhibitor, enalapril. Proc. Soc. Exp. Biol. Med., *175*:211, 1984.

70. Moncada, S., Gryglewski, R.J., Bunting, S., and Vane, J.R.: A lipid peroxide inhibits the enzyme in blood vessel microsomes that generates from prostaglandin endoperoxides the substance (prostaglandin X) which prevents platelet aggregation. Prostaglandins, *12*:715, 1976.

71. Lefer, A.M., Ogletree, M.L., Smith, J.B., Silver, M.J., Nicolaou, K.C., Barnette, W.E., and Gasic, G.P.: Prostacyclin: Profile of a potentially valuable agent for preserving jeopardized myocardial tissue in acute myocardial ischemia. Science, *200*:52, 1978.

72. Lefer, A.M., and Smith, E.F., III.: Protective action of prostacyclin in myocardial ischemia and trauma. *In* Prostacyclin. Edited by J.R. Vane and S. Bergstrom. New York, Raven Press, 1979.

73. Lefer, A.M., Sollott, S.L., and Galvin, M.J.: Beneficial actions of prostacyclin in traumatic shock. Prostaglandins, *17*:761, 1979.

74. Fletcher, J.R., and Ramwell, P.W.: The effects of prostacyclin (PGI₂) on endotoxin shock and endo-toxin-induced platelet aggregation in dogs. Circ. Shock, 7:299, 1980.

75. Lefer, A.M., Tabas, J., and Smith, E.F., III.: Salutary effects of prostacyclin in endotoxic shock. Pharmacology, 21:206, 1980.

76. Lefer, A.M., Trachte, G.J., Smith, J.B., Barnette, W.E., and Nicolaou, K.C.: Circulatory and platelet actions of 6,9-thiaprostacyclin (PGI₂-S) in the cat. Life Sci., 25:259, 1979.

77. Ogletree, M.L., Lefer, A.M., Smith, J.B., and Nicolaou, K.C.: Studies on the protective effect of prostacyclin in acute myocardial ischemia. Eur. J. Pharmacol., 56:95, 1979.

78. Araki, H., and Lefer, A.M.: Cytoprotective actions of prostacyclin during hypoxia in the isolated perfused cat liver. Am. J. Physiol., 238:H176, 1980.

79. Szczeklik, A., Gryglewski, R.J., Nizankowski, R., Szczeklik, J., Skawinski, S., and Gluszko, P.: Pros-tacyclin in the therapy of peripheral arterial disease. *In* Advances in Prostaglandin and Thrombox-ane Research. Vol. 7. Edited by B. Samuelsson, P.W. Ramwell, and R. Paoletti. New York, Raven Press, 1980.

80. Karim, S.M.M., and Adaikan, P.G.: Inhibition of platelet aggregation with oral administration of a stable prostacyclin analogue (carboprostacyclin) in baboons. IRCS Med. Sci., 8:338, 1980.

81. Morton, D.R., Bundy, G.L., and Nishizawa, E.E.: Five-membered ring-modified prostacyclin ana-logs. *In* Prostacyclin. Edited by J.R. Vane and S. Bergstrom. New York, Raven Press, 1979.

82. Lefer, A.M.: Role of prostaglandins and thromboxanes in shock states. *In* Handbook of Shock and Trauma. Vol. 1: Basic Sciences. Edited by B.M. Altura, A.M. Lefer, and W. Schumer. New York, Raven Press, 1983.

Chapter 2

VOLUME REPLACEMENT IN SHOCK

John Barrett • Lloyd M. Nyhus

Volume replacement is a problem that can be found in any form of shock, but it is a particular problem for the patient in hemorrhagic or hypovolemic shock. This chapter therefore concentrates particularly on the volume replacement necessary in these states.

To understand the rationale of fluid replacement in shock, it is necessary to recall how fluid is functionally lost to the patient in shock. As has been discussed in the previous chapter all shock states can be viewed as having a final common pathway at the cellular level. An impairment of cellular perfusion eventually resulting in some degree of cellular hypoxia is characteristic of all shock states.[1] The hypoxic cell undergoes alterations caused by a reduction in the level of energy available to the cell. There is uncoupling of oxidative phosphorylation[2] and the cell enters a phase of anaerobic metabolism. All energy-dependent functions of the cell are depressed. There are specific alterations in the sarcoplasmic reticulum in the mitochondria and the lysosomes.[1,3-5] There are also alterations that occur at the level of the cellular membrane.

The cellular membrane has an active transport mechanism and as such requires energy for its intact functioning. The membrane normally maintains a low intracellular sodium in comparison to the extracellular fluid by means of an energy-dependent "sodium pump." When the cell is subjected to a shock state, the active transport of sodium across the membrane is affected. The sodium leaks into the cell and the intracellular sodium concentration increases.[6,7] In effect, the sodium pump is "broken" because of a reduction in the level of the available energy. In a similar manner, potassium leaks out of the cell and there is a reduction in the intracellular potassium levels with a corresponding increase in levels in the interstitial fluid.[7,8] It is important to realize that as the sodium moves into the cell, it carries water with it and cellular swelling occurs. These fluid and ionic shifts are believed to be responsible for the alterations in potential differences across the membrane. It has been shown that the normal resting potential difference of -90 mV can be altered to values of -72 to -50 mV.[9-12] These alterations in transmembrane potential difference also appear to be related to the metabolic derangements in the cell.[13,14]

In addition to the fluid and ionic shifts across the cellular membrane, there is also a movement of extracellular fluid into the capillaries to replace the volume loss that occurs in hemorrhagic or hypovolemic shock. Transcapillary refilling of the circulating volume also occurs at the expense of the extracellular fluid. The net effect of these fluid movements is a reduction in the extracellular fluid volume.

Even though the patient may present in shock because of blood loss, what is functionally lost is not only the blood but the movement of extracellular fluid.

Fluid replacement in hemorrhagic shock can be viewed under two separate requirements. The first is that of volume replacement and the second is that of restoration of oxygen-carrying ability.

VOLUME REPLACEMENT

When considering volume replacement, two questions must be addressed: 1. What kind of fluid? and 2. How much to give a particular patient?

Both colloids and crystalloids have been proposed as suitable for fluid replacement in hemorrhagic shock. The difference between the two types of fluid is that the colloids are oncotically active. Proponents of colloid resuscitation argue that crystalloid dilutes the plasma proteins and reduces the plasma oncotic pressure. They further argue that these alterations result in an increased leakage of fluid across the capillary into the interstitium, hence creating interstitial edema. On the other hand, the proponents of crystalloid resuscitation argue that the colloid also leaks into the extravascular space and that the presence of colloid in the interstitium elevates the tissue oncotic pressure. They again argue that this elevation in the tissue oncotic pressure results in further fluid extravasation into the interstitium, thus creating even worse interstitial edema. At the center of the controversy are the effects that these various fluid combinations have on the lung, which is probably the most sensitive organ to this interstitial edema.

Although the "colloid-crystalloid controversy" still rages, to at least some extent there is a general agreement that in low-volume hemorrhagic shock, the losses can be replaced by crystalloid alone.[15] It has been shown that the reduction in colloid oncotic pressure (COP) produced by crystalloid resuscitation may not be detrimental to the lung. It has also been shown that if the COP is artificially reduced by plasmaphoresis, peripheral edema, ascites, and weight gain can be produced, but pulmonary edema does not occur. The reason that the lung is capable of protecting itself from this influx of fluid is that there is a marked increase in pulmonary lymph flow, which can increase by severalfold under these conditions.[16] In addition, radioisotope-labelled albumin has been shown to extravasate into the lung interstitium in baboons in hemorrhagic shock, and appears to correlate with increased lung water, while this increase does not occur in animals resuscitated by crystalloid.[17] Holcroft et al.[18], using a baboon model, also showed in a comparison of plasmanate to lactated Ringer's solution for resuscitation in hemorrhagic shock that there was more extravascular lung water in the plasmanate group. In a study of patients undergoing abdominal aortic operations Virgilio[19] compared the effects of lactated Ringer's solution resuscitation to those of albumin. Even though the lactated Ringer's group had a low COP and required much more volume, there was no difference in postoperative pulmonary shunting or respiratory failure. Moss[20] showed that crystalloid resuscitation tends to reverse the disruption of collagen fibrils in the lungs of baboons in shock and concluded that crystalloid resuscitation does not cause pulmonary failure. In a classic study by Lucas[21] conducted on severely injured patients, the effects of lactated Ringer's resuscitation were compared with those of lactated Ringer's solution plus albumin. He found that the albumin group required more ventilatory support and had a higher incidence of renal insufficiency, implying that colloid may even be detrimental. Studies in trauma patients by Lowe et al.[22], comparing lactated Ringer's solution with 5% albumin plus lactated Ringer's solution, failed to show any difference in the two groups.

It seems therefore that there is little evidence to support the contention that colloids are superior to crystalloids in fluid resuscitation of hemorrhagic shock, and there is at least some evidence that they may be worse. It is also certainly true that colloids are more expensive than crystalloids and hence their use can hardly be supported without good evidence of their superiority.

Crystalloids

Lactated Ringer's solution is probably the most commonly used resuscitative fluid in hemorrhagic shock and is in the resuscitative regimen recommended by the Committee on Trauma of the American College of Surgeons.[15] It is the closest available mimic of extracellular fluid and hence acts as an ideal substitute when extracellular fluid defects occur. Concern has been expressed over the "lactate" in "lactated" Ringer's solution. It has been argued that this will make the effects of anaerobic metabolism worse since it will exacerbate the pre-existing lactic acidosis. Even though it is true that lactated Ringer's solution does contain 28 mEq of lactate, this has not been shown to be a problem clinically. As has been pointed out by Mannix,[23] the lactate in the lactated Ringer's solution is the sodium salt, and it is the hydrogen ion that causes the problem in acidosis. In practice, if the patient is adequately resuscitated, the lactate levels will fall whether or not lactated Ringer's solution is used.[24] Finally, the lactate in Ringer's solution is converted in the liver into bicarbonate, adding an additional buffering effect.

Normal saline solution is probably as good a resuscitative fluid as lactated Ringer's solution, although it does suffer from the theoretic disadvantages of being less balanced from a physiologic point of view. The excessive concentration of chloride ions could cause a problem to the patient with impaired renal function. This is, however, difficult to prove, and studies on both animals[25] and humans[26] have shown little difference between lactated Ringer's and normal saline solution.

Colloids

The most widely used colloid plasma substitute in the United States is 5% albumin.[27] Disadvantages of its use include its high cost and the need for heat-treating to kill hepatitis virus. Two forms of dextran are available as colloid plasma substitutes. Dextran 70 (6% in isotonic saline solution, which has an intravascular retention of 30% after 24 hours) and dextran 40 (10% in isotonic saline solution), which has a shorter retention. Advantages of dextran include long shelf life, reasonable cost, and lack of hepatitis transmission. Concern has been expressed over dextran's possible interference with typing and cross-matching of the patient's blood. Possible advantages include the effects of dextrans on the rheologic properties of blood. At low flow rates, such as occur in the microcirculation, the viscosity of the blood increases and the ability of dextrans to alter viscosity may have some deficit.[28,29] Hydroxyethyl starch (HES) is a synthetic colloid with an intravascular retention similar to that of dextran 40.[30] After brief storage in the liver and kidney, HES is cleared without difficulty. Advantages include its low cost, nonantigenic nature, and little effect on clotting.

CLASSIFICATION OF HEMORRHAGIC SHOCK

Depending on the amount and rate of blood loss, specific physiologic alteration will be evident in the patient. Use can be made of these changes broadly to classify the patient as having one of four types of hemorrhagic shock.[15]

Class I

This consists of the acute loss of up to 15% of the estimated blood volume. In the average 70 kg man with a blood volume of 7% of body weight (5 liters) this would correspond to a loss of up to 750 ml of blood. Such small losses produce few physiologic alterations. There is minimal if any alteration in pulse. The blood pressure remains stable and there is no alteration in the capillary blanch test. This is performed by pressing on the nail bed to blanch the subungual capillary bed. The pressure is then released and the time taken for the capillaries to refill is noted. A normal filling response should be less than two seconds. Class I hemorrhage is well tolerated by the patient, corresponding as it does to the donation of a pint or so of blood. This small blood loss is easily replaced without significant overt physiologic alterations, by means of an alteration in venous capacitance. At any time approximately 75% of the total blood volume is on the venous side of the circulation and 25% is on the arterial side. A slight alteration in venous capacitance can therefore compensate for a class I hemorrhage. In theory, a class I hemorrhage requires no fluid replacement therapy.[31]

Class II

This is the acute loss of 15 to 30% of circulating volume, or approximately 750 to 1500 ml of blood. This is considered to be a moderate bleed. At this level of hemorrhage, overt physiologic alterations do begin to appear. There is a moderate increase in pulse rate, and an alteration in blood pressure is noted. The initial change is an increase in the diastolic pressure with subsequent narrowing of the pulse pressure. This alteration is caused by the initiation of sympathetic peripheral vasoconstriction. The subsequent increase in peripheral resistance causes the increase in diastolic pressure. Capillary refill is still present but is frequently delayed.

Blood loss of this magnitude requires volume replacement. Because of the alterations in capillary permeability and the fluid shifts mentioned earlier, it is necessary to replace each unit of blood loss with at least three units of crystalloid. A patient who presents after an acute hemorrhage with vital signs of 110/90 mm Hg blood pressure and pulse 110/min may well be suffering class II hemorrhage and can require as much as 2000 to 4000 ml of lactated Ringer's solution for adequate resuscitation.

Class III

This consists of acute loss of 30 to 40% of the circulating blood volume. It is a major bleed. Such patients present with reductions in systolic pressure and a low pulse pressure. In addition, at this level of acute blood loss there is evidence of impairment of organ function. The patient is often anxious and frequently confused. There is a reduction in urinary output, and the capillary blanch test may be positive. Blood losses of this magnitude require urgent replacement with large volumes of lactated Ringer's solution, perhaps as much as 4500 to 6000 ml. At this level of bleed there will also be a requirement for oxygen-carrying capacity, and such patients will require blood or blood components as part of their resuscitation.

Class IV

This consists in the acute loss of 40 to 50% of the circulating blood volume. This is a massive bleed, and such patients present in a state of profound shock. They are profoundly hypotensive with marked tachycardia. There is significant evidence of organ impairment. The patient has a negligible urinary output and is confused and lethargic. Resuscitation consists of massive fluid and blood replacement.

Acute losses of greater than 50% of the total volume of circulating blood usually result in irreversible shock unless the patient receives resuscitation during the course of the hemorrhage.

Use of this classification system allows some degree of estimation to be made concerning the volume of blood lost acutely. Care should be taken, however, not to administer fluid blindly to a patient in a state of shock according to any present formula. Measurements of resuscitation such as pulse, blood pressure, CVP, and even hemodynamic measurements from Swan-Ganz catheter placement, if needed, as well as evidence of organ perfusion—urinary output, capillary blanch, and sensorium and metabolic measurements (lactate and pH levels)—will also give assistance in judging the adequacy or otherwise of the resuscitation.

In addition, it must be remembered that some patients are bleeding at a rate that cannot be tolerated and will require definitive surgical control of the hemorrhage as part of their resuscitation. A patient who presents in hemorrhagic shock and who cannot be resuscitated despite adequate fluid replacement should be considered to be in this category and should undergo surgical control of the bleeding site if possible. A second, and more subtle class of patients also belongs in this group. This is the patient who presents a state of hemorrhagic shock but who is resuscitated after the initial fluid bolus. After the initial resuscitation is successful, the rate of fluid administration should be reduced. If the patient lapses back into the shock state when the rate of fluid administration is reduced, the bleeding is continuing, and early surgical intervention should be considered.

BLOOD AND BLOOD COMPONENTS

Although we do not normally consider it as such, blood is an organ, and if we are to consider blood transfusion, it should be to replace the loss of a particular organ function of the patient's native blood. Among the functions of blood are oxygen-carrying capacity, carbon dioxide removal, acid-base buffering availability, and transportation of hormones and antibodies. The most common initial indication for blood replacement in acute hemorrhage is a reduction in oxygen-carrying capacity.[31]

Oxygen is carried in the blood in two forms. The major portion of oxygen is carried bound to hemoglobin and a relatively small amount is carried in solution in the plasma. The total amount of oxygen carried in blood can be derived from the following equation.

$$(O_2) = (Hb \times 1.35 \times \% \text{ saturation}) + (Po_2 \times 0.0031)$$

where (O_2) = oxygen concentration in 100 ml of blood; Hb = hemoglobin concentration in $g/100$ ml; and Po_2 = partial pressure of oxygen.

Use of this equation results in a value of 20 ml/dl of O_2 on the arterial side of the circulation and 15 ml/dl on the venous side. Thus the normal arteriovenous oxygen difference of 5 ml/dl is derived. It is important to note that on the venous side there is a significant reserve of O_2 still available. Because of this, it is possible to reduce the total amount of Hb and not alter the amount of O_2 delivered to the tissues. Because of this reserve function, it is possible to allow a certain loss of blood (or of O_2 carrying-capacity) without replacement with blood. Such patients will still require volume replacement with crystalloid but because O_2 delivery to the tissues remains unimpaired, there is no indication for blood replacement.

This concept of an "allowable blood loss" has been explored by Bourke and Smith,[32] who have devised an equation that can be used to calculate the amount of blood that can be lost before blood replacement is required.

$$\text{Allowable blood loss} =$$
$$\text{estimated blood volume} \times \text{change in hematocrit} \times (3 - \text{average hematocrit})$$

Provided that volume is maintained, most patients can afford a reduction of their hematocrit value without undergoing significant physiologic compensation. Using the above equation for a 70 kg patient with a blood volume of 5 liters and an initial hematocrit reading of 45% and allowing a reduction of 34%, Bourke and Smith calculated the loss as

$$\text{Allowable blood loss} = 5000 \times (0.45 - 0.34) \times (3 - 0.45 + 0.34) = 1432 \text{ ml}$$

As will be recalled from our classification of hemorrhagic shock this would correspond to a class II bleed. Although such bleeds do require volume resuscitation, the reduction in oxygen-carrying capacity can be tolerated without depriving the tissues of O_2 delivery.[31]

It is possible therefore to classify patients who present with acute blood loss into three types:

	Blood Loss	Hemorrhage Class	Replacement
Type 1	0–700 ml	I	none
Type 2	700–1500 ml	II	fluid
Type 3	>1500 ml	III, IV	fluid, blood

Although some patients may require no replacement whatsoever and others require only asanguineous fluid replacement there is clearly a group (type 3) who will require blood as part of their resuscitation. Every effort should be made to maintain a hematocrit reading of 30% or greater in this group.

Autotransfusion

When confronted with a patient who does require blood replacement as part of resuscitation, the physician must decide which type of blood to use. Before resorting to the use of homologous (banked) blood some consideration should be given to the possibility of autologous blood transfusion or autotransfusion.

Autotransfusion offers several advantages. It can provide at least a partial solution to the problem of donor blood shortage, it is immediately available, and there is no need to type and cross-match the patient's blood. Blood group incompatibility is avoided. In addition, there is no risk of disease transmission from donor blood, and it provides a source of fresh warm blood. Liquid blood is stored in blood banks at 4°C. Transfusion of blood at this low temperature requires an energy expenditure by the patient to warm the blood to core temp (37°C). Furthermore blood at 4°C is considerably more viscous than at 37°C. For all of these reasons, therefore, autologous autotransfusions have advantages.[33]

METHODS

Simple methods of autotransfusion such as Trendelenburg positioning or air splints have been advocated. The most often used prehospital method is the application of an inflatable set of dungarees on the patient. Called either military antishock trousers (MAST) or pneumatic antishock garment (PASG), these can be inflated over both legs and abdomen. Although they have been advocated in a variety of situations, their most common clinical application is in the acutely traumatized patient in shock. Initially it was believed that the application of such garments produced an autotransfusion effect by emptying blood from the veins of the lower extremity and pelvis. More recent work has shown that the amount of blood autotransfused under these conditions is minimal, and that these garments appear to act by resistance and decreasing the volume of tissue perfused.[34-36]

COLLECTION AND REINFUSION

The most simple method of autotransfusion is that of collection of the lost blood and reinfusion. This can be done by a filter, or collection of the shed blood and separation of its components and then reinfusion of the packed cells.[37] Systems such as the Sorenson (Sorenson Research Company, Salt Lake City, Utah) are examples of the former; the Haemonetics system (Haemonetic Corp., Natick, Mass) is an example of the latter.

The decision as to which type of system to use depends on the particular needs of the patient. In the acutely traumatized patient with massive blood loss, the system will have to meet definite criteria. It should be easy and quick to assemble, easy to operate by available personnel, safe, transportable, and effective.[37] Such systems are becoming increasingly available.

PATIENT SELECTION

The first criterion that must be met by patients being considered for autotransfusion is that they do in fact require blood as part of their resuscitation. Patients who present with class III or greater hemorrhagic shock would qualify. The second criterion, and the more difficult, is that the blood must be available for autotransfusion. This implies that the blood should still be present within a body cavity, and should not be contaminated. The most common trauma patient who meets these requirements presents with blunt or penetrating chest trauma and a marked reduction in systolic pressure with evidence of a class III bleed. In addition, there must be presumed lack of contamination of the thoracic cavity. Such patients generally present with evidence of a massive hemothorax with hypotension, flat neck veins, and dullness to percussion over the involved side of the chest. As preparations are made for chest tube insertion in these patients, arrangements should also be made for autotransfusion.[38]

An additional group of patients who can be considered for autotransfusion are those with blunt abdominal trauma and class III hemorrhage. As the abdomen is opened during the exploratory laparotomy the contained blood can be evacuated into the autotransfusion device. The surgeon can then complete the abdominal exploration to ensure that there has been no contamination of the blood by associated injury to the gastrointestinal tract. If the blood proves to be uncontaminated, as is frequently the case in isolated splenic or liver injuries, the autotransfusion can proceed.

Major vascular procedures, such as abdominal aortic aneurysm resection, offer good possibilities for the use of autotransfusion, as do selected peripheral and orthopedic procedures.[39]

PROBLEMS

Infection.   The possibility of bacteremia is real with every autotransfusion, and antibiotic prophylaxis should be considered. A difficult decision may have to be made in the case of penetrating chest trauma when the integrity of the diaphragm and the presence of possible contamination are unknown. Such questions arise in penetrating trauma to the lower thorax in patients who would otherwise fulfill the criteria for autotransfusion. Such patients may have had diaphragmatic penetration and contamination from associated injuries to the gastrointestinal tract.

It is our policy to proceed with the autotransfusion in these patients, for although we agree that contaminated blood should not be deliberately autotransfused, should such occur the results are not as disastrous as one may suppose. One study showed that when contaminated blood was autotransfused into dogs, all the dogs had positive cultures, but all the infections resolved on antibiotic coverage.[40,41] In addition, human patients who received contaminated autotransfused blood had no complications.[42,43]

The amount of contamination can be reduced by washing the red blood cells before reinfusion. Certain autotransfusion systems now offer that capability.

Microemboli.   Autotransfused blood that has been exposed to a serosal surface contains microemboli of white cells and platelets. Considerable concern has been expressed over the infusion of such microparticulate matter into the circulation. These particles can be easily cleared by passing the autotransfused blood through micropore filters.[44–46] A number of such filters are currently available with effective pore sizes of 20 to 40 microns. In large-volume autotransfusion (greater than 2.5 liters) such filters should probably be used.

The practice of washing the red blood cells before transfusion will reduce the microembolic load, and in such circumstances micropore filters may not be as necessary.

Coagulopathy.   Blood that is exposed to several surfaces, although it may clot initially, soon is acted on by fibrinolysis and becomes defibrinated. Transfusion of large volumes (2.5 liters or more) will therefore produce coagulopathy in these patients and should be prevented by transfusion of specific component therapy. In addition, the platelet count may also be depressed and transfusion of platelets may be needed. In general, however, it takes autotransfusions of 4,000 ml or more to produce a drop in the patient's platelet count to 50,000.[44,47]

The most common coagulation abnormality, however, is a low fibrinogen level,[48–50] but the liver rapidly replaces the deficit, and many authors believe that this is not clinically significant.[46,47,49] Red blood cell hemolysis can also occur because of prolonged exposure of the cells to the serosal surface[51] and an elevated plasma free hemoglobin level is a common finding after autotransfusion.[48,52] Most elevations are in the 25 to 30 mg/dl range, and it is believed that levels below 100 mg/dl are well tolerated.[53]

Autotransfusion should be strongly considered in patients who are suitable candidates, but a final word of caution is in order. Patients who are being autotransfused continue to bleed. Any patient who has received in excess of one liter of autotransfused blood should be strongly considered for surgical control of the bleeding site.

Homologous Transfusion

The patient in class III hemorrhage who is unsuitable for autotransfusion must be considered for homologous blood transfusion.

The infusion of donor blood is not without its problems. Not only is banked blood expensive, but it is frequently unavailable. Additional difficulties include low pH, high potassium level, low platelet level, and risk of infection.[54,55] Microembolization of platelets and white cell aggregates poses an additional hazard.[56-58] Most blood is stored in liquid form in a mixture of citrate, phosphate buffer, and dextrose (CPD) at 4°C. Infusion of such a low-temperature fluid is not without its risks.[59]

An additional and often forgotten problem with such stored blood is the reduction in the levels of 2.3 diphosphoglycerate (DPG) in the stored cells. This reduction causes a left shift of the oxyhemoglobin dissociation curve with consequent reduction in available oxygen use in the tissues.[60-62] Although it seems obvious that the reduction of 2.3 DPG should be detrimental to the patient, this has proved difficult to demonstrate. Collins[63] exchange-transfused two groups of rats with fresh warm blood or with blood stored in anticoagulant citrate dextrose (ACD) for 14 to 20 days and showed that the survival time was the same provided that the hematocrit value was maintained at greater than 30%.

USE OF STORED BLOOD

Despite its disadvantages, stored blood is frequently the only available source of additional oxygen-carrying capacity for the patient in hemorrhagic shock. Group O blood is occasionally needed for the patient who presents in acute hemorrhagic shock in whom the transcapillary refill has resulted in an extremely low hematocrit reading. Even in these rare instances, every effort should be made to warm the blood before infusion.

Whenever possible, banked blood that has been properly grouped and crossmatched should be used. If time is a consideration, type-specific blood may be considered. Such blood can be available in 20 minutes, and this time can be put to good use in fluid resuscitation of the patient.

ALTERNATIVE METHODS OF IMPROVING OXYGEN-CARRYING CAPACITY

Stroma Free Hemoglobin Solutions

These solutions consist of red blood cells from which the cellular membranes have been removed and for which the hemoglobin is available for oxygen transport. The material does not have to be cross-matched before administration and since it can be prepared from old, out-dated blood, it is potentially inexpensive. It is the hemoglobin molecule that actively transports the oxygen, so such material has excellent possibilities as a method of oxygen transport and delivery.

A difficulty with these solutions is that there is a marked left shift of the oxy-hemoglobin dissociation curve with a P_{50} of 13 mm Hg. This, however, can be markedly improved by pyridoxylation with pyridoxal-5-phosphate.[64] Improved oxygen delivery has been demonstrated with this material in an exsanguinated baboon model.

Fluorocarbon Emulsions

These compounds are hydrocarbons with fluorine replacing the hydrogen atoms. The fluorocarbon that has received the most attention is perfluorode-calin.[66] In these emulsions, the oxygen is carried in solution rather than in chemical combination. The commercial preparation is Fluosol-DA (Green Cross Co., Osaka, Japan; U.S. Subsidiary, Alpha Therapeutics, Inc., Los Angeles, CA). Since the oxygen is carried in solution, the dissociation curve is linear. In order to achieve the normal 5 ml% of oxygen uptake in the tissues, the patient must be exposed to a high Po_2 either by increasing the F_{Io_2} or by the use of hyperbaric oxygen. Good organ function and animal survival have been reported using these emulsions.[67 69]

The correct administration of fluids to resuscitate the patient in hemorrhagic shock necessitates an understanding of the pathophysiologic process that exists in shock at a cellular level. Fluid resuscitation can be looked at from the two separate viewpoints of volume resuscitation or restoration of oxygen-carrying capacity. Currently it appears that crystalloid rather than colloid resuscitation for volume replacement is indicated. To restore oxygen-carrying capacity, blood component replacement is indicated. Every effort should be made to autotransfuse the blood of patients for whom this procedure is indicated. Rapid and effective volume resuscitation and restoration of oxygen-carrying ability are crucial to successful resuscitation of the patient in hemorrhagic shock.

REFERENCES

1. Lefer, A.M., and Spath, J.A., Jr.: Pharmacologic basis for the treatment of circulatory shock. *In* Cardiovascular Pharmacology, 2nd Ed. Edited by M. Antonaccio. New York, Raven Press, 1984.
2. Schumer, W., Das Gupta, T.K., Moss, G.S., and Nyhus, L.M.: Effect of endotoxemia on liver cell mitochondria in man. Ann. Surg., *71*:875, 1970.
3. Janoff, A., Weissmann, G., Zweifach, B.W., and Thomas, L.: Pathogenesis of experimental shock: IV. Studies on lysosomes in normal and tolerant animals subjected to lethal trauma and endotoxemia. J. Exp. Med., *116*:451, 1962.
4. Lefer, A.M.: The role of lysosomes in circulatory shock. A minireview. Life Sci., *19*:1803, 1976.
5. Lefer, A.M.: Lysosomes in the pathogenesis of circulatory shock. *In* Handbook of Shock and Trauma. Vol. 1. Edited by B.M. Altura, A.M. Lefer, and W. Schumer. New York, Raven Press, 1983.
6. Carrico, C.G., et al.: Fluid resuscitation following injury: Rationale for the use of balanced salt solutions. Crit. Care Med., *4*:46, 1976.
7. Shires, G.T.: Care of the Trauma Patient, New York, McGraw-Hill, 1979.
8. Haljamae, H.: Anatomy of the interstitial tissue. Lymphology, *11*:128, 1978.
9. Amundson, B., Bagge, U., Jennische, E., and Baranemark, P.I.: Pathophysiology of shock. Pathol. Res. Pract., *165*:200, 1979.
10. Sayeed, M.M., Adler, R.J., Chaudry, I.H., and Baue, A.E.: Resting membrane potential and ion distribution in the liver in hemorrhagic shock. Am. J. Physiol. *240*:R211, 1981.
11. Shires, G.T., et al.: Alterations in cellular membrane function during hemorrhagic shock in primates. Ann. Surg., *176*:288, 1972.

12. Trunkey, D.D., Illner, H., Wagner, G.Y., and Shires, G.T.: The effect of hemorrhagic shock on intracellular muscle action potentials in the primate. Surgery, 74:241, 1973.
13. Jennische, E., et al.: Co-relation between tissue pH, cellular transmembrane potentials and cellular energy metabolism during shock and during ischemia. Circ. Shock. 5:251, 1978.
14. Jennische, E., Medegard, K.A.E., and Haljamae, H.: Transmembrane potential changes as an indicator of metabolic deterioration in skeletal muscle during shock. Eur. Surg. Res., 10:125, 1978.
15. Subcommittee on advanced trauma life support (ATLS) of the American College of Surgeons (ACS) Committee on Trauma: Shock. *In* Advanced Trauma Life Support Course for Physicians. 1983–1984.
16. Staub, N.C.: Pulmonary edema. Chest, 74:559, 1978.
17. Holcroft, J.W., and Trunkey, D.D.: Pulmonary extravasation of albumin during and after hemorrhagic shock in baboons. J. Surg. Res., 18:91, 1975.
18. Holcroft, J.W., et al.: Extravascular lung water following hemorrhagic shock in the baboon; comparison between resuscitation with Ringer's lactate and plasmanate. Ann. Surg., 180:408, 1974.
19. Virgilio, R.W.: Balanced electrolyte solutions: experimental and clinical studies. Crit. Care Med., 7:98, 1979.
20. Moss, G.S.: The effects of saline resuscitation on pulmonary sodium and water distribution. Surg. Gynecol. Obstet., 136:934, 1973.
21. Lucas, C.E.: Effects of albumin versus nonalbumin resuscitation on plasma volume and renal excretory function. J. Trauma, 18:564, 1978.
22. Lowe, R.J., Moss, G.S., Gilek, J., and Levine, H.D.: Crystalloid versus colloid in the etiology of pulmonary failure after trauma: A randomized trial in man. Surgery, 81:676, 1977.
23. Mannix, F.L.: Hemorrhagic shock. *In* Emergency Medicine: Concepts and Clinical Practice. Edited by P. Rosen et al. St. Louis, C.V. Mosby Co., 1983.
24. Carey, L.C., et al.: Hemorrhagic shock. Curr, Probl. Surg., 8:1971.
25. Cervera, A.L., et al.: Dilutional reexpansion with crystalloid after massive hemorrhage: Saline versus balanced electrolyte solutions for maintenance of normal blood volume and arterial pH. J. Trauma, 15:498, 1975.
26. Safar, P.: Resuscitation in hemorrhagic shock, coma, and cardiac arrest. *In* Pathophysiology of Shock, Anoxia and Ischemia. Edited by R.A. Cowley and B.F. Trump. Baltimore, Williams & Wilkins, 1982.
27. Metcalf, W., et al.: Clinical physiological characterization of a new dextran. Surg. Gynecol. Obstet., 115:199, 1982.
28. Dawidson, I., Barrett, J., Miller, E., and Litwin, M.S.: Cellular aggregate dissolution in postoperative patients. Ann. Surg., 182:776, 1975.
29. Dawidson, I., Eriksson, B., Gecin, L.E., and Soderberg, R.: Oxygen consumption and recovery from surgical shock in rats; a comparison of the efficiency of different plasma substitutes. Crit. Care Med., 7:460, 1979.
30. Thompson, W.L., Fukushima, T., Rutherford, R.B., and Walton, R.P.: Intravascular persistence, tissue storage, and excretion of hydroxyethlyl starch. Surg. Gynecol. Obstet., 131:965, 1970.
31. Rice, C.L., and Moss, G.S.: Blood and blood substitutes. *In* Current Practice in Advances in Surgery. Vol. 13. Edited by G.L. Jordan. Chicago, Year Book, 1979.
32. Bourke, D.L., and Smith, T.C.: Estimating allowable hemodilution, Anesthesilogy, 41:609, 1974.
33. Young, G.P., and Purcell, T.B.: Emergency autotransfusion. Ann. Emerg. Med., 12:180, 1983.
34. Niemann, J.T.: Pneumatic antishock trousers: Safety, benefit and physiologic effect. Ann. Emerg. Med., 12:377, 1983.
35. Pelligra, R., and Sandberg, E.C.: Control of intractable abdominal bleeding by external counterpressure. J.A.M.A., 241:708, 1979.
36. Holcroft, J.W.: Impairment of venous return in hemorrhagic shock. Surg. Clin. North Am., 62:17, 1982.
37. MaHox, K.L.: Comparison of techniques of autotransfusion. Surgery, 84:700, 1978.
38. Symbas, P.N.: Autotransfusion from hemothorax. J. Trauma, 12:689, 1972.
39. Huth, J.F., Maier, R.V., Pavlin, E.G., and Carrico, J.: Utilization of blood recycling in non-elective surgery. Arch. Surg., 118:626, 1983.
40. Smith, R.N., Yaw, P.B., and Glover, J.L.: Autotransfusion of contaminated intraperitoneal blood: An experimental study. J. Trauma, 18:341, 1978.
41. Klebanoff, G., Phillips, J., and Evans, W.: Use of a disposable autotransfusion unit under varying conditions of contamination. Am. J. Surg., 120:351, 1970.
42. Griswold, R.A., and Ortner, A.B.: Use of autotransfusion in surgery of serous cavities. Surg. Gynecol. Obstet., 77:167, 1943.
43. Glover, J.L., et al.: Autotransfusion of blood contaminated by intestinal contents. J.A.C.E.P., 7:142, 1978.
44. Brewster, D.C., et al.: Intraoperative autotransfusion in major vascular surgery. Am. J. Surg., 137:507, 1979.

45. Raines, J., et al.: Intraoperative autotransfusion: Equipment, protocols, and guidelines. J. Trauma, *16*:616, 1976.
46. Reul, G.J., et al.: Experience with autotransfusion in the surgical management of trauma. Surgery, *76*:546, 1974.
47. Davidson, S.J.: Emergency unit autotransfusion. Surgery, *84*:703, 1978.
48. Mattox, K.L.: Autotransfusion in the emergency department. J.A.C.E.P., *4*:218, 1975.
49. Bell, W.: The hematology of autotransfusion. Surgery, *84*:695, 1978.
50. Symbas, P.N., et al.: A study on autotransfusion from hemothorax. South Med. J., *62*:671, 1969.
51. Stillman, R.N., et al.: The haematological hazards of autotransfusion. Br. J. Surg., *63*:651, 1976.
52. Symbas, P.N.: Extraoperative autotransfusion from hemothorax. Surgery, *84*:722, 1978.
53. Dyer, R.H., Alexander, J.T., and Brighton, C.T.: Atraumatic aspiration of whole blood for intraoperative autotransfusion. Am. J. Surg., *123*:510, 1972.
54. Howland, W.S., and Schweizer, O.: Physiologic compensation for storage lesion of banked blood. Anesth. Analg., *44*:8, 1965.
55. Bunker, J.P., et al.: Citric acid intoxication. J.A.M.A., *157*:1361, 1955.
56. Barrett, J., Tahir, A.H., and Litwin, M.S.: Increased pulmonary arteriovenous shunting in humans following blood transfusion; relation to screen filtration pressure of transfused blood and prevention by dacron wool (Swank) filtration. Arch. Surg., *113*:947, 1978.
57. Barrett, J., De Jonga, D.S., Miller, E., and Litwin, M.S.: Microaggregate formation in stored human packed cells: Comparison with formation in stored blood and a method for their removal. Ann. Surg., *153*:109, 1976.
58. Barrett, J., et al.: Pulmonary microembolism associated with massive transfusion. II. The basic pathophysiology of its pulmonary effects. Ann. Surg., *68*:273, 1975.
59. Boyan, C.P., and Howland, W.S.: Cardiac arrest and temperature of banked blood. J.A.M.A., *183*:144, 1963.
60. Valtis, D.J., and Kennedy, A.C.: Defective gas-transport function of stored red blood cells. Lancet, *1*:119, 1954.
61. Gullbring, B., and Strom, G.: Changes in oxygen-carrying function of human hemoglobin during storage in cold acid-citrate-dextrose solution. Acta Med. Scand., *155*:413, 1956.
62. Akerblom, O., De Verdier, C.H., Garry, L., and Hogman, C.F.: Restoration of defective oxygen transport function of stored red blood cells by addition of inosine. Scand. J. Clin. Lab. Invest., *21*:245, 1968.
63. Collins, J.A.: Abnormal hemoglobin-oxygen affinity and surgical hemotherapy. *In* Surgical Hemotherapy. Edited by J.A. Collins, and P. Lundsgaard-Hansen. Basel, S. Karger, 1980.
64. Messmer, K., Jesch, F., and Schaff, J.: Oxygen supply by stroma-free hemoglobin. Prog. Clin. Biol. Res., *19*:175, 1978.
65. Rosen, A.L., et al.: Cardiac output response to extreme hemodilution with hemoglobin solutions of various P_{50} values. Crit. Care. Med., *7*:380, 1979.
66. Clark, L.C., Jr.: Perflurodecalin as a red cell substitute. Prog. Clin. Biol. Res., *19*:69, 1978.
67. Geyer, P.: Fluorocarbon-polyol artificial blood substitutes. N. Engl. J. Med., *289*:1077, 1973.
68. Geyer, P., Monroe, R.G., and Taylor, K.: Survival of rats having red cells totally replaced with emulsified flurocarbon. Fed. Proc., *27*:384, 1968.
69. Clark, L.C., Jr.: Theoretical and practical considerations of fluorocarbon emulsions in the treatment of shock. *In* Pathophysiology of Shock, Anoxia, and Ischemia. Edited by R.A. Cowley, and B.F. Trump. Baltimore, Williams & Wilkins, 1982.

Chapter 3

MONITORING AND MEASUREMENT IN SHOCK

Loren D. Nelson

A patient in the state of shock presents the physician with a supreme clinical challenge. Shock so disrupts normal physiologic mechanisms that "traditional" clinical evaluation often leads the clinician to incorrect conclusions and inappropriate therapy. Patients are transferred to the intensive care unit (ICU) not only for intensive therapy but also for intensive monitoring to help avoid the pitfalls of clinical impression. The word monitor is derived from the Latin *monere,* meaning to warn. In the ICU patients are monitored with the hope of early warning of organ system dysfunction at a time when the dysfunction is potentially reversible. In this chapter we examine the role of monitoring and physiologic measurements in the diagnosis and treatment of shock. Special emphasis is placed on a global approach to monitoring and upon the multisystem effects of tissue hypoperfusion.

PHILOSOPHY OF MONITORING IN SHOCK

As was pointed out in Chapter 1, the very diagnosis of shock is often dependent upon discrete biochemical or physiologic measurements. Early in the shock state, before multiple system dysfunction has appeared, oliguria (urine output of less than 0.5 ml/kg/hour) may be the first sign of tissue (renal) hypoperfusion. However, in patients in shock for a period of time or those who are being actively resuscitated according to the principles discussed in Chapter 2, urine output may not accurately reflect inadequacies in renal perfusion. Obligatory urine losses caused by saline loading, hyperglycemia, or tubular dysfunction caused by ischemia or nephrotoxins may deceive the clinician into believing that tissue perfusion is improving when, in fact, it is not. Appropriate monitoring in the shock state should lead the clinician to the correct diagnosis, yield information regarding the relative magnitude of the tissue perfusion deficit, and suggest appropriate therapy to correct the inadequacy of tissue perfusion. Ideally, monitoring of the shock state would also produce prognostic information to aid the medical team in their decision to continue or withdraw treatment in what may be an unsalvageable situation. Because no single tool meets these criteria for an ideal monitor in shock, a global approach to these critically ill patients is preferred.[1]

A global approach to monitoring includes a detailed medical history of pertinent facts relating to the underlying disease and a meticulous physical examination, supplemented by physiologic, laboratory, and radiographic information for *each* organ system. The need for such a complete evaluation becomes apparent when the two major problems associated with the shock state are recognized:

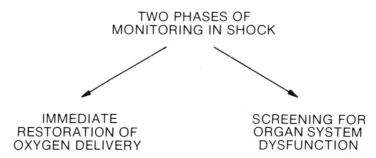

TWO PHASES OF
MONITORING IN SHOCK

IMMEDIATE
RESTORATION OF
OXYGEN DELIVERY

SCREENING FOR
ORGAN SYSTEM
DYSFUNCTION

Fig. 3-1.   The two phases of monitoring in shock may occur simultaneously or separately.

life-threatening physiologic imbalance created by acute hypoperfusion and ischemia and multisystem dysfunction resulting from end organ hypoxia (Fig. 3–1).
Two levels of monitoring are required—one to screen for signs of end organ dysfunction and another to evaluate specific end organ dysfunction if discovered. In
this way the severity of injury will determine the level of monitoring so that the
level of observation as well as therapy will be most efficient in terms of risks,
benefits, and costs.

With the concept in mind of a global approach and graded levels of monitoring
tailored to the magnitude of illness, we must consider which organ systems are
at risk for failure in critically ill patients. Most physicians dealing with acute illness
or injury are keenly aware of the cardiovascular, pulmonary, and renal effects of
shock. However, other systems must be reviewed in a serial manner to allow
early detection of potentially life threatening problems: the gastrointestinal tract
for mucosal bleeding and ischemia related to low flow; the hepatobiliary system
for hepatocyte dysfunction, cholestasis, and cholecystitis; the pancreas for acute
inflammation, infection, and endocrine dysfunction; the hematologic system for
hemolysis, anemia, abnormal white cell count or differential, or thrombocytopenia; the coagulation system for dysfunction of the intrinsic, extrinsic, or platelet
phases of hemostasis; the central and peripheral nervous systems, including
assessment for acute psychiatric disturbances; the endocrine system for adrenal
insufficiency and failure of glucose control. Other items that need careful attention in critically ill patients include: nutrition, care of the skin and integument, and
a daily evaluation of the necessity of invasive tubes, lines, and drains, which may
become a source of complications in themselves. The admonition to monitor the
monitors cannot be overstressed. Careful assessment of the indications for initiation of invasive monitoring and prompt removal of invasive devices when they
are no longer needed is the cornerstone of a plan to reduce the complications
associated with invasive monitoring.

CONCEPT OF OXYGEN TRANSPORT MONITORING

The complex milieu of pathophysiologic processes which we identify as clinical
shock has as its common denominator inadequate perfusion to meet the metabolic needs of the tissue. The maldistribution of blood flow at the microcirculatory
level cannot be evaluated clinically with currently available technology. Therefore
it is not possible to evaluate organ by organ the adequacy of oxygen delivery to
meet that particular tissue's oxygen requirement. It is possible, however, to evaluate the overall balance between oxygen supply and demand for a patient. Using

Table 3–1. Definitions of Oxygen Transport Terms.

Term	Definition	Units
O_2 transport	Overall balance between O_2 supply and demand	none
O_2 delivery	Arterial O_2 content times cardiac output	ml/min
O_2 demand	Volume of O_2 required by tissue for normal function	ml/min
O_2 consumption/uptake	Measurable volume of O_2 metabolized for tissue function	ml/min
O_2 utilization/extraction	Ratio of O_2 consumption to O_2 delivery (i.e., a quantitation of O_2 transport balance)	%

Many sources use the terms O_2 delivery and O_2 transport synonymously; here, however, transport is used to indicate a supply/demand balance. Also many sources use O_2 demand to mean O_2 consumption. Here consumption is the measurable O_2 uptake and demand is the O_2 requirement of tissue. Normal values are: O_2 delivery = 800 to 1800 ml/min; O_2 demand = O_2 consumption; O_2 consumption = 180 to 280 ml/min; O_2 utilization = 22 to 33%.

this information along with an understanding of the pathophysiology of shock and a knowledge of pharmacologic agents that alter distribution of blood flow the clinician may make interventions which help to reverse the shock state and improve outcome. **Since outcome following shock is dependent upon a prompt restoration of tissue oxygenation, monitoring in shock requires the evaluation of the oxygen transport balance to the tissue.**

Although somewhat arbitrary, some definitions are necessary to discuss oxygen transport monitoring (Table 3–1). Oxygen transport or oxygen transport balance is used to refer to the dynamic balance between the oxygen supply available to the tissue and the oxygen demand created by the tissue (Fig. 3–2). As stated previously, this balance currently cannot be assessed organ by organ but rather only as a total body balance. Oxygen supply to the tissues is assessed by measuring oxygen delivery (O_2 Del). Oxygen delivery is defined as the mathematical product of cardiac output (CO) in liters per minute times arterial oxygen content (Ca_{O_2}) in ml of oxygen per dl of blood. O_2 Del tells the clinician the volume of oxygen (bound to hemoglobin and dissolved in plasma) that is pumped from the left side of the heart each minute. Oxygen demand is a value that cannot be measured but refers to the amount of oxygen needed by the tissue to supply its current metabolic needs. On the other hand, oxygen consumption (O_2 Con) or uptake refers to the volume of oxygen taken up and actually used by the patient

O2 Supply   O2 Demand

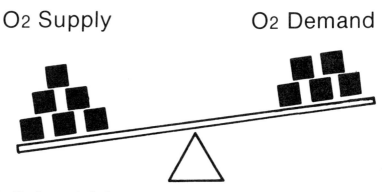

Fig. 3–2. The "economics" of oxygen transport balance is based upon principles of supply and demand.

each minute. When oxygen demand exceeds oxygen consumption, lactic acidosis ensues.[2] The oxygen utilization (O_2 Util) or extraction ratio is the mathematical representation of oxygen transport balance, i.e., the quotient between O_2 Con and O_2 Del. With this background we will now examine the supply side (O_2 Del) of the oxygen transport balance.

The determinants of oxygen delivery to tissue are the determinants of arterial oxygen content and of cardiac output. The hemoglobin concentration and the degree of saturation of the hemoglobin are the primary determinants of arterial oxygen content. Approximately 98% of the oxygen delivered to the tissue (assuming near-normal hemoglobin concentration) is bound to hemoglobin. The other 2% is dissolved in the plasma (Table 3–2). From this it is obvious that one of the best ways to improve oxygen delivery is to increase the hemoglobin concentration by transfusing packed red blood cells. Oxygen delivery may also be increased by increasing the arterial oxygen saturation. This is a very effective way of improving delivery when arterial hypoxemia is present, but the utility decreases as the saturation increases above 95%. Similarly, increasing arterial oxygen tension after the hemoglobin is fully saturated does little to increase oxygen delivery.

Tissue oxygen delivery is also directly affected by changes in cardiac output, which in turn is determined by heart rate and stroke volume. Since therapeutic interventions to improve cardiac output by altering heart rate are usually ineffective (except at the extremes of tachycardia or bradycardia), cardiac output is usually increased by raising stroke volume. The determinants of stroke volume are preload (the volume of blood presented to the ventricle for ejection), afterload (the impedence to the ejection of blood created by the mass and viscosity of blood and systemic vascular resistance), and contractility. For practical purposes

Table 3-2. Cardiorespiratory Formulae Derived from Analysis of Gases.

Term	Formula	Units	Normal Range
Arterial O_2 content	Ca_{O_2} (Hb × 1.39 × Sa_{O_2}) + (.0031 × Pa_{O_2})	ml O_2/dl	16–22
Mixed venous O_2 content	Cv_{O_2} = (Hb × 1.39 × Sv_{O_2}) + (.0031 × Pv_{O_2})	ml O_2/dl	12–17
Pulmonary capillary O_2 content	Cc_{O_2} = (Hb × 1.39) + (.0031 × PA_{O_2})	ml O_2/dl	(varies with FI_{O_2})
Alveolar O_2 tension	$PA_{O_2} = (PB - PH_2O) FI_{O_2} - \dfrac{Pa_{CO_2}}{RQ}$	mm Hg	(varies with FI_{O_2})
Arterial-venous O_2 content difference	C (a − v) Do_2 = Ca_{O_2} − Cv_{O_2}	ml O_2/dl	3–5
Respiratory quotient	$RQ = \dfrac{Vco_2}{Vo_2}$	fraction	0.7–1.0
CO_2 production	Vco_2 = VE × FE_{CO_2}	ml/min	140–250
O_2 consumption (Fick)	Vo_2 = C (a − v) Do_2 × CO × 10	ml/min	180–280
O_2 consumption (measured)	$Vo_2 = VE \left(\dfrac{FI_{O_2} - FE_{O_2} - (FI_{O_2} \times FE_{CO_2})}{1 - FI_{O_2}} \right)$	ml/min	180–280
Physiologic right-to-left shunt (venous admixture)	$Q_{sp}/Q_T = \dfrac{Cc_{O_2} - Ca_{O_2}}{Cc_{O_2} - Cv_{O_2}}$	fraction	0.03–0.05

Cardiorespiratory measurements derived from the analysis of blood and expired gases form the basis for understanding oxygen transport balance (see text for interpretation of these data). Hb = hemoglobin concentration; Sa_{O_2} = arterial O_2 saturation; Pa_{O_2} = arterial O_2 tension; Sv_{O_2} = mixed venous O_2 saturation; Pv_{O_2} = mixed venous O_2 tension; PB = barometric pressure; PH_2O = partial pressure of water vapor (47 mm Hg at 37° C); VE = expired minute ventilation, FE_{CO_2} = mixed expired CO_2 fraction; CO = cardiac output; FI_{O_2} = inspired O_2 fraction; FE_{O_2} = expired O_2 fraction.

these factors are independent and the magnitude and direction of change of one value cannot be inferred from changes in others. To make matters worse, clinicians skilled in the evaluation of these parameters are unable from clinical assessment to predict reliably even the direction of deviation from normal.[3] This emphasizes the need for invasive hemodynamic montoring in patients with suspected decreases in oxygen delivery.

Finally we must consider the demand side of the oxygen transport balance. The measurement of oxygen consumption in critically ill patients is a relatively new practice begun because of dissatisfaction with oxygen consumption calculated by the Fick equation. A number of factors (temperature, activity, acid-base status, stress level, sepsis, and injury) are known to affect oxygen consumption. In patients with limited cardiopulmonary reserves an increase in oxygen consumption may not be compensated by an increase in oxygen delivery and may result in disruption of the oxygen transport balance. If unchecked this may result in tissue hypoxia, that is, shock.

TECHNICAL ASPECTS OF OXYGEN TRANSPORT MONITORING

Arterial Catheterization

The placement of an indwelling arterial catheter is one of the first steps of the critical care monitoring of a patient in shock. There are two primary indications for arterial catheterization: a need for continuous blood pressure monitoring, and a need for frequent arterial blood sampling. Although there are no specific contraindications to arterial catheterization, bleeding diatheses (including thrombolytic and anticoagulant therapy) increase the risk of hemorrhagic complications. Arterial occlusive disease, the presence of vascular prostheses, and local infection are contraindications to specific sites for catheterization.

The choice of site (Fig. 3–3) for arterial catheterization remains a parochial issue,[4] but specific advantages and disadvantages have been discussed and should be considered when selecting the most appropriate site for a particular patient. The dual blood supply to the hand and the superficial location of the vessel make the radial artery the most commonly used site for arterial catheterization.[5] Since digital ischemia is one of the most significant complications of radial catheterization, the assessment of adequate ulnar collateral flow should be confirmed by an Allen test before cannulation. When the radial artery is not suitable, the dorsalis pedis artery may be used in a similar manner. Collateral flow through the posterior tibial artery should be confirmed to be adequate. The major disadvantages of this vessel are its small size and (later in the clinical course) problems related to the patient's walking. Both of these vessels may be difficult to cannulate if the shock state is accompanied by hypotension or profound vasoconstriction. Since both of these conditions are common in the shock state, alternative catheterization sites must be reviewed.

The axillary artery offers the advantages of a larger size, abundant collateral circulation, and freedom of movement of the extremity.[6] The major disadvantage is the technical difficulty of catheter insertion because of the rather deep location and mobility of the vessel and its proximity to the brachial plexus. Cannulation of the axillary artery is usually performed at the axillobrachial junction with the patient's arm abducted and externally rotated and the hand placed beneath the patient's head. The catheter is placed percutaneously using either an over-the-needle catheter or a modified Seldinger technique.[1,6]

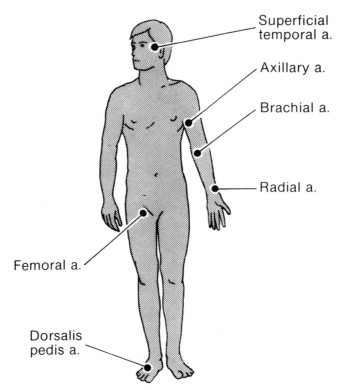

Superficial
temporal a.

Axillary a.

Brachial a.

Radial a.

Femoral a.

Dorsalis
pedis a.

Fig. 3-3. Multiple sites are available for arterial catheterization for hemodynamic monitoring. (Modified from Beal, J.M.: Critical Care for Surgical Patients. New York, Macmillan Publishing Co., 1982.)

Femoral arterial catheterization is regaining popularity in the treatment of critically ill patients. Advantages of this vessel are its large size, high blood flow, and superficial location. Major disadvantages are the presence of atherosclerotic disease in older patients and potential septic complications in the presence of draining abdominal wounds and ostomies. The concern over septic complications arose from a report reviewing a small number of femoral catheters,[7] and since then at least two larger prospective studies have shown the incidence of local and systemic infection to be equal to that of other sites.[8,9] The femoral artery is usually cannulated using a modified Seldinger technique.[8]

The superficial temporal artery (because of its small size) and the brachial artery (because of potential limb loss from thrombotic complications) are rarely used as sites for indwelling catheters to monitor patients in shock.

An indwelling arterial catheter in a patient in shock allows for frequent analysis of arterial blood gases and for continuous monitoring of the arterial pressure waveform. Frequent blood gas analysis is necessary in the resuscitation phase of shock to monitor the adequacy of the therapy. A progressive metabolic acidosis would suggest that the hypoperfusion is not responding and oxygen transport remains inadequate. Hypoxemia may indicate that pulmonary function is deteriorating or that there is a moderate degree of intrapulmonary shunting and a high degree of peripheral oxygen extraction resulting in marked venous desaturation. Only further monitoring of mixed venous oxygen saturation will allow the clinician to distinguish between these possibilities.

Analysis of the pressure waveform yields information regarding the systolic, diastolic, and mean arterial pressures. Accurate data are necessary for the calculation of systemic vascular resistance, coronary perfusion pressure, and the rate-pressure product. These numbers may be important in determining appropriate therapeutic changes in the shock state. Waveform analysis may also give the clinician useful information regarding the dynamic response characteristics of the monitoring system. If the response of the system is adequate, the rate of rise of the systemic pressure gives information about left ventricular contractility and impedance to flow, and the rate of fall of diastolic pressure will reflect changes in systemic vascular resistance. The area under each pulse curve is proportional to that stroke volume.

Potential problems associated with arterial catheterization include: failure to cannulate the vessel, local bleeding and hematoma, disconnection with bleeding, thrombosis, antegrade or retrograde arterial embolism, local inflammation or infection, and systemic catheter-related sepsis.[10] Prompt removal of the catheter is indicated if these problems are noted.

Central Venous Catheterization

Central venous catheterization has become one of the most frequently performed procedures in critically ill patients. Its primary indication is to provide secure access to the venous circulation, which may be necessary for fluid therapy, drug infusion, parenteral nutrition, frequent venous blood sampling, or measurement of central venous pressure. There are no absolute contraindications to central venous catheterization, but bleeding diatheses increase the risk of hemorrhagic complications. Thrombosed vessels and areas of local inflammation should be avoided. The most commonly used sites are the subclavian,[11] internal[12,13] and external[14] jugular, femoral, and brachiocephalic veins (Fig. 3–4). The high incidence of thrombotic complications of the femoral vein[13] and problems relating to catheter malpositioning[15] and thrombosis[16] of arm veins make them unacceptable except in unusual circumstances. The central veins may be cannulated using over-the-needle, through-the-needle, or modified Seldinger techniques. New technology now allows the placement of multipurpose, multiple-lumen central venous catheters,[17] which permit simultaneous infusions of vasoactive medications, blood products, and nutrition solutions, and have an additional lumen available for measurement of central venous pressure (Fig. 3–5). These catheters may decrease the risk to patients of multiple line-insertion procedures when more than one access route is required. They also may prove to be cost effective in that only one chest roentgenogram is required rather than a separate one for each line insertion.

While central venous lines are placed primarily for access into the venous circulation, occasionally useful information can be obtained by measuring the central venous pressure (CVP). CVP may be helpful in the differentiation between hypotension caused by pericardial tamponade versus hypovolemia following trauma. A properly placed CVP catheter can be used to measure right atrial pressure, which, in the absence of tricuspid valve disease, will reflect the right ventricular end diastolic pressure. This pressure gives the clinician information regarding the relationship between intravascular volume and right ventricular function. CVP does not give information about either of these factors independently nor does it give information concerning left ventricular function.[18] It is important to note that

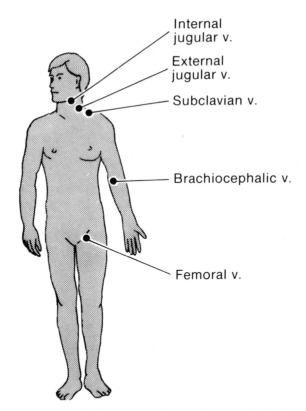

Internal
jugular v.

External
jugular v.

Subclavian v.

Brachiocephalic v.

Femoral v.

Fig. 3–4. Multiple sites are available for access to the central venous circulation.

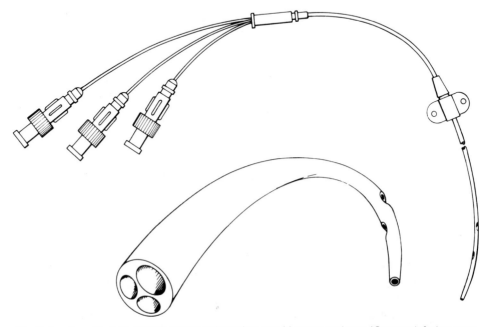

Fig. 3–5. A multilumen central venous catheter has one 16-gauge and two 18-gauge infusion ports.

CVP cannot be used as an indicator of intravascular volume replacement in shock,[19] nor does it reliably predict left-sided filling pressures in any identifiable population of critically ill patients.[1]

The incidence of complications following central venous catheterization is significant[20] and may be even higher when these lines are placed in emergency situations.[21] A detailed description of the types of complications recorded and recommendations to avoid them is available elsewhere.[1,22] Suffice it to say here that the lines should be placed for specific indications and by established techniques. It is important to remember in the treatment of shock that intravenous fluids usually may be infused more safely and rapidly through large bore lines in peripheral veins than by longer and smaller bore lines in central veins. As resuscitation progresses central venous lines may be necessary for the administration of vasoactive drugs or as introducers for pulmonary artery catheters.

Pulmonary Artery Catheterization

Widespread clinical use of pulmonary artery (PA) catheterization has opened new dimensions not only in hemodynamic monitoring but also in monitoring oxygen transport in patients in shock. For the first time at the bedside, pressure measurements can now be supplemented by blood flow and mixed venous gas analysis. Specific indications for PA catheterization in shock may be debated, but most clinicians would agree that it should be performed when the cause of the shock state is unclear, when the patient does not respond to judicious volumes of intravenous fluid, or when there are signs of progressive end organ (especially lung and kidney) dysfunction. There are no specific contraindications to PA catheterization; however, the same cautions regarding central venous catheterizations should be observed.

Complete hemodynamic monitoring, i.e., arterial and PA catheterization, is indicated whenever precise information can replace the uncertainty of clinical impressions.[15]

Civetta describes the technique for PA catheterization in detail.[15] An important development in catheter technology was the availability of the side-arm catheter introducer (Fig. 3–6). This is a large bore (8.5 French) central venous catheter that may be placed by a modified Seldinger technique and used for rapid administration of blood or intravenous fluids to the patient in shock. When indicated, the catheter may be used as an introducer sheath for the placement of PA line without the risk of another central venipuncture. With a PA catheter in place the side arm may still be used as an infusion port (although the lumen size is significantly decreased) for medications or fluids into the central circulation.

Once the position of the PA catheter is confirmed by the pressure tracing and portable chest roentgenogram, a vast amount of data regarding hemodynamics and oxygen transport is available to the clinician. Directly measured parameters include pulmonary artery systolic, diastolic, and mean pressures, CVP, pulmonary artery occlusion ("wedge") pressure (PAOP), and cardiac output (CO). With the addition of systemic blood pressure data recorded from the arterial catheter, a multitude of derived hemodynamic parameters may be calculated (Table 3–3). These are useful and even necessary to select the optimal cardiovascular interventions for a patient in shock.

Perhaps even more important is the utility of the PA catheter to evaluate the

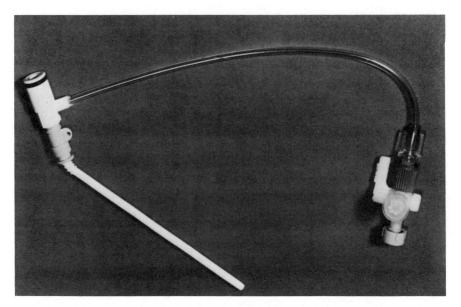

Fig. 3-6. The side arm catheter introducer sheath may be used for large volume blood and fluid administration, and if necessary provide access for PA catheter placement while still providing an additional infusion port. (Photo compliments of Arrow International, Inc., Reading, PA.)

adequacy of the hemodynamic state to provide oxygen to the tissue. The adequacy of tissue oxygenation can be best assessed by the analysis of venous blood gases and calculation of the derived oxygen transport parameters (Table 3–2). The interpretation of these parameters will be discussed in detail later in this chapter.

The complications of PA catheterization include all of the complications of any

Table 3-3. Derived Hemodynamic Parameters.

Term	Formula	Units	Normal Range
Cardiac index	$CI = \dfrac{CO}{BSA}$	liter/min/m$_2$	2.8–4.2
Stroke volume	$SV = \dfrac{CO}{HR}$	ml/beat	(varies with size)
Stroke index	$SI = \dfrac{SV}{BSA}$	ml/beat/m^2	30–65
Mean arterial pressure	$MAP = DP + \dfrac{(SP - DP)}{3}$	mm Hg	70–105
Systemic vascular resistance	$SVR = \dfrac{MAP - CVP}{CO} \times 80$	dyne $\times$ sec x cm^{-5}	900–1400
Pulmonary vascular resistance	$PVR = \dfrac{MPAP - PAOP}{CO} \times 80$	dyne $\times$ sec x cm^{-5}	150–250
Left ventricular stroke work index	$LVSWI = SI(MAP - PAOP) \times 0.0136$	g $\times$ m/m^2	43–61
Right ventricular stroke work index	$RVSWI = SI(MPAP - CVP) \times 0.0136$	g $\times$ m/m^2	7–12
Coronary perfusion pressure	$CPP = DP - PAOP$	mm Hg	60–90

Hemodynamic parameters derived from intravascular pressure and flow measurements are used to select the optimal management for patients with inadequate cardiac output. CO = cardiac output; BSA = body surface area; HR = heart rate; DP = diastolic pressure; SP = systolic pressure; CVP = central venous pressure; MPAP = mean pulmonary artery pressure; PAOP = pulmonary artery occlusion pressure.

form of central venous catheterization plus others related to the unique intracardiac and intrapulmonary position of the catheter. Because PA catheters must be maintained as "open" systems (i.e., stopcocks available for blood sampling, drug infusions, cardiac output thermal indicator injection, etc.), the incidence of bacterial colonization is likely to be higher than with simple central lines. When the tips of catheters removed from critically ill patients are cultured, as many as 35% are positive for bacteria.[23] The clinical importance of this bacterial colonization is uncertain because less than 2% of patients with positive catheter tip cultures have bacteremia with the same organism. In patients with a defined septic focus, 25% were found to have positive blood cultures drawn through the PA catheter within 72 hours of insertion. After 72 hours all patients had positive PA blood cultures.[24] While the clinical importance is again uncertain, these patients have an increased risk for catheter-related bacteremia, and the catheters should be removed as soon as they are no longer necessary; perhaps, in septic patients, they should be changed to another site every 72 hours.

Mechanical complications caused by PA catheters include cardiac arrhythmias during insertion,[25] right bundle branch block,[25] left fascicular blocks,[26] central vein thrombosis,[27] thrombotic endocardial vegetations,[28] pulmonary artery rupture,[29] intracardiac knotting,[30] pulmonary infarction,[31] and balloon rupture.[31] The risk of complications resulting from the insertion and maintenance of PA catheters may be lessened by meticulous attention to detail and careful evaluation of the data obtained.[23]

PITFALLS IN INVASIVE HEMODYNAMIC MONITORING

One of the most common pitfalls of invasive hemodynamic monitoring in shock is the often crucial therapeutic time lost while monitoring devices are being placed. While the placement of these lines normally may take only a few minutes each, the technical challenges may be greater when a patient is suffering profound vasoconstriction or hypotension. Therapy and clinical evaluation may be interrupted while the patient is "lost" under the drapes. And since time is of the essence early in the resuscitation from shock, even a few minutes of continued organ hypoperfusion may have disastrous outcomes.

Another common pitfall of hemodynamic monitoring is blind reliance upon electronically displayed data. A pressure monitoring system consists of an intravascular catheter, connecting tubing, a continuous flow flush device, an electromechanical transducer, an amplifier, a cathode ray tube display, a digital display, and perhaps a strip chart recorder or electronic trend recorder (Fig. 3–7). The complexity of this system may cause the displayed pressure to differ considerably from the true intravascular pressure. The dynamic response of the system is determined by the frequency response of the electronic portion of the system and by the adequacy of damping of the mechanical or hydraulic portion of the system. Most modern electronic systems have an adequate frequency response of greater than 10 times the biologic frequency generated; i.e., a maximum heart rate of 120 to 180 beats/min or 2 to 3 c/sec $\times$ 10 = 20 to 30 c/sec response. Pressure measurement artifacts more commonly occur because of inappropriate damping of the system.[32] Overdamping is the result of high resistance or compliant tubing or, most commonly, because of air bubbles in the tubing or transducer dome. The result of overdamping is that the systolic and diastolic pressure changes are overly blunted and tend toward the mean pressure, i.e., a significant decrease in systolic

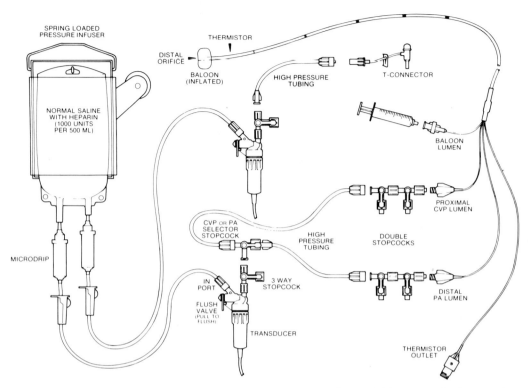

Fig. 3-7. The components of a hemodynamic monitoring system allow multiple sources for inappropriate dynamic responses to pressure changes. (Modified from Sprung, C. L.: The Pulmonary Artery Catheter. Baltimore, University Park Press, 1983.)

pressure and an increase in diastolic pressure resulting in little change in the measured mean pressure. Obviously only the most severe overdamping can be detected by the digital display of pressures, but observation of the displayed waveform may be very helpful in detecting overdamping. The characteristics of the overly damped tracing are a slower rate of rise to systolic and fall to diastolic pressures, blunting of the wave peak, and loss of the dicrotic notch (Fig. 3–8, left).

Equally important to overdamping is the problem of underdamping. Underdamping is caused by factors that reduce the natural frequency of the monitoring system toward the frequencies generated by the biologic system. When the natural frequency is significantly reduced, oscillations may occur at harmonics to the frequencies produced by the patient. These harmonic waves may be greatly amplified, producing increases in the displayed pressure variance and thereby greatly overestimating the systolic pressure and underestimating the diastolic pressure. This phenomenon may be better understood when one considers a musical instrument such as a flute. When air passes over the mouthpiece a number of low amplitude (inaudible) frequencies are generated, causing the column of air in the instrument to oscillate. The flutist may change the natural frequency of the instrument by changing the functional length of the air column, thereby producing high amplitude (audible) tones at harmonic frequencies to those produced at the mouthpiece. This "harmonic amplification" causes artifactually large fluc-

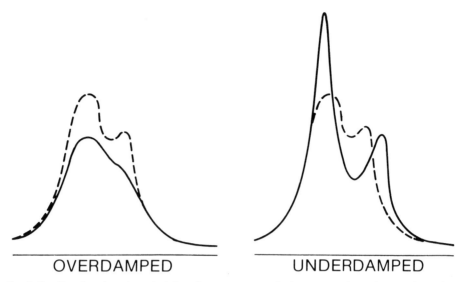

OVERDAMPED   UNDERDAMPED

Fig. 3-8. The damping characteristics of a pressure monitoring system determine to a large degree the dynamic response of the system. Normal arterial pressure wave forms are shown with dashed lines. On the left the characteristics of an overdamped tracing are shown by the solid line. On the right the characteristics of an underdamped wave are demonstrated.

tuations in the recorded pressures, i.e., overestimation of systolic pressure and slight underestimation of diastolic pressure.

The clinical importance of underdamping in the shock state is that the clinician may be lulled into complacency by the display of an "adequate" systolic pressure that in fact is artifactually high because of underdamping. An underdamped signal cannot be detected by the digital pressure display but may be detected by observation of the pressure waveform. The characteristics of an underdamped waveform are a narrow, peaked systolic curve with a low but prominent dicrotic notch (Fig. 3-8, right).

Overdamping occurs most commonly when tubing connecting the catheter to the transducer is too long. The length of the tubing and the extravascular portion of the catheter determine, for the most part, the natural frequency of the system and should be kept less than three feet whenever feasible. Other suggestions to minimize dynamic response problems are to eliminate meticulously all air bubbles from the system, use low compliance tubing, minimize the number of components (such as stopcocks) in the system, achieve the proper dome-to-transducer interface, and record electronic mean pressures rather than systolic and diastolic pressures since the mean is affected least by damping artifacts.[32,33]

Yet another common pitfall with invasive hemodynamic monitoring is misinterpretation of ventricular filling pressures. Since filling pressures are influenced by intrapleural pressure, the point in the ventilatory cycle when the measurement is made may have a profound impact on the value obtained. This is especially true when patients have respiratory distress, and fluctuations in airway pressure (and therefore intrapleural pressure) are greater than normal. The most commonly accepted convention is to measure the PAOP at end-exhalation immediately before the next spontaneous or mechanical breath. At that point the pleural pressure should have the least effect on PAOP.[34]

The other area of great concern regarding PAOP measurement during mechanical ventilatory support is in patients on positive end-expiratory pressure (PEEP). Since PEEP may increase pleural pressure, it may also alter the observed PAOP independent from changes in left ventricular function and intravascular volume. It is known that the effect of airway pressure on PAOP is least when the PA catheter tip is in West's zone III. Fortunately, zone III segments have the highest blood flow, and since the PA catheter is "flow directed" it tends to preferentially enter zone III on insertion.[35] However, when patients are repositioned after catheter insertion, the zone III segments may change, leaving the catheter tip in zone I or II where the influence of airway pressure is more pronounced. Perhaps the most efficient way to determine the effect of PEEP on PAOP is transiently to disconnect the patient from the ventilator (recognizing that this maneuver may cause significant arterial hypoxemia) and immediately assess the PAOP.[36] Since significant hemodynamic changes may occur after only a few seconds off the ventilator, the immediate "pop-off" PAOP may most accurately reflect the hemodynamic status of PEEP support.[37]

INTERPRETATION OF OXYGEN TRANSPORT DATA IN SHOCK

The interpretation of oxygen transport data in shock can be viewed on two levels, the adequacy of oxygen transport and evaluation of therapy to improve oxygen transport balance. The adequacy of oxygen transport can be evaluated in clinical terms of vital signs and evidence of end organ perfusion. Marked hypotension in a patient with previously normal blood pressure usually is a sign associated with tissue hypoperfusion. Hypotension is a very late sign, however, and may not occur at all in a patient with profound shock. Similarly, cold mottled extremities, oliguria, and mental confusion all may be present or absent for a variety of reasons in patients with or without clinical shock. For these reasons the adequacy of oxygen transport in patients with these signs or those who for other reasons are suspected of having inadequate tissue perfusion (such as an unexplained metabolic acidosis) should have a physiologic evaluation of oxygen transport parameters by PA catheterization and sampling of mixed venous blood gases.

Care must be taken during mixed venous blood sampling not to draw back blood too rapidly because of the possibility of aspirating pulmonary capillary blood rather than, or in addition to, the mixed venous sample that is desired. A high venous oxygen saturation or tension should alert the clinician to evaluate the sample further. The venous carbon dioxide tension should be at least 3 to 5 mm Hg greater than the arterial sample drawn at the same time.[38]

When an adequate mixed venous sample is obtained, the most important number to assess the adequacy of oxygen transport is the oxygen saturation (Sv_{O_2}). Low Sv_{O_2} values indicate increased oxygen extraction, i.e., an imbalance of oxygen supply and demand.[39] While low Sv_{O_2} indicates that an oxygenation imbalance exists, it does not give information regarding the source of the imbalance. The possibilities include severe anemia, arterial oxygen desaturation, low cardiac output, and high oxygen consumption. Anemia and arterial hypoxemia are easily ruled out by determining the hemoglobin concentration and arterial oxygen saturation. The absolute value of cardiac output can be determined by the thermodilution technique using the PA catheter. Finally the arterial-venous oxygen content difference may be calculated and used in the Fick equation to estimate total body oxygen consumption. The mathematical quotient between oxygen consumption and oxygen delivery is the oxygen utilization or extraction ratio (Table 3–1). This value is the numeric expression of oxygen transport balance and may be useful to estimate the magnitude of the perfusion deficit in shock. Since the Sv_{O_2} is inversely related to this number (Fig. 3–9), it also may prove to be a useful indicator of therapeutic responses in shock.[39]

The mixed venous oxygen tension is also a measurement useful in assessing the adequacy of oxygen transport. It must be remembered, however, that Pv_{O_2} is a variable dependent upon the Sv_{O_2} and the position of the oxyhemoglobin dissociation curve. Since Sv_{O_2} is determined by hemoglobin concentration, arterial oxygen content, cardiac output, and oxygen consumption, it is the primary determinant of Pv_{O_2}. In critically ill patients, when one is rarely certain of the position of the oxyhemoglobin dissociation curve, both Sv_{O_2} and Pv_{O_2} must be measured to calculate precisely venous oxygen content. Sv_{O_2} should not be determined from the Pv_{O_2} using a nomogram or a program in a blood gas analyzer. In fact for clinical purposes, Pv_{O_2} can be grossly estimated to be near the normal physiologic value (35 to 40 mm Hg) since it contributes so little (less than 1%) to venous oxygen content. The importance of Pv_{O_2} is that it provides the driving force for the diffusion of oxygen from the vasculature to the mitochondria for cellular energy production. When the Pv_{O_2} is less than 20 mm Hg, the mitochondria do not receive the 1 to 2 mm Hg driving pressure necessary for aerobic metabolism. Low values of Pv_{O_2} correlate with the severity of tissue hypoxia and the development of lactic acidosis.[40]

If the underlying deficit causing the shock state is one of inadequate oxygen

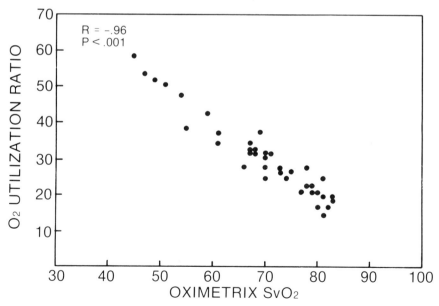

Fig. 3–9. The graph demonstrates a high degree of inverse correlation between calculated O_2 utilization and measured Sv_{O_2}.

delivery and if adequate arterial oxygen content has been obtained, the therapeutic challenge is to improve cardiac output. Hemodynamic monitoring can
guide the clinician to the most appropriate of the four ways (preload augmentation, afterload reduction, contractility enhancement, or alteration of heart rate) to
increase cardiac output.

Preload may be defined as the volume of blood presented to the ventricle for
ejection. The end diastolic volume which determines myocardial sarcomere
length cannot be readily or repeatedly measured at the bedside, so a series of
assumptions must be made to evaluate changes in left ventricular preload. The
first assumption is that over short periods of time ventricular compliance is constant so that changes in volume are reflected by changes in pressure. Next, in the
absence of mitral valve disease, the left atrial pressure is assumed to equal the left
ventricular end diastolic pressure. Finally, as is the case in most clinical circumstances (bearing in mind the cautions noted previously), the PAOP is assumed to
equal the left atrial pressure. When these assumptions are true, changes in PAOP
may be considered to reflect changes in preload and therefore may be used as a
guide for volume replacement to optimize cardiac output by the Frank-Starling
mechanism. Since intravascular volume deficiencies are common in most shock
states, the utility of PAOP measurement should be self-evident.

Afterload may be defined as the impedance to the ejection of blood from the
ventricle during systole. Impedance to blood flow is the result of the interplay
between several factors which cannot be modified by current therapy but the
major impedance to flow is the systemic vascular resistance (SVR). SVR may be
calculated (Table 3–3), and if it is found to be elevated, in the presence of adequate filling pressure, it may be lowered by vasodilators in order to reduce impedance to left ventricular outflow and increase stroke volume. It is important to note
that repeated hemodynamic measurements are necessary after therapeutic interventions for two reasons. First it must be determined if progress was made
toward improving the oxygen transport balance. Second, an intervention aimed
at affecting one of the determinants of oxygen transport may have the opposite
effect on other factors so that the net result is that the two effects cancel one
another. For example, vasodilator administration to improve stroke volume by
afterload reduction may also cause venodilation and reduce preload and yield a
net effect of no change in cardiac output. It must be remembered when treating
patients in shock that preload must be optimized before afterload reduction is
used to improve stroke volume. SVR is often increased in shock to compensate
for a relative deficit in intravascular volume. Vasodilation would block the compensation and may have disastrous effects on blood pressure.

The final factor affecting stroke volume is myocardial contractility. Myocardial
contractility may be assessed in the cardiac catheterization lab by indirect measurement of the maximum velocity of contraction or by measuring the rate of the
change in ventricular pressure over time. Neither of these techniques has application for repeated or continuous measurement in shock patients in the ICU. Contractility may be assessed in terms of the work performed by the ventricle at different volume loads. Frank-Starling ventricular function curves (Fig. 3–10) plot a
factor representing preload against work performed by the ventricle. As ventricular function (contractility) is improved, the curve will shift up and to the left. In
a critically ill patient, when filling pressure (PAOP) is maintained at some optimal

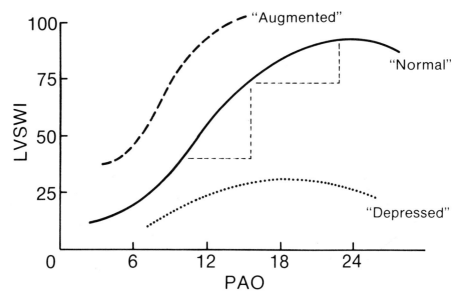

Fig. 3-10. The graph demonstrates typical relationships between left ventricular filling pressure (as an indicator of changes in preload) and left ventricular stroke work index. Changes in the position of the curve up and to the left indicate increased contractility. A shift in the curve downward and to the right indicates decreased contractility.

value, an increase in the left ventricular stroke work index (Table 3-3) indicates increased contractility.

So far, our consideration of oxygen transport monitoring of patients in shock has looked only at the net oxygen supply and demand to the entire body. It is important to remember that different vascular beds have different oxygen requirements. Although the kidneys have a high blood flow, the oxygen consumption per gram of tissue is relatively low. On the other hand, while the coronary circulation of normal hearts has the ability to markedly increase blood flow during times of increased demand, the oxygen extraction is near maximum at all times. Patients with coronary artery occlusive disease, whose coronary vascular resistance is relatively fixed, cannot respond to increased metabolic demands by increasing coronary blood flow. Interventions aimed to increase cardiac output by increasing contractility may fail since these interventions will increase the demand for oxygen in excess of the increase in myocardial oxygen supply. If, however, the interventions result in an increase in coronary perfusion pressure by raising diastolic pressure more than PAOP, myocardial oxygen delivery may be improved more than consumption is increased, and the oxygen transport balance across the myocardium will improve. These individual organ system changes in oxygen transport balance are difficult to predict and therefore re-emphasize the need for serial monitoring of cardiopulmonary and other end organ function.

NEW DEVELOPMENTS IN MONITORING THE PATIENT IN SHOCK

One of the most important advances in monitoring patients in shock since the development of routine PA catheterization is the incorporation of fiberoptic bundles into the catheter, allowing the continuous measurement of mixed venous oxygen saturation (Fig. 3–11). Mixed venous saturation gives the clinician an on-line indication of the balance between oxygen consumption and delivery.[39] This measurement serves two useful functions in patients in shock: first, one as an early warning of the need for more complete oxygen transport assessment,[41] and second, as an on-line indicator of the efficacy of therapeutic interventions to improve oxygen transport. A normal or supranormal value (> .75) does *not* indicate that hypoperfusion is not occurring in some vascular beds, but a low value does indicate a global derangement in oxygen transport balance that requires further evaluation and, likely, therapy.

It is important to realize that disturbances in the balance of oxygen transport do not always occur because of a decrease in oxygen delivery but at times may be caused by an increase in oxygen demand that cannot be supplied because of poor cardiopulmonary reserves. The assessment of metabolic demands in critically ill patients has not gained wide acceptance because of technologic limitations. Investigations have shown that the stress of trauma, shock, major surgical procedures, and nutritional support may increase oxygen consumption and carbon dioxide production.[42] New technology is available that allows continuous moni-

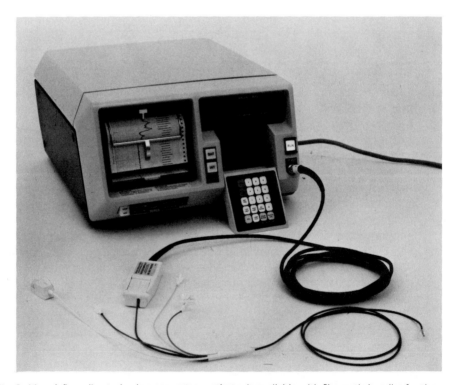

Fig. 3-11.   A flow-directed pulmonary artery catheter is available with fiberoptic bundles for the continuous in vivo measurement of mixed venous oxygen saturation by reflectance spectrophotometry. Also shown is the electronic processor used to display and record the Sv_{O_2} continuously. (Photograph compliments of Oximetrix, Inc., Mountainview, CA.)

toring of these measurements in critically ill patients.[43] It is not unreasonable to hope that further understanding of the demand side of the oxygen transport balance in patients in shock may lead to new forms of therapy, which may ultimately improve survival.

A variety of new gas analysis techniques have been demonstrated to be somewhat dependent upon blood flow (transcutaneous oxygen and carbon dioxide tension,[44] ear oximetry and digital pulse oximetry,[45] transconjunctival oxygen tension,[46] intravascular gas tension analysis[47]) and may someday have a role for less invasive monitoring of oxygen delivery.

A large effort to develop noninvasive forms of hemodynamic monitoring has been put forth in the last several years. This is a laudable goal since all forms of invasive monitoring have associated morbidity. While noninvasive means to estimate blood pressure[48] and cardiac output[49] are available today, the devices have major shortcomings when applied to critically ill patients in shock. Noninvasive measurement of blood pressure is intermittent rather than continuous and is notoriously inaccurate in hypotensive patients with abnormal vascular resistance. Similarly, while noninvasive cardiac output determinations may be accurate by some techniques, without information about filling pressures (and therefore resistances), therapy to improve cardiac output by modification of preload, afterload, and contractility would be by trial and error. Finally, the most important information obtained from hemodynamic monitoring is based on mixed venous blood sampling, which requires PA catheterization. With present technology, noninvasive hemodynamic monitoring may find a role as a screening tool to detect which patients need further invasive monitoring, but it has little role in the management of patients in shock.

The monitoring technology explosion of the last decade can present the clinician caring for patients in shock with such an overwhelming amount of information that the patient can truly be "lost in the numbers." Computer systems capable of collecting, recording, analyzing, and presenting data in a usable form show promise. Some of these systems are capable of compiling data from a variety of sources to formulate diagnoses and suggest therapeutic alternatives.[50] These systems should not be developed only as sophisticated data storage devices but rather as clinical tools to alert the physician to early changes in the patient's status so that clinical decisions may be made in a timely manner and outcome improved.

Invasive hemodynamic monitoring is an essential part of the diagnosis and treatment of patients with refractory shock syndromes. Placement of monitoring devices should not delay therapy in shock but should proceed concomitantly with therapy. It is only with precise and complete data that optimal therapy directed toward specific physiologic goals can be accomplished. A global, system-oriented approach is necessary for the early detection of end organ dysfunction related to hypoperfusion. Early detection with prompt treatment of organ dysfunction is our only hope to prevent progressive system failure and death. The monitoring devices are not amulets which by themselves protect the patient. Data obtained must be processed by the health care team and used to supplement rather than replace clinical judgment. Monitoring is not a goal in itself, but rather a means of reaching the goal of optimal patient care.

REFERENCES

1. Nelson, L.D., and Civetta, J.M.: Surgical intensive care and perioperative monitoring. *In* Textbook of Surgery. Edited by A.P. Monaco, R.S. Jones, P. Elbert, and R. Simmons. New York, Macmillan Publishing Co., 1985.
2. Aberman, A.: Fundamentals of oxygen transport in a hemodynamic monitoring context. *In* Continuous Measurement of Blood Oxygen Saturation in the High Risk Patient. Edited by J.F. Schweiss. San Diego, Beach International, Inc., 1983.
3. Connors, A.F., McCaffree, D.R., and Gray, B.A.: Evaluation of right heart catheterization in the critically ill patient without acute myocardial infarction. N. Engl. J. Med., *308*:263, 1983.
4. Civetta, J.M.: Invasive catheterization. *In* Critical Care: State of the Art. Vol. 1. Edited by W.C. Shoemaker, and W.L. Thompson. Fullerton, Ca., Society of Critical Care Medicine, 1980.
5. Bedford, R.F.: Long term radial artery cannulation: effects on subsequent vessel function. Crit. Care Med., *6*:64, 1978.
6. Bryan-Brown, C.W., et al.: The axillary artery catheter. Heart Lung, *12*:492, 1983.
7. Band, J.D., and Maki, D.G.: Infections caused by arterial catheters used for hemodynamic monitoring. Am. J. Med., *67*:735, 1979.
8. Thomas, F., et al.: The risk of infection related to radial versus femoral sites for arterial catheterization. Crit. Care Med., *11*:807, 1983.
9. Russell, J.A., et al.: Prospective evaluation of radial and femoral artery catheterization sites in critically ill adults. Crit. Care Med., *11*:936, 1983.
10. Puri, V.K., et al.: Complications of vascular catheterization in the critically ill. Crit. Care Med., *8*:495, 1980.
11. Borja, A.R.: Current status of infraclavicular subclavian vein catheterization. Ann. Thorac. Surg., *13*:615, 1972.
12. Defalque, R.J.: Percutaneous cannulation of the internal jugular vein. Anesth. Analges., *53*:116, 1974.
13. Jernigan, W.R., et al.: Use of the internal jugular vein for placement of central venous catheter. Surg. Gynecol. Obstet., *130*:520, 1970.
14. Blitt, C.D., et al.: Central venous catheterization via the external jugular vein. J.A.M.A., *229*:817, 1974.
15. Civetta, J.M.: Pulmonary artery catheter insertion. *In* The Pulmonary Artery Catheter. Edited by C.L. Sprung. Baltimore, University Park Press, 1983.
16. Qureshi, G.D., and Lilly, E.L.: Complications of CVP catheter insertion in cubital vein. J.A.M.A., *209*:1906, 1969.
17. Duval, A: The Multi-lumen catheter—a new concept in infusion therapy. Nutr. Supp. Serv., *4*:22, 1984.
18. Civetta, J.M., Gabel, J.C., and Laver, M.B.: Disparate ventricular function in surgical patients. Surg. Forum, *22*:136, 1971.
19. Wilson, R.F., Sarver, E., and Birks, R: Central venous pressure and blood volume determinations in clinical shock. Surg. Gynecol. Obstet., *132*:631, 1971.
20. Herbst, C.A.: Indications, management, and complications of percutaneous subclavian catheters: an audit. Arch. Surg., *113*:1421, 1978.
21. Abraham, E., Shapiro, M., and Podolsky, S.: Central venous catheterization in the emergency setting. Crit. Care Med., *11*:515, 1983.
22. Feliciano, D.V., et al.: Major complications of percutaneous subclavian vein catheters. Am. J. Surg., *138*:869, 1979.
23. Elliot, C.G., Zimmerman, G., and Clemmer, T.P.: Complications of pulmonary artery catheterization in the care of critically ill patients. Chest, *76*:647, 1979.
24. Applefield, J.J., et al.: Assessment of the sterility of long-term cardiac catheterization using the thermodilution Swan-Ganz catheter. Chest, *74*:377, 1978.
25. Thompson, I.R., Dalton, B.C., Lappas, D.G., and Lowenstein, E.: Right bundle branch block and complete heart block caused by the Swan-Ganz catheter. Anesthesiology, *51*:359, 1979.
26. Castellanos, A., et al.: Left fascicular blocks during right heart catheterization using the Swan-Ganz catheter. Circulation, *64*:1271, 1981.
27. Chastre, J., et al.: Thrombosis as a complication of pulmonary artery catheterization via the internal jugular vein. N. Engl. J. Med., *307*:278, 1982.
28. Pace, N.L., and Horton, W.: Indwelling pulmonary artery catheters: their relationship to aseptic thrombotic endocardial vegetations. J.A.M.A., *233*:893, 1975.
29. Kelly, T.F., et al.: Perforation of the pulmonary artery with Swan-Ganz catheters: diagnosis and surgical management. Ann. Surg., *193*:686, 1981.
30. Schwartz, K.V., and Garcia, F.G.: Entanglement of Swan-Ganz catheter around an intracardiac structure. J.A.M.A., *237*:1198, 1977.

31. Pace, N.L.: A critique of flow-directed pulmonary arterial catheterization. Anesthesiology, *47*:455, 1977.
32. Gardner, R.M.: Direct blood pressure measurement—dynamic response requirements. Anesthesiology, *54*:227, 1981.
33. Bruner, J.M.R., et al.: Comparison of direct and indirect methods of increasing arterial blood pressure: parts I, II, III. Med. Instrum., *15*:11, *15*:97, *15*:182, 1981.
34. Cengiz, M., Crapo, R.O., and Gardner, R.M.: The effect of ventilation on the accuracy of pulmonary artery and wedge pressure measurements. Crit. Care Med., *11*:502, 1983.
35. Shatsby, D.M., et al.: Swan-Ganz catheter location and left atrial pressure determine the accuracy of the wedge pressure when positive end-expiratory pressure is used. Chest, *80*:666, 1981.
36. DeCampo, T., and Civetta, J.M.: The effect of short term disconnection of high level PEEP in patients with acute respiratory failure. Crit. Care Med., *7*:47, 1979.
37. Carter, R.S., Snyder, J.V., and Pinsky, M.R.: "Pop-off" wedge as a reflection of left ventricular filling pressure. Crit. Care Med., *12*:297, 1984.
38. Shapiro, H.M., et al.: Errors in sampling pulmonary artery blood with a Swan-Ganz catheter. Anesthesiology, *40*:291, 1974.
39. Nelson, L.D., and Norwood, S.H.: The clinical utility of continuous venous oximetry in the care of critically ill patients. Crit. Care Med., *12*:295, 1984.
40. Krasnitz, P., et al.: Mixed venous oxygen tension and hyperlactatemia—survival in severe cardiopulmonary disease. J.A.M.A., *236*:570, 1976.
41. Watson, C.B.: The PA catheter as an early warning system. Anesthesiol. Rev., *10*:34, 1983.
42. Cuthbertson, D.P.: Alterations in metabolism following injury. Injury, *11*:175, 1980.
43. Westenskow, D.R., Cutler, C.A., and Wallace, W.D.: Instrumentation for monitoring gas exchange and metabolic rate in critically ill patients. Crit. Care Med., *12*:183, 1984.
44. Shoemaker, W.C., and Tremper, K.K.: Transcutaneous P_{O2} and P_{CO2} monitoring in the adult. *In* Textbook of Critical Care. Edited by W.C. Shoemaker, W.L. Thompson, and P.R. Holbrook. Philadelphia, W. B. Saunders Co., 1984.
45. Yelderman, M., and New, W.: Evaluation of pulse oximetry. Anesthesiology, *59*:349, 1983.
46. Fatt, I., and Deutsh, T.A.: The relation of conjunctival P_{O2} to capillary bed P_{O2}. Crit. Care Med., *11*:445, 1983.
47. Ledingham, I.M., Macdonald, A.M., and Douglas, I.H.S.: Monitoring of ventilation. *In* Critical Care: State of the Art. Vol. 2. Edited by W.C. Shoemaker, and W.L. Thompson. Fullerton, Ca., Society of Critical Care Medicine, 1981.
48. Paulus, D.A.: Non-invasive blood pressure measurement. Med. Instrum., *15*:91, 1981.
49. Huntsman, L.L., et al.: Noninvasive Doppler determinations of cardiac output in man: clinical validation. Circulation *67*:593, 1983.
50. Gardner, R.M., et al.: Computer-based ICU data acquisition as an aid to clinical decision making. Crit. Care Med., *10*:823, 1982.

Part II
SUPPORTING THE VITAL ORGANS

Chapter 4
THE LUNG IN SHOCK

Neil S. Yeston • Marc Palter

In response to the various precipitating factors producing shock in the surgical patient, the lung behaves in a predictable manner, often with devastating results. Although contributory events may differ, the end result has been categorized in the all-inclusive "adult respiratory distress syndrome." This chapter explores the precipitating events, the pathophysiology, and current therapy of this syndrome complex.

The adult respiratory distress syndrome (ARDS) continues to pose a major complicating event in the care of critically ill patients. Approximately 150,000 patients die of acute respiratory failure each year. Despite the various precipitating causes, sepsis and trauma prevail. Although the mortality remains greater than 50% in most cases, only a few patients die as a result of hypoxemia.[1,2] It would appear, therefore, that the major cause of death is related to associated organ dysfunction, sepsis or renal failure, for example, rather than to the pulmonary injury per se. It has been suggested that if the patient can survive the morbidity of the associated injury, the pulmonary dysfunction should improve and recover in time, providing appropriate supportive therapy is administered in a timely manner. The final common denominator appears to be a diffuse capillary leak. Only recently has the proposed mechanism of this altered vascular permeability state been revealed.[3,4]

ARDS is a term widely used to describe the syndrome characterized by a derangement in blood gas exchange, resulting from injury to the alveolar capillary membrane. Causes generally associated with this syndrome include sepsis, aspiration, thoracic trauma, pancreatitis, and intravenous drug abuse, as well as various metabolic and hematologic causes. After events such as those listed in Table 4–1, a latent period usually exists between the initiating event and onset of clinical symptoms. As a result of specific mediators, a capillary injury prevails and results in a diffuse leak of proteinaceous fluid from the intravascular to the interstitial space, producing the well described, non-hydrostatic pulmonary edema.[5]

Initially, the interstitial space is quite compliant and compensates for the increase in extravascular lung water. Simultaneously, the pulmonary lymphatic flow dramatically increases. As ingress proves greater than egress, compliance worsens, at which point there is encroachment of the interstitial fluid on the terminal airways. Subsequently, alveolar flooding ensues, causing loss of surfactant, an alteration of alveolar surface tension, and reduced lung volumes. This phenomenon is manifested by progressive alveolar collapse and loss of functional residual capacity (FRC). Consequently, areas of inadequate ventilation adjacent to normal perfusion that produce a right-to-left intrapulmonary shunt and ultimate hypoxemia are identified. As a consequence, the work of breathing, which often heralds

Table 4-1.   Causes of ARDS.

Thoracic and nonthoracic trauma
Gram negative sepsis
Fat embolism—fractures
Aspiration
Pancreatitis
Intestinal infarction
Burns
Cardiopulmonary bypass
Viral and bacterial pneumonia
Oxygen toxicity
Neurogenic factors
Massive blood transfusion

---

the necessity for mechanical ventilation, increases. At this point, despite often subtle radiographic changes of increased interstitial densities, or mild bilateral pulmonary infiltrates, the patient usually demonstrates the triad of hypoxemia, hypocarbia, and tachypnea—alerting the physician to the diagnoses. Ultimately, hypoxemia (resistant to oxygen therapy) worsens, pulmonary hypertension in the face of a normal pulmonary capillary wedge pressure develops, and a decrease in pulmonary compliance is noted. Radiographic changes consistent with the diagnosis become more obvious and the full blown syndrome evolves.

PATHOGENESIS AND PATHOPHYSIOLOGY

Pathology

The pathologic findings of ARDS in humans, following sepsis or trauma, correlate well with experimental models.[6-9] The earliest histologic change observed appears to be pulmonary microvascular engorgement and plugging with aggregates of leukocytes, platelets, and fibrin.[10] The accumulation of these blood elements in the lungs is associated with peripheral leukopenia and thrombocytopenia.[11] Initially, this stage is followed by the migration of leukocytes into the pulmonary interstitium. Varying degrees of degranulation and fragmentation of neutrophils are observed, followed by capillary endothelial edema and separation of the basement membrane.[10] Consequently, interstitial edema forms in perivascular and peribronchial connective tissue. As fluid accumulation continues, edema appears first in the alveolar septum and finally within the alveoli themselves.[12] This finding of pulmonary edema correlates with the diffuse infiltrates seen on roentgenograms and with the markedly decreased lung compliance seen clinically. The widespread atelectasis and severe pulmonary congestion observed have given rise to the description of ARDS as "congestive atelectasis."[13] Damage to alveolar epithelium leading to necrosis, coupled with the accumulation of fibrin and protein exudates, results in the formation of hyaline membranes. Interstitial fibrosis of varying degrees may occur in later stages of ARDS as a result of the reparative processes and is dependent upon the severity and duration of the syndrome.[14]

Pulmonary Edema in ARDS

The pulmonary edema that occurs in ARDS is a direct consequence of increased pulmonary endothelial permeability.[4] This alters the fluid balance normally present

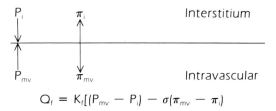

$$Q_f = K_f[(P_{mv} - P_i) - \sigma(\pi_{mv} - \pi_i)]$$

Q_f = transvascular flow of fluid
K_f = fluid filtration coefficient
P_{mv} = microvascular hydrostatic pressure
P_i = interstitial hydrostatic pressure
σ = fluid reflection coefficient
π_i = plasma osmotic pressure
π_{mv} = interstitial osmotic pressure

Fig. 4-1.   The Starling equation favors a small net transvascular flow of fluid into the interstitium. This fluid is removed by pulmonary lymphatics. When the capacity of the lymphatics is exceeded, edema forms.

in the lung, described by the Starling equation (Fig. 4–1), and results in an accumulation of extravascular lung water.

In normal lungs, the pulmonary capillary endothelium is only semipermeable to oncotically active substances which consist mostly of proteins. Capillary permeability is represented in the Starling equation by the fluid reflection coefficient, which is normally closer to a value of one than to zero. The plasma osmotic pressure can be easily measured and is thought to be slightly higher than the interstitial osmotic pressure. The latter cannot be measured clinically, but in various experimental models it is estimated by measuring the composition of lymph drained from the lungs.[15,16] The lymph, therefore, is thought to reflect accurately interstitial fluid composition.

If there is increased permeability, as hypothesized in ARDS, then the fluid reflection coefficient falls toward zero, and the osmotic gradient decreases because of the free flow of protein across the endothelium. Transvascular fluid flux is then dependent on the hydrostatic pressure gradient, which favors flow into the interstitium. Especially in ARDS, it is often associated with elevated pulmonary artery pressures.[17] Several "edema safety factors" can accommodate some increase in flow into the interstitium.[18] Extravascular lung water can be significantly increased with the radiographic appearance of edema without affecting gas exchange.[19–21] This is probably caused in part by the accumulation of fluid in collagen-rich areas of the alveolar septum away from the alveolar-capillary interface.[21] Additionally, the lymphatics afford a significant degree of protection by dramatically increasing flow.[18] Once these safety factors are overcome, gas exchange will deteriorate and intra-alveolar fluid will begin to accumulate.

Sepsis: Endotoxin

Since most patients with ARDS manifest sepsis as an associated disorder, much interest in the role of endotoxin has evolved. An infusion of endotoxin derived from *Escherichia coli* into awake sheep creates both an early dramatic increase in airway resistance and a marked decrease in pulmonary compliance similar to that seen in ARDS.[22] A marked increase in pulmonary artery pressure is also observed, which correlates well with the deterioration in lung mechanics (phase I).[23] Since these events occur within 20 minutes of endotoxin infusion, and they are not associated with an increase in lymph protein concentration, the early changes observed in pulmonary mechanics are not believed to be the result of edema formation. Later, endotoxin was shown to cause an increase in pulmonary capillary permeability by endothelial injury (phase II), which is the proposed mechanism for hypoxemia in ARDS. *E. coli* endotoxin infusion in awake sheep results in an increase in lung lymph flow and a protein clearance without an elevation in pulmonary capillary wedge pressure. This suggests an increase in capillary permeability.[23] Extravascular lung water is also increased, confirming the presence of pulmonary edema.[22] This is in contrast to the response associated with elevated left atrial pressure whereby lymph flow increases, but protein concentration decreases.[24]

Pathologic changes associated with endotoxin infusion can be seen paralleling the physiologic alterations observed. Focal endothelial cell damage associated with mild interstitial edema is observed at one hour after endotoxin infusion. Two hours subsequent to endotoxin infusion, disruption of the endothelium and perivascular and intra-alveolar edema evolve. Hypoxemia ultimately ensues.[25]

Hypoxemia may be worsened as a result of endotoxin ablation of hypoxic pulmonary vasoconstriction. Normally, hypoxic pulmonary vasoconstriction is a mechanism by which the lung reduces blood flow to poorly ventilated areas and consequently shunts blood toward alveoli that are better oxygenated. Endotoxin infusion, even in sublethal doses, will abolish this pulmonary pressor response to hypoxia, resulting in perfusion of hypo-oxygenated areas and worsening shunt.[26]

The Role of the Granulocyte

An increasing body of clinical and experimental evidence has implicated the granulocyte in the pathogenesis of the capillary leak phenomenon in ARDS.[27] Pathologic evidence during early ARDS demonstrates pulmonary sequestration of granulocytes within the pulmonary microcirculation.[25] These same granulocytes can be later shown to have migrated into the pulmonary interstitium.[25] Moreover, [111]indium oxide-tagged granulocytes are observed to be sequestered within the lung fields in patients with ARDS as compared to normal volunteers.[28]

Experimental evidence for granulocyte involvement in the capillary leak phenomenon is demonstrated by the following: 1. Endothelial destruction results from incubation of endothelial cells with activated granulocytes and plasma;[29] 2. levels of elastase and collagenase (proteolytic enzymes derived from granulocytes and thought to be responsible for the interstitial destruction in ARDS) are elevated in patients with this syndrome;[30] 3. the infusion of endotoxin into awake sheep causes peripheral leukopenia of variable duration, attributed to the sequestration of leukocytes in the pulmonary capillary bed, and correlates with the magnitude of lymph protein clearance;[31] 4. activation of granulocytes by complement or endotoxin in awake sheep results in the syndrome of pulmonary hypertension, hypoxemia, hypocarbia, and tachypnea in the face of nonhydrostatic pulmonary edema (similar if not identical to ARDS);[7,22,25] 5. the depletion of granulocytes by hydroxyurea in the same model does not prevent pulmonary hypertension, although pulmonary edema measured by lymph flow and lymph protein was significantly reduced,[32] or attenuation of dynamic compliance and total lung resistance;[33] and 6. activated granulocytes recovered from pulmonary arterial blood in patients with ARDS have been identified.[34]

Granulocytes cause endothelial damage by the release of toxic oxygen radicals, such as superoxide, hydrogen peroxide, and hydroxyl radicals.[29] They also contain an abundance of proteolytic enzymes, among them elastase, collagenase, and myeloperoxidase. There is experimental evidence to show that activated granulocytes, which are sequestered in the microcirculation, can cause endothelial damage by the generation of toxic free radicals.[35] Phorbol myristate acetate-activated granulocytes appear to cause pulmonary vascular injury by this mechanism, since infusion of dimethylthiourea (a hydroxyl radical scavenger) will inhibit edema formation.[35-37] Toxic free radicals perfused through an isolated lung preparation can cause permeability edema that can be inhibited by dimethylsulfoxide or dimethylthiourea.[38] If N-acetylcysteine (another free radical scavenger) is infused it will reduce the effects of endotoxin infusion, although it will not block them entirely.[39] Granulocytes collected from pulmonary artery blood in patients with ARDS have been shown to be in the activated state and therefore are more likely to release inflammatory mediators.[34] It would follow that either prevention of granulocyte sequestration within the pulmonary microvasculature or neutralization of toxic free oxygen radicals may ultimately be therapeutic in this syndrome.

Complement

The notion that activated complement may be largely responsible for ARDS has evolved through a circuitous series of observations. Earliest of these was the discovery that leukopenia and hypoxemia developed during early hemodialysis whereas pulmonary fibrosis and calcification occurred after prolonged therapy.[40,41] The leukopenia and hypoxemia were attributed to activation of complement (C5a) by the dialyzer coil with subsequent aggregation, margination, and sequestration of granulocytes in the pulmonary microvasculature.[40,42] This phenomenon can be experimentally reproduced by the infusion into experimental animals of autologous exposed plasma to a dialyzer coil.[42]

Reasoning that complement may be activated by endotoxin in sepsis and lipopolysaccharides in trauma, fat emboli, pancreatitis, and burns, it was suggested that as a result of this activation granulocytes aggregate and embolize to the pulmonary microvascular tree, ultimately marginating onto endothelial surfaces, accounting for the disappearance of these cells from the circulation.[3] Subsequently, toxic free oxygen radicals are liberated, producing endothelial damage and the diapedesis of protein-rich fluid through the capillary leak into the interstitial space and the resultant nonhydrostatic pulmonary edema. The eventual encroachment of this fluid upon terminal airway causes alveolar collapse and increases intrapulmonary shunt and hypoxemia. In support of this concept, it has been shown that: 1. Complement (C5a) will cause granulocytes to aggregate and marginate in vitro and granulocytes to embolize in vivo;[43-45] 2. infusion of activated complement into awake unanesthetized sheep results in a syndrome pathologically and clinically identical to ARDS;[7,46] 3. elevated levels of C5a complement have been prospectively observed in patients at risk for and subsequently developing ARDS, with some patients noted to have elevated levels before any clinical manifestation of the syndrome;[47] and 4. neutralization or absence of complement prevents endothelial destruction and reduces toxic free radical oxygen levels.

The discovery of a potential "early warning marker" (C5a) has significant therapeutic implications inasmuch as early intervention with modulators of the potential noxious mediators may prove beneficial.[29,48]

Platelets

Platelets have also been implicated in the development of ARDS. Endotoxin, collagen infusion, or soft tissue injury associated with shock will all result in a sharp fall in circulating platelets, accompanied by intravascular platelet aggregation and sequestration of platelets in the pulmonary microcirculation, and this occurs simultaneously with a rise in pulmonary artery pressure and pulmonary vascular resistance.[49-51] Pulmonary hypertension is not observed in animals made thrombocytopenic before endotoxin infusion, but the development of interstitial edema is not prevented.[52] Similarly, in a model of increased lung vascular permeability resulting from microembolization, thrombocytopenia prevented the pulmonary hypertension, yet had no effect on the formation of increased microvascular permeability.[53] Thrombocytopenia has been observed clinically in patients with ARDS for whom administration of labelled platelets revealed pulmonary sequestration.[54] Platelets appear to be involved with the development of pulmonary hypertension during the early phase of ARDS.

Arachidonate Metabolites

PROSTAGLANDINS

Arachidonic acid metabolites are produced by platelets, leukocytes, and vascular endothelium and play a prominent role in the evolution of ARDS (Fig. 4–2). Infusion of complement-activated plasma associated with an ARDS-like syndrome in animals is accompanied by increased prostaglandin production.[55] The infusion of arachidonate or several of its cyclo-oxygenase derivatives has been shown to cause a worsening in respiratory mechanics and an increase in pulmonary vasoconstriction, but it is not associated with an increase in lung permeability.[56,57] Prostaglandins E_2, F_2, G_2, and H_2, and an analog of thromboxane A_2 cause elevated pulmonary artery pressure and airway constriction when infused into various experimental animals.[58,59] A number of experimental ARDS models, such as soft tissue trauma with shock or endotoxin infusion, will result in elevated levels of stable metabolites of thromboxane A_2 (thromboxane B_2) and prostacyclin (6-keto-PGF1α) in plasma and lung lymph.[55,60,61] Thromboxane B_2 levels peak early, concomitant with the early changes in pulmonary artery pressure and lung mechanics, while 6-keto-PGF$_{1\alpha}$ peaks later, closer to the stage of increased permeability.[59,61] Cyclo-oxygenase inhibitors, such as meclofenamate, ibuprofen, and indomethacin, prevent the early endotoxin and complement-induced changes in lung mechanics[31,61,62] and severe increase in pulmonary hypertension, but not the later, smaller increase in pulmonary vascular resistance, deterioration of lung compliance, or increase in lung permeability believed to be related to granulocytes.[61-64]

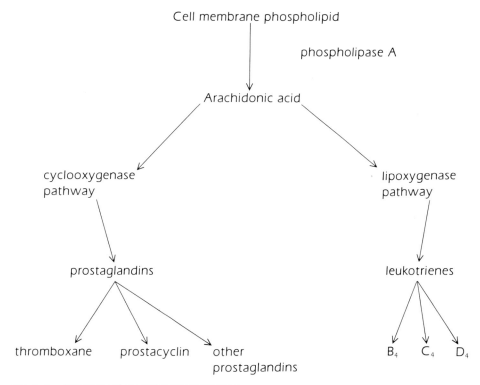

Fig. 4-2. Pathways of arachidonate metabolism.

Evidence also exists for involvement of metabolites of the lipoxygenase pathway of arachidonic acid. These include products that are released by granulocytes and that cause chemotaxis and granulocytic aggregation.[65,66] The leukotrienes C_4 and D_4 cause intense vasoconstriction, increased permeability, and leukocyte adhesion to the systemic endothelium.[67] They have been shown to cause bronchoconstriction and pulmonary vasoconstriction and are thought to be involved in a variety of pathophysiologic mechanisms involving the lung.[65,68,69] The concentration of the lipoxygenation products 5-HETE and 12-HETE increases in lung lymph after endotoxemia in sheep during the phase of increased permeability.[25,70] The leukotriene concentration increases in lung lymph more slowly than the prostaglandin concentration. The highest concentration is reached at the time of maximum leukopenia, just before the physiologic changes that indicate increased permeability and histopathological changes that demonstrate endothelial injury.[25,70] Further studies using specific lipoxygenase blockers are needed to clarify their participation in the development of ARDS.

Histamine, Bradykinin, Angiotensin-Converting Enzyme, Serotonin

Various other substances may also be involved in the pathogenesis of ARDS. Histamine is a potent bronchoconstrictor and can cause increased vascular permeability.[71,72] Infusions of histamine in sheep can cause increased lung lymph flow at doses that do not elevate pulmonary vascular pressure.[73] Diphenhydramine, an antihistamine, will reduce the magnitude of the response to endotoxin, but will not eliminate it.[74]

Bradykinin is normally metabolized by angiotensin-converting enzyme (ACE), derived from the pulmonary endothelium. Hypoxia decreases the effectiveness of ACE, and, if bradykinin is infused into sheep in the presence of hypoxia, there is an increase in lung lymph flow attributed to increased permeability.[75] Decreased serum levels of ACE have been observed in patients with ARDS.[76]

Serotonin has been suggested as a mediator of pulmonary hypertension and bronchoconstriction, but it does not cause increased vascular permeability.[71,77] Septic patients developing ARDS have been reported to have elevated serotonin levels.[78]

Reticuloendothelial System

The reticuloendothelial system (RES) clears from the blood particulate matter such as bacteria, debris from soft tissue trauma, and leukocyte-platelet-fibrin aggregates. Fibronectin is a serum opsonic protein that is essential for phagocytic function of the RES.[79] This protein is depleted in many clinical situations, among them trauma and sepsis.[80]

It is thought that activated leukocytes destroy fibronectin; as a result particulate matter circulates longer. Therefore, blunting of RES clearance of intravascular debris leads to increased microembolization and lung injury.[81,82] It has been shown that blockade of the RES enhances the effects of intravenous thrombin on the formation of pulmonary edema and associated pulmonary hypertension.[83] The infusion of cryoprecipitate (which is rich in fibronectin) into septic patients has been reported to improve pulmonary function.[84]

Disseminated Intravascular Coagulation

Disseminated intravascular coagulation (DIC) is often associated with ARDS, but its exact role in causing pulmonary dysfunction is still unclear.[85] The fibrin degradation products (FDP) are higher in patients with ARDS than in similar patients without respiratory dysfunction.[86] The FDP fragment D is often increased after trauma.[87] Fragment D infused into experimental animals has been observed to cause thrombocytopenia, pulmonary dysfunction, and increased capillary permeability, suggesting a mediator role in ARDS.[87] Others have indicated that intravascular coagulation induced in dogs does not produce ARDS.[83] However, in the presence of RES blockade, intravascular coagulation produces an elevation in pulmonary vascular resistance, hypoxemia, dead space, and shunt. In a study identifying 30 patients with ARDS, 23% had DIC, all of whom died and were found to have microthrombi within the pulmonary circulation.[88] However, 4 of 5 patients with ARDS who did not manifest DIC and who died of the syndrome, demonstrated microthrombi in their lungs. Others have identified patients with trauma or sepsis who were followed for the development of ARDS concomitantly with conventional laboratory evidence of DIC.[89] Patients in whom ARDS developed exhibited no differences in the observed laboratory variables compared with patients without pulmonary dysfunction. It is therefore difficult to determine whether FDPs are markers or mediators of ARDS, and further work is needed for clarification.

Transfusion

Massive transfusions, often required in severely injured patients, have been implicated as a cause of ARDS. Stored blood is known to form microaggregates consisting of platelets, leukocytes, and fibrin that resemble the pulmonary microemboli found in patients who have received large volumes of blood and have subsequently died of respiratory failure.[90] In an experimental model, exchange transfusion through standard (200μ) blood filters produced an increase in intrapulmonary shunt and a decrease in pulmonary diffusing capacity; this was associated with pulmonary microemboli and alveolar congestion on microscopic examinations.[91] These changes could be prevented by the use of micropore (40 μ) filters.[92] In other studies, however, shocked baboons were resuscitated with stored blood, and no significant changes in pulmonary, hemodynamic, or ventilatory functions were observed.[93]

Clinical studies have also produced conflicting results. In one study, increases in intrapulmonary shunt and alveolar-arterial oxygen gradient developed in patients who had greater than 20% of their blood volume transfused through standard filters.[94] These changes were not observed in patients who received transfusions through micropore filters or who had less than 20% of their blood volume transfused. Other studies, however, have failed to confirm any differences in pulmonary function with respect to comparing standard or micropore filters.[95,96] Retrospective studies have failed to show any correlation between the amount of blood transfused and the occurrence of respiratory dysfunction.[93,97] Because of the inconsistent results in animal and human studies, the role of massive transfusion in the pathogenesis of ARDS remains unclear.

Fat Embolism

The fat embolism syndrome resulting in acute respiratory failure has been reported to occur in 5 to 15% of patients with pelvic or multiple long bone fractures, particularly if shock is present.[98-100] In fact, 50 to 70% of patients with extremity fractures and no pre-existing lung disorders have asymptomatic pulmonary changes, such as respiratory alkalosis or mild hypoxemia.[101] Fat droplets are thought to emoblize to the lung from fracture sites, where they are then broken down by pulmonary lipase into free fatty acids toxic to the pulmonary endothelium.[102,103] Evidence also indicates that fat emboli may occur through trauma-induced alterations in fat metabolism as a result of increased plasma levels of free fatty acids (rather than the escape of fat from a marrow source).[104,105]

Thrombocytopenia is associated with fat embolism and has been attributed to tissue thromboplastin activation of platelets and their adhesion to fat emboli resulting in embolization of fibrin-platelet microaggregates. This may correlate with the hypoxemia and pulmonary hypertension observed.[106] Infusion of fat emulsion into sheep causes pulmonary hypertension, which can be blocked by indomethacin, suggesting a prostaglandin mediator.[107] Early internal fixation of long bone fractures has been reported to decrease the incidence of the fat embolism syndrome.[108]

Hemorrhagic Shock

Early studies of hemorrhagic shock in canine models initially seemed to indicate that a state of shock followed by resuscitation was sufficient for the development of ARDS.[109,110] Increased transvascular flux of albumin was interpreted as evidence for increased capillary permeability. However, subsequent studies in other animal models found no increase in extravascular lung water, and the albumin flux was attributed to elevated microvascular pressure.[111] In fact, hemorrhagic shock alone does not cause lung injury in human or animal models except (perhaps) in dogs.[111-113]

It now appears that the combination of hemorrhagic shock associated with soft tissue injury is required for the development of ARDS.[114] The various factors involved in the pathogenesis of ARDS are summarized in Figure 4–3.

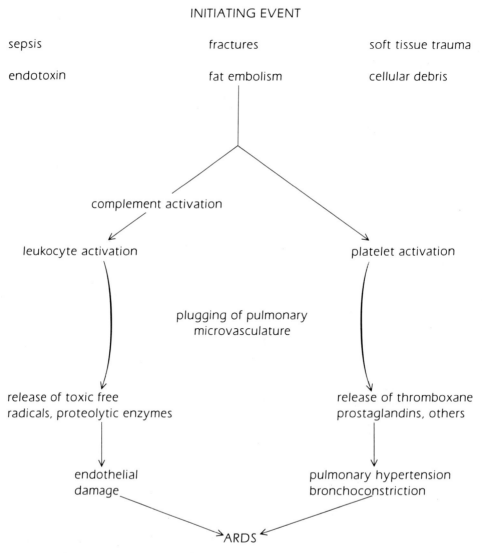

Fig. 4-3.   Summary of pathogenesis of ARDS.

CLINICAL COURSE AND TREATMENT

The presence of a latent period following the initial insult, during which time the patient's condition appears stable, requires the physician to have a high index of suspicion of individuals whose conditions are predisposing to the development of ARDS. Initially the physical examination is unremarkable, except perhaps for moderate tachypnea. Roentgenograms of the chest are often normal, but may show a slight increase in interstitial markings. Arterial blood gases obtained at this time often reveal a normal or increased pH, normal or minimally decreased Po_2, and moderate hypocapnia, indicating compensation by hyperventilation. This constellation of moderate hypoxemia, hypocarbia, and tachypnea should alert the physician to the pathophysiologic sequence that has been set in motion.

As hypoxemia progresses, attempts by the patient to compensate for a decreased tidal volume and functional residual capacity by further hyperventilation lead to increased work of breathing. The patient's condition continues to deteriorate until acute respiratory distress develops manifested by severe dyspnea and tachypnea, basilar rales on lung exam, and diffuse bilateral interstitial and alveolar infiltrates on chest roentgenogram. The fraction of inspired oxygen (F_{IO_2}) must be increased as hypoxemia worsens, and intubation and mechanical ventilation are eventually necessary as the patient finally decompensates.

Assisted mechanical ventilation notwithstanding, there is often refractory hypoxemia with a Pa_{O_2} less than 50 mm Hg, despite an F_{IO_2} greater than 60%.[115] The presence of a pulmonary capillary wedge pressure less than 18 mm Hg confirms the presence of nonhydrostatic pulmonary edema, which defines ARDS and excludes a cardiogenic cause.[116]

Since arterial blood gases early in the syndrome complex may appear deceptively normal, measurements of the alveolar-arterial oxygen difference ($AaDo_2$) may be helpful (see Appendix). In the early stages of ARDS, $AaDo_2$ may rise 30 to 40 mm Hg, and in patients with severe ARDS, $AaDo_2$ may exceed 300 mm Hg. The use of $AaDo_2$ is limited, however, because it is affected by changes in F_{IO_2}, mechanical ventilation, venous oxygen content, and cardiac output, all of which may change frequently in the patient with ARDS.

A more accurate method of assessing the severity of pulmonary dysfunction is the measurement of pulmonary venous admixture or shunt (QSP/QT) (see Appendix). Significant increase in intrapulmonary shunt and physiologic deadspace reflect the ventilation-perfusion ($\dot{V}/\dot{Q}$) mismatch that occurs in ARDS. Intrapulmonary shunt, a measure of the alveoli perfused but not ventilated, is sufficiently elevated in patients with ARDS. In order to measure shunt accurately, a pulmonary artery catheter must be in place to obtain mixed venous blood samples (Pv_{O_2}). This is the only accurate method of obtaining Pv_{O_2}, which is necessary for the shunt calculation. Intrapulmonary shunt should not be measured with the patient breathing 100% oxygen because increasing the F_{IO_2} to 100% will worsen pulmonary venous admixture by causing absorptive atelectasis and release of hypoxic pulmonary vasoconstriction.[117]

Indirect measurements of lung vascular permeability are both difficult and often of little help, as insertion of a pulmonary artery catheter can usually distinguish cardiogenic from noncardiogenic pulmonary edema. Several methods, however, have been evaluated for this indirect measurement. The ratio of alveolar fluid to plasma protein concentrations may help distinguish permeability from hydrostatic pulmonary edema. In one study, all patients with a pulmonary capillary wedge pressure less than 20 mm Hg and diagnosed as having ARDS exhibited an edema fluid to plasma protein ratio that exceeded 0.6.[118] Others have observed ratios greater than 0.7, indicative of noncardiac edema, and less than 0.5, characteristic of cardiogenic edema.[119] However, values between these ratios were nondiagnostic. Radioisotopic studies may be used to assess the permeability of pulmonary capillary endothelium.[120] The clearance into bronchial aspirates of ^{131}I-labelled ablumin is significantly greater in patients with ARDS-induced pulmonary edema than those with cardiac causes.[121]

Improved oxygenation is the most immediate goal of therapy in patients with ARDS. Mechanical ventilation is inevitable in most instances since oxygen therapy alone often fails because the patient cannot generate the work of breathing required to maintain adequate oxygenation. Use of high levels of oxygen has been shown to have toxic effects on the lung and are therefore undesirable.[122] These effects include alteration of type I and type II pneumocytes,[122] decrease in surfactant production,[123] promotion of mucociliary depression,[124] sensitization of terminal airways to gram-negative bacteria,[125] and the development of pulmonary fibrosis.[126] Absorptive atelectasis may also occur as a result of an elevated F_{IO_2}, leading to worsening hypoxemia.[117] Absorptive atelectasis occurs as a result of the diminished nitrogen tension in the alveoli, as nitrogen is displaced by a high concentration of oxygen. With the loss of the partial pressure of nitrogen, alveolar collapse ensues (as perfusion continues to remove oxygen molecules, ultimately lowering intra-alveolar pressure). Additionally, increased levels of F_{IO_2} will negate hypoxic pulmonary vasoconstriction.[117] This is a protective reflex that is postulated to occur as the result of contraction of the precapillary sphincter adjacent to hypo-oxygenated alveoli. Therefore, mixed venous blood is directed toward alveoli, which are well aerated. Administration of high concentrations of oxygen has been reported to prevent the contraction of the capillary adjacent to the hypo-oxygenated alveoli. As a consequence intrapulmonary shunt increases and hypoxemia ensue. The first goal in the treatment of ARDS, therefore, is to decrease the F_{IO_2}, while maintaining an adequate Pa_{O_2}. Although considerable debate exists as to what level is safest, most would agree that in F_{IO_2} below 50% is clinically acceptable.

Since hypoxemia in ARDS is the result of a reduction in functional residual capacity, the goal of mechanical ventilatory support is to restore this lost volume. Although intermittent positive pressure ventilation (IPPV) will expand collapsed alveoli, it alone has failed to be an effective therapeutic tool in most patients.[127] Considering that the positive pressure breath delivery by the ventilator lasts for only one second during the inspiratory cycle, and expiration endures 2 to 3 times longer, unless expiration is met with a counter-force adequate to maintain the recently opened alveoli in the patent state, alveolar collapse ensues, and gas exchange is not improved (Fig. 4–4).[128] Positive end-expiratory pressure (PEEP) delivered at adequate levels will restore the functional residual capacity by maintaining persistently expanded alveoli and subsequently will improve oxygenation.[129]

The use of PEEP has been shown to produce a significant improvement in mortality in patients suffering from the adult respiratory distress syndrome.[130] How-

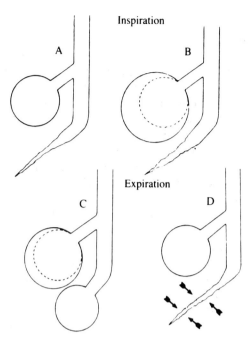

Fig. 4-4. Limitation of intermittent positive pressure ventilation (IPPV). Suggested events occurring in two adjacent lung segments (or alveoli), one of which (A) is normally inflated and the other collapsed or fluid-filled. Initial inflation tends to increase volume in the normal area preferentially (B). Later in the cycle, continued gas delivery may partially inflate the abnormal area (C). During exhalation, whatever forces were predisposing to airway closure are again unopposed, and a return to the baseline abnormal condition results (D). (Reproduced with permission from Kirby, R.R.: Mechanical ventilation in the newborn: pitfalls and practice. Perinatol. Neonatol., 5:47, 1981.)

ever, numerous authors have debated the optimal level of PEEP necessary to produce significant clinical improvement. In one series, optimal, or best PEEP, was defined as that level immediately preceding a worsening in pulmonary compliance.[131] Essentially, this was the level of PEEP associated with optimal oxygen delivery. Increasing PEEP beyond this point was believed potentially to reduce oxygen delivery as a consequence of the decreased cardiac output. The level of PEEP often associated with a fall in cardiac index was 15 cm of water. Others have advocated increasing the level of PEEP to reduce the intrapulmonary shunt to less than 15%, while augmenting cardiac output, with volume resuscitation or pharmacologic agents as necessary.[132,133] This practice of "splinting the lung in the position of function," i.e., reducing the intrapulmonary shunt to less than 15% in contrast to hypoxic-hyperoxic therapy, in which PEEP is increased to a level at which hypoxemia is corrected (Po_2 greater than 60 mm Hg) on nontoxic levels of oxygen, has been untested in prospective clinical trials. At the least, PEEP should be administered to that level where the F_{IO_2} can be lowered to nontoxic ranges, while oxygenation is maintained in an acceptable range.

The effect of PEEP on myocardial function has received much attention. Multiple causes for a reduction in cardiac output have been proposed. They include: 1. a reduction in venous return, as a result of increased intrathoracic pressure;[134] 2. humerally mediated cardiac depression;[135] 3. reduced diastolic filling caused by compression of the heart by distended lungs; and 4. leftward shifting of the intraventricular septum (as a consequence of an elevated right ventricular end diastolic pressure), causing a reduced left ventricular stroke volume.[136] Because PEEP or increased intrathoracic pressure caused by mechanical ventilation above a critical level will depress cardiac output, it is essential that accurate hemodynamic monitoring be used to ensure appropriate oxygen delivery. The use of the pulmonary artery catheter provides the data necessary to make accurate therapeutic decisions. For example, since increased intrathoracic pressure may reduce cardiac output as a consequence of a decrease in preload, restoration of an adequate filling pressure by volume infusion is often corrective. In addition, the pulmonary artery catheter can distinguish hypoxemia resulting from pulmonary dysfunction (large intrapulmonary shunt) from hypoxemia as a consequence of a reduced cardiac output superimposed on a moderate intrapulmonary shunt. The presence of a low mixed venous oxygen tension associated with a normal hemoglobin concentration is consistent with hypoxemia resulting from a depressed cardiac output. Correction of cardiac output and improvement in mixed venous oxygen tension often improves arterial oxygenation. If a reduction in cardiac output is suspected as a consequence of increased intrathoracic pressure (PEEP exceeding 15 cm of water), hemodynamic monitoring is essential.

The use of intermittent manditory ventilation (IMV) as compared to controlled mechanical ventilation (CMV) has been reported to facilitate weaning in patients with ARDS.[137] Advocates of IMV suggest that this mode of mechanical ventilation 1. prevents the discordant breathing often seen with controlled mechanical ventilation; 2. avoids respiratory alkalosis and the leftward shift of the oxygen dissociation curve, thus favoring oxygen delivery; 3. improves the ventilation to perfusion ratio; 4. avoids paralytic drugs; and 5. provides a progressive decremental method for weaning from the ventilator.[137] However, to date no prospective trials comparing IMV to controlled mechanical ventilation are available.

Although most patients with ARDS do not die of hypoxemia as the terminal event, there are those who are resistant to all forms of conventional therapy. It was hoped that extracorporeal membrane oxygenation would improve the survival rate in this group. However, the results of a recent study have been unable to demonstrate any significant clinical benefit, and the mortality in this group continues to exceed 90%.[138]

With this apparent limitation of technology the focus of investigation has shifted toward the potential pharmacologic modulation of the mediators of permeability edema as a mechanism of improved survival.

Corticosteroids

The use of corticosteroids in the treatment of ARDS has remained controversial, although there are experimental and theoretic rationales for their use. High dose corticosteroids will prevent damage to endothelial cells exposed to endotoxin and granulocytes in vivo.[134] Steroids can inhibit complement-induced granulocyte aggregation, sequestration in the lungs, and toxic free oxygen radical production.[139] Administration of corticosteroids to sheep before endotoxin infusion can diminish, but not eliminate, the early pulmonary hypertension usually observed.[140] More important, several studies have shown that steroids can prevent the late increase in vascular permeability.[141] Unfortunately, these effects are seen only if the drug is administered before, or just after, endotoxin infusion. Once the increase in permeability has occurred, steroids will not alter its course. Steroids could limit the production of leukotrienes and prostaglandins since they prevent release of arachidonic acid from cell membranes by inhibition of phospholipase A_2.[142] An improvement in capillary permeability has been seen in patients with ARDS given steroids, as evidenced by an increase in the airway fluid-plasma protein ratio.[143] However, no change in pulmonary artery pressure, shunt, compliance, or oxygenation has been observed. In a series observing trauma patients receiving high-dose steroids, a transient improvement in oxygenation was seen, but no significant difference in mortality was observed.[144] Since C5a may prove promising as an early marker of ARDS, before the onset of increased permeability, administration of pharmacological doses of corticosteroids at that juncture may prove beneficial. Large clinical trials are necessary before this therapeutic effort can be recommended.

Nonsteroidal Antiinflammatory Drugs

Inhibition of the formation of arachidonic acid metabolites may also be of benefit in ARDS. Several studies using indomethacin have shown that inhibitors of the cyclo-oxygenase pathway can block endotoxin-induced pulmonary hypertension.[145] However, indomethacin does not prevent later increases in pulmonary hypertension, and permeability may actually worsen.[146] This phenomenon has been attributed to the blocking of prostacyclin formation and the diversion of arachidonic acid to the lipoxygenase pathway. More specific thromboxane inhibitors (imidazole, OXY 1581) will prevent pulmonary hypertension, but will have no effect on permeability.[147,148] Infusion of prostacyclin has been shown to decrease significantly pulmonary hypertension and lung lymph flow, and to reduce mortality following endotoxin infusion.[149,150] Further studies are needed to evaluate the usefulness of these nonsteroid agents in the treatment of ARDS.

Fluid Resuscitation (ARDS)

Controversy still exists as to the choice of resuscitation fluid for the patient at risk for or during the development of ARDS. Proponents of colloid resuscitation argue that a fall in the osmotic gradient, as a result of a reduced plasma colloid osmotic pressure (COP) after resuscitation with large volumes of crystalloid, promotes the accumulation of interstitial fluid and subsequent pulmonary edema. In several studies evaluating colloid and crystalloid resuscitation, the risk of pulmonary edema in the crystalloid group was found to be higher when there was a lower colloid osmotic pressure and an associated fall in COP-PCWP gradient.[151,152] However, in these studies pulmonary edema was defined only roentgenographically, rather than hemodynamically, and no difference between Pa_{O_2} and intrapulmonary shunt could be found between groups. In addition there was no evidence that the COP-PCWP gradient was reflective of the transcapillary osmotic gradient, since interstitial osmotic pressure was not measured. Indeed, experimental evidence exists to show that transvascular fluid flow and accumulation of extravascular lung water do not correlate with the COP-PCWP gradient.[153] Since the osmotic pressure gradient develops passively, any change in intravascular osmotic pressure will be reflected by a change in interstitial osmotic pressure, and therefore no change in the gradient will occur.[154] In addition, hemodilution causes a rise in pulmonary lymph flow, which counteracts any increase in transvascular fluid flow.[155] Resuscitation with crystalloids will cause a fall in plasma COP, but the associated increase in transvascular fluid flux will wash out interstitial proteins, thereby lowering interstitial osmotic pressure and maintaining the same osmotic gradient.[156] A reduction of plasma COP by plasmapheresis is not associated with the development of pulmonary edema in the absence of elevated hydrostatic pressure.[155,157] In a primate model of hemorrhagic shock, in which fluid was given to restore intravascular pressure to baseline, no correlation between the use of crystalloid or colloid and the development of pulmonary edema was observed.[158]

In a series of studies using a sheep model of hemorrhagic shock, a chronic lymph fistula was constructed to assess lung lymph flow and protein concentration following resuscitation.[16,159–161] In studies comparing blood vs crystalloid resuscitation, plasma colloid osmotic pressure fell significantly in the crystalloid group. However, lymph flow increased equally following resuscitation with either fluid. In addition, there was a fall in the lymph protein concentration indicating a decrease in interstitial COP parallel to that seen in plasma. Therefore, the increase in transvascular fluid flux was caused by higher intravascular pressures seen after resuscitation and not to a change in the osmotic gradient.[16,159–161]

Many clinical studies fail to demonstrate any difference in survival rate or incidence of respiratory failure or pulmonary dysfunction following resuscitation with crystalloid or colloid.[162–165] In patients undergoing aortic aneurysm operations, the therapeutic endpoint of a pulmonary capillary wedge pressure was maintained within 5 mm Hg of baseline using crystalloid or colloid resuscitation. Although there was a 40% fall in plasma COP and an 80% fall in the COP-PCWP gradient in the crystalloid resuscitated group, intrapulmonary shunt was the same for both groups and there was no evidence of pulmonary edema.[165] Postmortem studies have shown minimal capillary endothelial and alveolar injury in trauma patients following resuscitation with crystalloid.[9] In addition, severely injured trauma patients resuscitated from shock with large volumes of blood and crystalloid have not demonstrated an increase in measured extravascular lung water, despite a fall in plasma COP and COP-PCWP gradient.[164,166] Accordingly, as long as hydrostatic pressure is not excessive, resuscitation with crystalloid appears safe and economically attractive in patients with ARDS.[167]

SUMMARY

Major advances in therapy for patients suffering from the adult respiratory distress syndrome have evolved as a result of improved understanding and technology in respiratory care. Unfortunately, the diagnosis is often made after a pathophysiologic cascade of noxious events has been set into motion, hampering our ability to employ aggressive pharmacologic modulation of the various mediators now known to play a significant role in this event. Thus, the institution of mechanical ventilatory support must be considered to be a failure of early recognition of the syndrome and effective chemotherapy. Identification of patients at risk, as well as early warning markers are necessary before elective drug therapy can be evaluated.

REFERENCES

1. Fowler, A.A., et al.: Adult respiratory distress syndrome: risk with common predispositions. Ann. Intern. Med. *98*:593, 1983.
2. Gallagher, T.J., and Civetta, J.M.: Goal directed therapy of acute respiratory failure. Anesth. Anal., *59*:831, 1980.
3. Jacob, H.S., Craddock, P.R. Hammerschmidt, D.E., and Moldow, C.F.: Complement induced granulocyte aggregation: An unsuspected mechanism of disease. N. Engl. J. Med., *320*:789, 1980.
4. Rinaldo, J.E., and Rogers, R.M.: Adult respiratory distress syndrome: changing concepts in lung injury and repair. N. Engl. J. Med., *306*:900, 1982.
5. Pontappidon, H., Geffin, B., and Lowenstein, E.: Acute respiratory failure in the adult (first of three parts). N. Engl. J. Med., *287*:690, 1977.
6. Pratt, P.C.: Pathology of adult respiratory distress syndrome: implications regarding therapy. Sem. Resp. Med., *4*:79, 1982.
7. Craddock, P.R., et al.: Complement and leukocyte mediated pulmonary dysfunction in hemodialysis. N. Engl. J. Med., *296*:769, 1977.
8. Demling, R.H.: The pathogenesis of respiratory failure after trauma and sepsis. Surg. Clin. North Am., *60*:1373, 1980.
9. Pietra, G.G., Ruttner, J.R., Wust, W. and Glinz, W.: The lung after trauma and shock—fine structure of the alveolar-capillary barrier in 23 autopsies. J. Trauma, *21*:454, 1981.
10. Coalson, J.J.: Pathophysiologic responses of the subhuman primate in experimental septic shock. Lab. Invest., *32*:561, 1975.
11. Corrin, B.: Lung pathology in septic shock. J. Clin. Path., *33*:891, 1980.
12. Greenberg, S.D., Schweppe, H.I., and Harness, M.: Shock lung: disruption of alveolar capillary walls. Texas Med., *72*:45, 1976.
13. Schramel, R., Hyman, A., Keller, C.A., and Woolverton, W.: Congestive atelectasis. J. Trauma, *8*:821, 1968.
14. Marisco, S.A., Sereri, B., Grillone, G., and Zanoni, A.: Ultrastructural changes in the noncardiogenic pulmonary edema. Bronchopneumologie, *30*:111, 1980.
15. Brigham, K.L., Woolverton, W.C., Blake, L.H., and Staub, N.C.: Increased sheep lung vascular permeability caused by pseudomonas bacteremia. J. Clin. Invest., *54*:792, 1974.
16. Demling, R.H., Selinger, S.L., Bland, R.D., and Staub, N.C.: Effect of acute hemorrhagic shock on pulmonary microvascular fluid filtration and protein permeability in sheep. Surgery, *77*:512, 1975.
17. Zapol, W.M., and Snider, M.T.: Pulmonary hypertension in severe acute respiratory failure. N. Engl. J. Med., *296*:476, 1977.
18. Civetta, J.M.: A new look at the Starling equation. Crit. Care Med., *7*:84, 1979.
19. Rodman, G.H., and Kirby, R.R.: Post-traumatic respiratory failure: role of fluid therapy. Contemp. Anesth. Pract. *6*:119, 1983.
20. Cooper, J.D., Maeda, M., and Lowenstein, E.: Lung water accumulation with acute hemodilution in dogs. J. Thorac. Cardiovasc. Surg. *69*:957, 1975.
21. Staub, N.C., Nagano, H., and Pearce, M.L.: Pulmonary edema in dogs especially the sequence of fluid accumulation in lungs. J. Appl. Physiol. *22*:227, 1967.
22. Esbenshade, A.M., et al.: Respiratory failure after endotoxin infusion in sheep: lung mechanics and lung fluid balance. J. Appl. Physiol., *53*:967, 1982.
23. Brigham, K., Bowers, R., and Haynes, J.: Increased sheep lung vascular permeability caused by E. coli endotoxin. Circ. Res. *45*:292, 1979.
24. Parker, R.E., Roselli, R.J., Harris, T.R., and Brigham, K.L.: Effects of graded increases in pulmonary vascular pressures on lung fluid balance in unanesthetized sheep. Circ. Res., *49*:1164, 1981.
25. Meyrick, B., and Brigham, K.L.: Acute effects of E. coli endotoxin on the pulmonary microcirculation of anesthetized sheep. Lab. Invest., *48*:458, 1983.
26. Weir, E.K., Miczoch, J., Reeves, J.T., and Grover, K.F.: Endotoxin and prevention of hypoxic pulmonary vasoconstriction. J. Lab. Clin. Med., *88*:975, 1981.
27. Tate, R.M., and Repine, J.E.: Neutrophils and the adult respiratory distress syndrome. Am. Rev. Resp. Dis., *128*:552, 1983.
28. Powe, J.E., Short, A., Sibbald, W.J., and Driedger, A.A.: Pulmonary accumulation of polymorphonuclear leukocytes in the adult respiratory distress syndrome. Crit. Care Med., *10*:712, 1982.
29. Sacks, T., Moldow, C.F., Craddock, P.R., Bowers, T.K., and Jacob, H.S.: Oxygen radicals mediate endothelial cell damage by complement-stimulated granulocytes. J. Clin. Invest., *61*:1161, 1978.
30. Cochrane, C.G., et al.: The presence of neutrophil elastase as evidence of oxidation activity in bronchoalveolar lavage of patients with adult respiratory distress syndrome. Am. Rev. Resp. Dis., *127*:S25, 1983.
31. Snapper, J.R., et al.: Endotoxemia-induced leukopenia in sheep. Am. Rev. Resp. Dis., *127*:306, 1983.

32. Heflin, A.C., and Brigham, K.L.: Prevention by granulocyte depletion of increased vascular permeability of sheep lung following endotoxemia. J. Clin. Invest., *68*:1253, 1981.

33. Hinson, J.M., et al.: Effect of granulocyte depletion on altered lung mechanics after endotoxemia in sheep. J. Appl. Physiol. *55*:92, 1983.

34. Zimmerman, G.A., Renzetti, A.D., and Hill, H.R.: Functional and metabolic activity of granulocytes from patients with adult respiratory distress syndrome. Am. Rev. Resp. Dis., *127*:290, 1983.

35. Till, G.O., Johnson, K.J., Kunkel, R., and Ward, P.A.: Intravascular activation of complement and acute lung injury. J. Clin. Invest., *69*:1126, 1982.

36. Shasby, D.M., et al.: Granulocytes mediate acute edematous lung injury in rabbits and in isolated rabbit lungs perfused with phorbol myristate acetate: role of oxygen radicals. Am. Rev. Resp. Dis., *125*:443, 1982.

37. Shasby, D.M., Shasby, S.S., and Peach, M.J.: Granulocytes and phorbol myristate acetate increase permeability to albumin of cultured endothelial monolayers and isolated perfused lung. Am. Rev. Resp. Dis., *127*:72, 1983.

38. Tate, R.M., et al.: Oxygen radical-induced pulmonary edema. Chest, *81*:Suppl 57S, 1982.

39. Lucht, W.D., et al.: Effect of N-acetyl cysteine on the pulmonary response to endotoxin in awake sheep. Fed. Proc., *42*:1107, 1983.

40. Kaplow, L.S., and Goffinet, J.A.: Profound neutropenia during early hemodialysis. J.A.M.A., *203*:133, 1968.

41. Conger, J.D., et al.: Pulmonary calcification in chronic dialysis patients: clinical and pathological studies. Ann. Intern. Med., *83*:330, 1975.

42. Craddock, P.R., et al.: Hemodialysis leukopenia. J. Clin. Invest., *59*:879, 1977.

43. Craddock, P.R., et al.: Complement (C5a)-induced granulocyte aggregation in vitro. J. Clin. Invest., *60*:260, 1977.

44. Hammerschmidt, D.E., et al.: Complement-induced granulocyte aggregation in vivo. Am. J. Pathol., *102*:146, 1981.

45. O'Flaherty, J.T., Craddock, P.R., and Jacob, H.S.: Effect of intravascular complement activation on granulocyte adhesiveness and distribution. Blood, *51*:731, 1978.

46. Jacobs, H.S.: Damaging role of activated complement in myocardial infarction and shock lung. *In* Critical Care: State of the Art. Edited by W.C. Shoemaker, and W.L. Thompson, Fullerton, CA, Society of Critical Care Medicine, 1980.

47. Hammerschmidt, D.E., et al.: Association of complement activation and elevated plasma-C5a with adult respiratory distress syndrome. Lancet, *947*: May 3, 1980.

48. Goldstein, J.M., et al.: Influence of corticosteroids on human PMN leukocyte function in vitro: reduction of lysosomal enzyme release and superoxide production. Inflammation, *1*:305,1976.

49. Vaage, J.: Intravascular platelet aggregation and acute respiratory insufficiency. Circ. Shock, *4*:279, 1977.

50. Myrrold, H.E., Svalander, C.: Pulmonary microembolism in early experimental septic shock. J. Surg. Res., *23*:65, 1977.

51. Thorne, L.J., Kuenzig, M., McDonald, H.M., and Schwartz, S.I.: Effect of denervation of a lung on pulmonary platelet trapping associated with traumatic shock. Surgery, *88*:208, 1980.

52. Bredenberg, C.E., Taylor, G.A., and Webb, W.R.: The effect of thrombocytopenia on the pulmonary and systemic hemodynamics of canine endotoxin shock. Surgery, *87*:59, 1980.

53. Binder, A.S., et al.: Effect of platelet depletion on lung vascular permeability after microemboli in sheep. J. Appl. Physiol., *48*:414, 1980.

54. Schneider, R.C., Zapol, W.M., and Carvalho, A.C.: Platelet consumption and sequestration in severe acute respiratory failure. Am. Rev. Resp. Dis., *122*:445, 1980.

55. Cooper, J.D., et al.: Prostaglandin production associated with the pulmonary vascular response to complement activation. Surgery, *88*:215, 1980.

56. Ogletree, M.L., and Brigham, K.L.: Arachidonate raises vascular resistance but not permeability in lungs of awake sheep. J. Appl. Physiol., *48*:581, 1980.

57. Kadowitz, P.J., Gruetter, C.A., Spannhake, E.W., and Hyman, A.L.: Pulmonary vascular responses to prostaglandins, Fed. Proc., *40*:1991, 1981.

58. Brigham, K.L., and Ogletree, M.L.: Effects of prostaglandins and related compounds on lung vascular permeability. Bull. Europ. Physiopathol. Resp., *17*:703, 1983.

59. Bowers, R.E., Ellis, E.F., Brigham, K.L., and Oates, J.A.: Effects of prostaglandin cyclic endoperoxides on the lung circulation of unanesthetized sheep. J. Clin. Invest., *63*:131, 1979.

60. Demling, R.H.: Pulmonary injury and prostaglandin production during endotoxemia in conscious sheep. Am. J. Physiol., *240*:H348, 1981.

61. Snapper, J.R., Hutchison, A.A., Ogletree, M.L., and Brigham, K.L.: Effects of cyclooxygenase inhibitors on the alterations in lung mechanics caused by endotoxemia in the unanesthetized sheep. J. Clin. Invest., *72*:63, 1983.

62. Brigham, K.L.: Mechanisms of lung injury. Clin. Chest Med., *3*:9, 1982.

63. Kerstein, M.D., and Crivello, M.: Reversal of histopathologic pulmonary changes with indomethacin. Surg. Gynecol. Obstet., *151*:786, 1980.

64. Ogletree, M.L., and Brigham, K.L.: Effects of cyclooxygenase inhibitors on pulmonary vascular responses to endotoxin in unanesthetized sheep. Prost. Leuk. Med., *8*:489, 1982.

65. Ford-Hutchinson, A.W., et al.: Leukotriene B, a potent chemokinetic and aggregating substance released from polymorphonuclear leukocytes. Nature, *286*:241, 1980.

66. O'Driscoll, B.R.C.: Editorial: Leukotrienes and lung disease. Thorax, *37*:241, 1982.

67. Dahlen, S., Hedquist, P., Hammerstrom, D., and Samuelsson, B.: Leukotrienes are potent constrictors of human bronchi. Nature, *288*:484, 1980.

68. Dahlen, S., et al.: Leukotrienes promote plasma leakage and leukocyte adhesion in postcapillary venules. Proc. Natl. Acad. Sci. U.S.A., *78*:3887, 1981.

69. Ogletree, M.L., Snapper, J.R., and Brigham, K.L.: Immediate pulmonary vascular and airway responses after intravenous leukotriene D_4 injections in awake sheep. Physiologist, *25*:275, 1982.

70. Ogletree, M.L., Oates, J.A., Brigham, K.L., and Hubbard, W.C.: Evidence for pulmonary release of 5-hydroxyeicosatetraenoic acid during endotoxemia in unanesthetized sheep. Prostaglandins, *23*:459, 1982.

71. Parrat, J.R., and Sturgess, R.M.: The possible roles of histamine, 5-hydroxytryptamine and prostaglandin F_2 as mediators of the acute pulmonary effects of endotoxin. Br. J. Pharmacol. *60*:209, 1977.

72. Pietra, G.G., Szidon, J.P., Leventhal, M.M., and Fishman, A.P.: Histamine and interstitial pulmonary edema in the dog. Circ. Res., *29*:323, 1971.

73. Brigham, K.L., and Owen, P.J.: Increased sheep lung vascular permeability caused by histamine. Circ. Res., *37*:647, 1975.

74. Brigham, K.L., et al.: Diphenhydramine reduces endotoxin effects on lung vascular permeability in sheep. J. Appl. Physiol., *49*:516, 1980.

75. Pang, L.M., O'Brodovich, H.M., Mellins, R.B., and Stalcup, S.A.: Bradykinin induced increase in pulmonary vascular permeability in hypoxic sheep. J. Appl. Physiol., *52*:370, 1982.

76. Casey, L., et al.: Decreased serum angiotensin converting enzyme in adult respiratory distress syndrome associated with sepsis. Crit. Care Med., *9*:651, 1981.

77. Brigham, K.L., and Owen, P.J.: Mechanism of the serotonin effect on lung transvascular fluid and protein movement in awake sheep. Circ. Res., *36*:761, 1975.

78. Sibbald, W., Peters, S., and Lindsay, R.M.: Serotonin and pulmonary hypertension in human septic ARDS. Crit. Care Med., *8*:490, 1981.

79. Saba, T.M., and Jaffe, E.: Plasma fibronectin: its synthesis by vascular endothelial cells and role in cardiopulmonary integrity after trauma as related to reticuloendothelial function. Am. J. Med., *68*:577, 1980.

80. Blumenstock, F.A., and Saba, T.M.: Fibronectin: a mediator of phagocytosis and its potential in treating septic shock. Adv. Exp. Med. Biol., *155*:613, 1982.

81. Niehaus, G.D., Shumacker, P.R., and Saba, T.M.: Reticuloendothelial clearance of blood-borne particles. Ann. Surg., *191*:479, 1980.

82. Niehaus, G.D., Saba, T.M., Edmonds, R.H., and Dillon, B.C.: Leukocyte involvement in pulmonary localization of blood-borne microparticulates. Circ. Shock, *12*:95, 1984.

83. Schumacker, P.R., and Saba, T.M.: Pulmonary gas exchange abnormalities following intravascular coagulation. Ann. Surg., *192*:95, 1980.

84. Saba, T.M., Blumenstock, F.A., Scovill, W.A., and Bernard, H.: Cryoprecipitate reversal of opsonic alpha 2 binding glycoprotein deficiency in septic surgical and trauma patients. Science, *201*:622, 1978.

85. Blaisdell, F.W., Lim, R.C., and Stallone, R.J.: The mechanism of pulmonary damage following traumatic shock. Surg. Gynecol. Obstet., *130*:15, 1970.

86. Haynes, J.B., et al.: Elevated fibrinogen degradation products in the adult respiratory distress syndrome. Am. Rev. Resp. Dis., *122*:841, 1980.

87. Manwaring, D., and Curreri, P.W.: The role of platelet aggregation and release in fragment D-induced pulmonary dysfunction. Am. Surg., *192*:103, 1980.

88. Bone, R.C., Francis, P.B., and Pierce, A.K.: Intravascular coagulation associated with the adult respiratory distress syndrome. Am. J. Med., *61*:585, 1976.

89. Modig, J.: The value of variables of disseminated intravascular coagulation in the diagnosis of adult respiratory distress syndrome. Acta Anesthesiol. Scand., *27*:369, 1983.

90. Bredenberg, C.E.: Acute respiratory distress. Surg. Clin. North Am., *54*:1043, 1974.

91. Barrett, J., et al.: Pulmonary microembolism associated with massive transfusion. Ann. Surg., *182*:56, 1975.

92. Brown, C., et al.: Progression and resolution of changes in pulmonary function and structure due to pulmonary microembolism and blood transfusion. Ann. Surg., *185*:92, 1977.

93. Rosario, M.D., et al.: Blood microaggregates and ultrafilters. J. Trauma, *18*:498, 1978.

94. Barrett, J., Tahir, A.H., and Litwin, M.S.: Increased pulmonary arteriovenous shunting in humans following blood transfusion. Arch. Surg., *113*:947, 1978.
95. Virgilio, R.W., et al.: To filter or not to filter? Inten. Care Med., *3*:144, 1977.
96. Snyder, E.L., et al.: An in vivo evaluation of microaggregated blood filtration during total hip replacement. Ann. Surg., *190*:75, 1979.
97. Collins, J.A., et al.: The relationship between transfusion and hypoxemia in combat casualties. Ann. Surg., *188*:513, 1978.
98. Peltier, L.F., Collins, J.A., Evarts, C.M., and Sevitt, S.: Fat embolism. Arch. Surg., *109*:112, 1974.
99. Peltier, L.F.: Fat embolism syndrome. Clin. Ortho., *66*:241, 1969.
100. Pollack, R., and Myers, R.A.M.: Early diagnosis of the fat embolism syndrome. J. Trauma, *18*:121, 1978.
101. Wilson, R.F., McCarthy, B., LeBlanc, P., and Mammen, F.: Respiratory and coagulation changes after uncomplicated fractures. Arch. Surg., *106*:395, 1973.
102. Meek, R.N., Woodruft, B., and Allardyce, D.B.: Source of fat macroglobules in fractures of the lower extremity. J. Trauma, *12*:432, 1972.
103. Oh, W.H., and Mital, M.A.: Fat embolism: current concepts of pathogenesis, diagnosis, and treatment. Ortho. Clin. North Am., *9*:769, 1978.
104. McNamara, J.J., et al.: Lipid metabolism after trauma. J. Thorac. Cardiovasc. Surg., *63*:968, 1972.
105. Nixon, J.R., and Brock-utne, J.G.: Free fatty acid and arterial oxygen changes following major injury. J. Trauma, *18*:73, 1978.
106. Shier, M.R., and Wilson, R.F.: Fat embolism syndrome: traumatic coagulopathy with respiratory distress. Surg. Annu., *12*:139, 1980.
107. McKeen, C.R., Brigham, K.L., Bowers, R.E., and Harris, T.R.: Pulmonary vascular effects of fat emulsion infusion in unanesthetized sheep. J. Clin. Invest., *61*:1291, 1978.
108. Riska, E.B., and Myllynen, P.: Fat embolism in patients with multiple injuries. J. Trauma, *22*:891, 1982.
109. Northrup, W.F., and Humphrey, E.W.: The effect of hemorrhagic shock on pulmonary vascular permeability to plasma proteins. Surgery, *83*:264, 1978.
110. Todd, T.R.J., Baile, E., and Hogg, J.C.: Pulmonary capillary permeability during hemorrhagic shock. J. Appl. Physiol., *45*:298, 1978.
111. Demling, R.H., Niehaus, G., and Will, J.A.: Pulmonary microvascular response to hemorrhagic shock, resuscitation and recovery. J. Appl. Physiol., *46*:498, 1979.
112. Meyers, J.R., Meyer, J.S., and Baue, A.E.: Does hemorrhagic shock damage the lung? J. Trauma, *13*:509, 1973.
113. Michel, R.P., LaForte, M., and Hogg, J.C.: Physiology and morphology of pulmonary microvascular injury with shock and reinfusion. J. Appl. Physiol., *50*:1227, 1981.
114. Porcelli, R., et al.: Pulmonary circulatory changes in pathogenesis of shock lung. Am. J. Med. Sci., *268*:250, 1974.
115. Petty, T.L., and Fowler, A.A.: Another look at ARDS. Chest, *82*:98, 1982.
116. Pepe, P.E., et al.: Clinical predictors of the adult respiratory distress syndrome. Am. J. Surg., *144*:124, 1982.
117. Suter, P.M., Fairley, H.B., and Schlobohm, R.M.: Shunt, lung volume, and perfusion during short periods of ventilation with oxygen. Anesthesiology, *43*:617, 1975.
118. Fein, A., et al.: The value of edema fluid protein measurement in patients with pulmonary edema. Am. J. Med., *67*:32, 1979.
119. Sprung, C.L., et al.: The spectrum of pulmonary edema: differentiation of cardiogenic, intermediate and noncardiogenic forms of pulmonary edema. Am. Rev. Resp. Dis., *124*:718, 1981.
120. Gorin, A.B., Kohler, J., and DeNardo, G.: Noninvasive measurement of pulmonary transvascular protein flux in normal man. J. Clin. Invest., *66*:869, 1980.
121. Anderson, P.R., et al.: Documentation of pulmonary capillary permeability in the adult respiratory distress syndrome accompanying human sepsis. Am. Rev. Resp. Dis., *119*:868, 1979.
122. Winter, P.M., and Smith, G.: The toxicity of oxygen. Anesthesiology, *37*:210-235, 1982.
123. Giammona, S.T., Kerner, D., and Bondurant, S.: Effect of oxygen breathing at atmospheric pressure on pulmonary surfactant. J. Appl. Physiol., *20*:855, 1965.
124. Wolfe, W.G., Abert, P.A., and Sabiston, D.C.: Effect of high oxygen tension on mucociliary function. Surgery, *72*:246, 1976.
125. Higuchi, J.H., Coalson, J.J., and Johanson, W.G.: Effect of hyperoxia on tracheal mucosal adherence, lower respiratory tract colonization and infection. Am. Rev. Resp. Dis., *121(suppl)*:353, 1980.
126. Bowden, D.H., Adamson, P.R., and Wyatt, J.P.: Reaction of lung cells to high concentrations of oxygen, Arch. Pathol., *20*:835, 1965.
127. Sands, J.H., et al.: A controlled study using routine intermittent positive pressure breathing in the postsurgical patient. Dis. Chest, *40*:128, 1961.

128. Smith, R.H.: PEEP-CPAP historical and theoretical considerations, Part I. Current Reviews in Respiratory Therapy. Miami, Frank Moya, 1978.
129. Tyler, D.C.: Positive end-expiratory pressure: a review. Crit. Care Med., *11*:300, 1983.
130. Ashbaugh, D.G., Petty, T.L., Bigelow, D.B., and Harris, T.M.: Continuous positive pressure breathing in adult respiratory distress syndrome. J. Thorac. Cardiovasc. Surg., *57*:31, 1969.
131. Suter, P.M., Fairley, H.B., and Isenberg, M.D.: Effect of tidal volume and positive end-expiratory pressure on compliance during mechanical ventilation. N. Engl. J. Med. *292*:284, 1975.
132. Walkinshaw, M., and Shoemaker, W.C.: Use of volume loading to obtain preferred levels of PEEP. Crit. Care Med., *8*:81, 1980.
133. Gallagher, T.J., Civetta, J.M., and Kirby, R.R.: Terminology update: optimal PEEP. Crit. Care Med., *6*:323, 1978.
134. Cournard, A., Motley, H.L., Werko, L., and Richards, D.W.: Physiological studies of the effects of intermittent positive pressure breathing on cardiac output in man. Am. J. Physiol., *52*:162, 1948.
135. Patten, M.T., Liebman, P.R., and Hechtman, G.B.: Humorally mediated decreases in cardiac output associated with positive end expiratory pressure. Microvasc. Res., *13*:137, 1979.
136. Jardin, F., et al.: Influence of positive end expiratory pressure on left ventricular performance. N. Engl. J. Med., *304*:387, 1981.
137. Downs, J.B., Perkins, H.M., and Modell, J.H.: Intermittent mandatory ventilation. Arch. Surg., *109*:519, 1974.
138. National Heart, Lung and Blood Institute, Division of Lung Diseases: Extracorporeal support for respiratory insufficiency. 243.5, 1979.
139. Hammerschmidt, D.E., White, J.G., Craddock, P.R., and Jacob, H.J.: Corticosteroids inhibit complement-induced granulocyte aggregation. J. Clin. Invest., *63*:798, 1979.
140. Brigham, K.L., Bowers, R.E., and McKeen, C.R.: Methylprednisolone prevention of increased lung vascular permeability following endotoxemia in sheep. J. Clin. Invest. *67*:1103, 1981.
141. White, G.L., Archer, L.T., Beller, B.H., and Hinshaw, L.B.: Increased survival with methylprednisolone treatment in canine endotoxic shock. J. Surg. Res., *25*:357, 1978.
142. Hyman, A.L., Mathe, H.A., Lippton, H.L., and Kadowitz, P.J.: Prostaglandins and the lung. Med. Clin. North. Am., *65*:789, 1981.
143. Sibbald, W.J., et al.: Alveo-capillary permeability in human septic ARDS. Chest, *79*:133, 1981.
144. Lucas, C.E., and Ledgerwood, A. M.: Pulmonary response of massive steroids in seriously injured patients. Ann. Surg., *194*:256, 1981.
145. Demling, R.H.: Role of prostaglandins in acute pulmonary microvascular injury. Ann. N.Y. Acad. Sci., *384*:517, 1982.
146. Ogletree, M.L., and Brigham, K.L.: Indomethacin augments endotoxin induced increased lung vascular permeability in sheep. Am. Rev. Resp. Dis., 119:383, 1979.
147. Smith, E.F., Tabas, J.H., and Lefer, A.M.: Beneficial actions of imidazole in endotoxin shock. Prostagland. Med., *4*:215, 1980.
148. Casey, L.C., Fletcher, J.R., Zmudka, M.I., and Ramwell, P.W.: Prevention of endotoxin induced pulmonary hypertension in primates by the use of a selective thromboxane synthetase inhibitor. J. Pharm. Exp. Therapeut., *222*:441, 1982.
149. Demling, R.H., et al.: The effect of prostacyclin infusion on endotoxin-induced lung injury. Surgery, *89*:257, 1981.
150. Fletcher, J.R., and Ramwell, P.W.: The effect of prostacyclin on endotoxin shock and endotoxin induced platelet aggregation in dogs. Circ. Shock, *7*:299, 1980.
151. Da Luz, P.L., et al.: Pulmonary edema related to changes in colloid osmotic and pulmonary artery wedge pressures in patients after acute MI. Circulation, *51*:350, 1975.
152. Weil, M.H., Henning, R.J., Morissette, M., and Michaels, S.: Relationship between colloid osmotic pressure and pulmonary artery wedge pressure in patients with cardiorespiratory failure. Am. J. Med., *64*:643, 1978.
153. Levine, O.R., Mellins, R.B., Senior, R.M., and Fishman, A.P.: The application of Starling's law of capillary exchange to the lungs. J. Clin. Invest., *46*:934, 1967.
154. Staub, N.C.: Pulmonary edema due to increased microvascular permeability. Annu. Rev. Med., *32*:291, 1981.
155. Zarins, C.K., Rice, C.L., Peters, R.M., and Virgilio, R.W.: Lymph and pulmonary response to isobaric reduction in plasma oncotic pressure in baboons, Circ. Res., *43*:925, 1978.
156. Zarins, C.K., et al.: Role of lymphatics in preventing hypo-oncotic pulmonary edema. Surg. Forum, *27*:257, 1976.
157. Rice, C.L., et al.: Effect of sepsis and reduced colloid osmotic pressure on pulmonary edema. J. Surg. Res., *27*:342, 1979.
158. Holcroft, J.W., and Trunkey, D.D.: Extravascular lung water following hemorrhagic shock in the baboon. Ann. Surg., *180*:408, 1974.

159. Demling, R.H., Manohar, M., Will, J.A., and Belzer, F.O.: The effect of plasma oncotic pressure on the pulmonary microcirculation after hemorrhagic shock. Surgery, *86*:323, 1979.
160. Demling, R.H., Manohar, M., and Will, J.A.: Response of the pulmonary microcirculation to fluid loading after hemorrhagic shock and resuscitation. Surgery, *87*:552, 1980.
161. Demling, R.H.: Lung fluid and protein dynamics during hemorrhagic shock, resuscitation and recovery. Circ. Shock, *7*:149, 1980.
162. Moss, G.S., et al.: Comparison of asanguineous fluids and whole blood in the treatment of hemorrhagic shock. Surg. Gynecol. Obstet., *129*:1247, 1969.
163. Moss, G.S.: Argument in favor of electrolyte solution for early resuscitation. Surg. Clin. North Am., *52*:3, 1972.
164. Lowe, R.J., Moss, G.S., Jilek, J., and Levine, H.D.: Crystalloid vs. colloid in the etiology of pulmonary failure after trauma. Surgery, *81*:676, 1977.
165. Virgilio, R.W., et al.: Crystalloid vs. colloid resuscitation: Is one better? Surgery, *85*:129, 1979.
166. Tranbaugh, K.F., Elirgs, V.B., Christensen, J., and Lewis, F.R.: Determinants of pulmonary interstitial fluid accumulation after trauma. J. Trauma, *22*:820, 1982.
167. Guyton, A.C., and Lindsey, A.W.: Effect of left atrial pressure and decreased plasma protein concentration on the development of pulmonary edema. Circ. Res., *7*:649, 1959.

APPENDIX

Equations for calculating alveolar-arterial oxygen difference and intrapulmonary shunt.

$$\text{Eq. 1. } AaDo_2 = (713 \text{ mm Hg} \times F_{IO_2}) - (1.25 \times Pa_{CO_2}) - Pa_{O_2}$$

$$\text{Eq. 2. } QS/QT = \frac{Cc_{O_2} - Ca_{O_2}}{Cc_{O_2} - Cv_{O_2}}$$

where Ca_{O_2} = arterial O_2 content; Cv_{O_2} = venous O_2 content; and Cc_{O_2} = capillary O_2 content.

$Ca_{O_2} = (Hb \times 1.34 \times Sat) + (Pa_{O_2} \times 0.003)$
$Cv_{O_2} = (Hb \times 1.34 \times Sv) + (Pv_{O_2} \times 0.003)$
$Cc_{O_2} = PA_{O_2} = (713 \times F_{IO_2} - (1.25 \times Pa_{O_2})$
Hb = hemoglobin
Sat = arterial saturation
Pa_{O_2} = arterial oxygen tension
Sv = mixed venous saturation
Pv_{O_2} = mixed venous oxygen tension
PA_{O_2} = alveolar oxygen content

Chapter 5
THE BRAIN IN SHOCK

Glenn C. Hamilton • Blaine C. White

ANATOMY OF THE BRAIN

The brain is a complex collection of neurons (gray matter), nerve fibers (white matter), and interconnections (synapses). It is subdivided into an anatomic hierarchy of function, the cerebral cortex being the highest level—consciousness—and the spinal cord the lowest—reflex. Cell bodies are grouped at the cortex or gray matter. Densely arranged axon tracts make up much of the central white matter. Neurons, which constitute 60 to 70% of brain tissue, are synthesizers and secreters of neurotransmitters. They are most sensitive to changes in cellular perfusion and have no mitotic capability. Once destroyed, they are gone. Glial cells, which make up 20 to 30% of the brain, provide mechanical and metabolic support and may be important in forming the blood brain barrier. Vascular tissues and interstitial spaces make up the remainder.

The blood brain barrier (BBB) is anatomically made up of the vascular wall and perivascular glial membrane.[1] Its exact location is still controversial, but functionally it includes a carrier-mediated mechanism, an active transport process, and physiochemical properties.[2] It maintains homeostasis of the brain's fluid and solute milieu,[2,3] although its effectiveness varies with animal species, brain region, nature of insult, and substance used for measurement.[2] This variability has important implications in interpreting brain research.

The brain is protected by the scalp, skull, and supporting meninges. The cranium is a rigid structure with three major compartments. Brain tissue occupies 80% of the cranium, with the remaining space filled by blood (12%) and cerebrospinal fluid (8%), the latter averaging 130 to 150 ml in the adult. The brain is bathed and buffered by cerebrospinal fluid (CSF) in the subarachnoid space. This space lies between the closely vested pia mater and the highly vascular subarachnoid membrane. The third layer of the meninges is the dura mater, which fuses with the periosteum of the skull.

The vascular supply consists of the paired carotid and vertebral arteries joined at the circulus arteriosus (circle of Willis). From this circle, branches pass anteriorly, laterally, and posteriorly to supply the cortex from the surface. Anastomatic channels exist between the principle arterial branches at superficial and deep levels. Still, the penetrating vessels are primarily end-arteries, resulting in a structurally limited collateral circulation and increased ischemic vulnerability.

PHYSIOLOGY OF THE BRAIN

The brain can be viewed physiologically as a high-consumption, finicky eater with minimal storage. Accounting for only 2% of the total body weight, it consumes 20% of total oxygen used by the body, and up to 66% of the liver's glucose production.[2] The cerebral metabolic rate for oxygen is a very high 3.0 to 3.5 ml/100 g of tissue/min.[4] Its main substrate for energy production is glucose, with the exception of selected ketones in starvation states. Oxidative metabolism is essential, since anaerobic glycolysis cannot satisfy the brain's energy demands. Therefore mitochondria play a particularly critical yet vulnerable role in maintaining cerebral energy balance.[5] These characteristics, combined with lack of energy substrate storage, make the brain particularly vulnerable to slowing or cessation of blood flow (ischemia). Within 10 sec of complete ischemia, oxygen is consumed; within 4 min ATP is depleted; and disruption of cellular function can begin at 5 min.[5] Compensation for circulatory insufficiency is directed toward increasing cardiac output and shifting blood flow away from other organs toward the brain in an attempt to maintain cerebral blood flow.

The normal cerebral blood flow (CBF) averages 50 ml/100g of tissue/min with a range of 20 to 80 ml depending on the region.[6,7] Flows are higher in the frontal cortex and lower in temporal and parietal areas.[8] This flow is closely related to the cerebral perfusion pressure (CPP), by the following equations: 1. CPP = mean arterial pressure (MAP) — intracranial pressure (ICP); and 2. Pouiselle's law, which relates flow to pressure over resistance. Therefore, arterial blood pressure, intracranial pressure, and cerebral vascular resistance have critical influences over cerebral perfusion.

Defined as decreased perfusion, ischemia in the brain can occur in shock or with normal blood pressure, dependent on the ICP and vascular resistance. The ICP is directly related to the fluid volume and compliance within the unyielding skull.[9] Recognition of this relationship is essential in understanding the therapeutic concerns and interventions in caring for the brain-injured patient.

One mechanism used by the brain to maintain a constant blood flow is autoregulation. Be it neurogenic, myogenic, or both, autoregulation allows a change in cerebral vascular resistance proportional to the brain's metabolic demands[10,11] (Fig. 5–1). This link of flow to nerve activity and metabolism occurs both regionally and globally.[12] Normally, a constant CBF is maintained by variable vascular resistance between mean arterial pressures of 60 and 150 mm Hg. This pressure-sensitive autoregulation protects the brain in high and low CPP states[10] (Fig. 5–2). Acute hemorrhagic shock may raise the limits of these pressure measurements as the result of adrenergic vasoconstriction.[13] Autoregulation is a sensitive phenomenon and may be easily altered or lost during CNS ischemia. It is useful to view the brain as being unable to respond protectively to levels of MAP below 60 mm Hg. The cerebral vasculature is also very sensitive to changes in Pa_{CO_2} levels. The response is rapid; a change from Pa_{CO_2} of 40 to 60 mm Hg almost doubles the CBF.[14] Maximal vasodilation occurs at 60 mm Hg Pa_{CO_2}, while below 20 mm Hg ischemia may occur.[12] CO_2-responsiveness remains but may be decreased after anoxic-ischemic arrest.[15]

The normal ICP is 5 to 10 mm Hg.[9] Compliance of the brain allows ICP to remain within normal range in the early phases of volume increase from tumors, hematomas, hemorrhage, or edema. As the volume increases, a point is reached whereby the brain is minimally compliant, and a small increase in volume significantly increases ICP (Fig. 5–3). Depending on the insult, this change in ICP may occur early or late but, if not controlled, is almost always associated with eventual

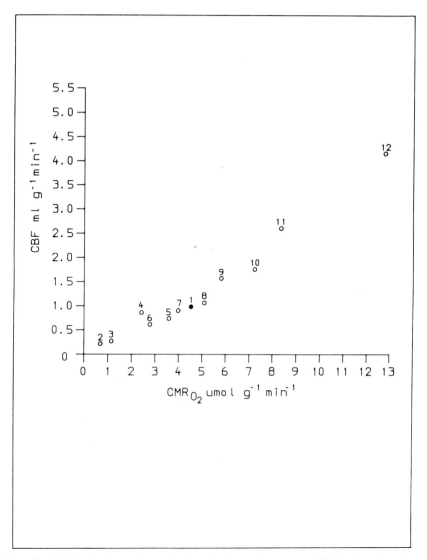

Fig. 5-1. The CBF in relation to the cerebral metabolic rate for oxygen CMR-O_2 in various situations. 1 = N_2O-analgesia; 2 = phenobarbital anesthesia [150 mg/kg(−1)] combined with hypothermia (23°C); 3–5 = hypothermia at 22°C, 27°C, and 32°C, respectively; 6 and 7 = phenobarbital anesthesia, 150 mg/kg(−1), and 50 mg/kg(−1), respectively; 8 and 9 = hyperthermia at 40°C and 41.5°C, respectively; 10 = homocystine-induced seizures; 11 = immobilization stress; 12 = bicuculline-induced seizures. All experiments were performed in rats during steady state conditions. (Modified from Nilsson, B., Rehncrona, S., and Siesjo, B.K.: Coupling of cerebral metabolism and blood flow in epileptic seizures, hypoxia and hypoglycemia. *In* Cerebral Vascular Smooth Muscle and Its Control. Ciba Foundation Symposium No. 56. Amsterdam, Elsevier/Excerpta Medica, 1978.)

caudal displacement of the brain stem and microhemorrhagic infarcts in this structure caused by shearing of the penetrating branches of the basilar artery.

MECHANISM OF BRAIN INJURY

Brain injury usually evolves from the functional (reversible) to the structural (irreversible). Unfortunately, the dividing line between the two is poorly understood

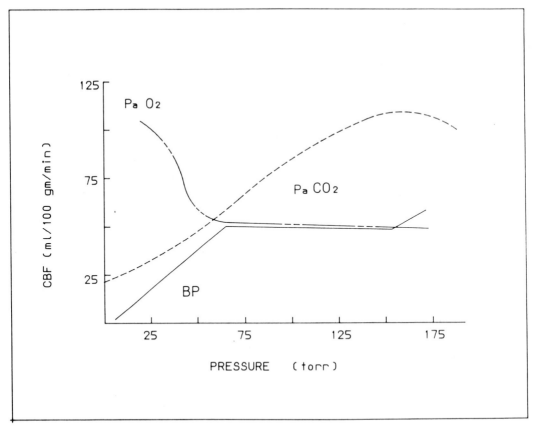

Fig. 5–2. Cerebral blood flow varies with changes in blood pressure, in arterial oxygen tension (Pa_{O_2}), and in arterial carbon dioxide tension (Pa_{CO_2}). (Reprinted with permission from Grenvik, A., and Safar, P.: Brain Failure and Resuscitation. Vol. 2. Clinics in Critical Care Medicine. New York, Churchill Livingstone, 1981.)

and clinically blurred. Confronted by the rapid progression from insult to irreversible damage, the clinician must consider the often interwoven mechanisms of injury in an organized manner.

In discussing cerebral trauma, Langfitt and Obrist[16] divided all brain injuries into five categories of mechanism: 1. mechanical, 2. ischemic (substrate deficiency), 3. hemorrhagic, 4. edematous, and 5. toxic. With some rearrangement, these mechanisms can apply to all forms of injury and be used as a differential diagnostic approach to therapy (Table 5–1). Obviously, these mechanisms may lead to one another or occur simultaneously.

Primary injury by any mechanism includes tissue destruction and damage. It represents lost tissue because, at present, irreversibly injured central neural tissue heals with scarring and does not regenerate. Damaged tissue may recover in irregular patterns but is often associated with altered function and seizure potential.

Secondary injuries should be viewed as potentially preventable, and are the major thrust of brain resuscitation research and therapy. They are the most com-

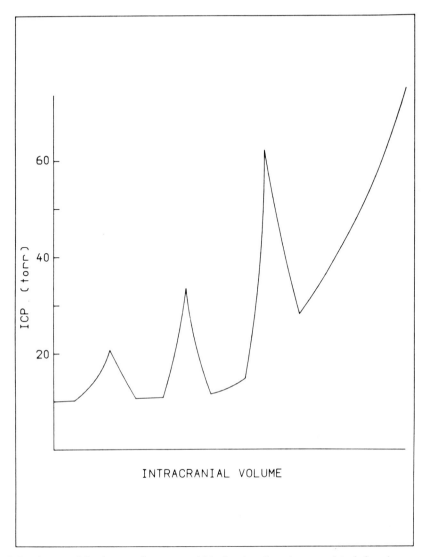

Fig. 5-3.   Intracranial volume and pressure within the closed cranium are related. As volume expands progressively, compliance is reduced so that each additional increment in volume causes a more marked rise in intracranial pressure (ICP). When ICP is already elevated, even a small increase in intracranial volume (as from an increase in CBF) may induce a tremendous surge in ICP before returning to the expected points on the compliance curve. Such an increase in ICP may also result in a plateau curve with the pressure remaining at a dangerously high level for several minutes. (Reprinted with permission from Grenvik, A., and Safar, P.: Brain Failure and Resuscitation. Vol. 2. Clinics in Critical Care Medicine. New York, Churchill Livingstone, 1981.)

mon factors increasing brain morbidity and mortality.[17] Each of the five categories can occur as a secondary injury that can alter cerebral function or structure directly or through elevated ICP. Each tier of the medical system, from prehospital care to neurologic ICU, must repetitively consider and prevent each of these secondary mechanisms.

Table 5-1. Classifications of Mechanisms of Brain Injury.

Primary—not reversible
  Mechanical damage/destruction of tissue
Secondary—potentially reversible
  Substrate deficiency
  Hematoma/mass formation
  Altered metabolism
  Toxins
  Edema
  Ischemia
Tertiary—potentially reversible
  Elevated intracranial pressure

Substrate deficiencies may include oxygen, glucose, and thiamine. Because 40 to 60% of head-injured patients present with hypoxemia, early optimum airway and ventilatory management is mandatory in the obtunded patient with head trauma.[18] The selective preference of the brain for glucose makes it an essential element. Hypoglycemia has long been known to have potentially damaging effects on cerebral function and structure.[19] Recently, hyperglycemia has been implicated in poor neurologic outcome in both global and focal ischemia animal models.[20,21]

Mass formation is most commonly from epi- or subdural hematoma secondary to trauma.[17] Timely intervention in these lesions has shown a significant improvement in neurologic outcome.[22] Intracranial hemorrhage from hemorrhagic stroke has less of a favorable recovery. Mass formation leads to compensatory structure shifts which may result in ICP rise, tentorial herniation of the uncus, or stem devascularization. This progression of neurologic injury can be potentially reversed by early diagnostic (CT scan) and surgical intervention.[17,22,23]

Altered metabolism from either hyperthermia or seizure activity has been shown to increase CMR O_2 demand at a time when supply may be limited.[5] Both seizures and hypothermia can accentuate the damaging processes set in motion by the insult. Anticipation and control are necessary.

Toxins may be endogenous or exogenous. Since metabolic disorders are the most common cause of coma, a search for these complicating factors must be made.[24] Toxic products derived from either endogenous metabolic derangements or exogenous sources may suppress the level of consciousness and compromise evaluation. Disorders of sodium, calcium, or magnesium homeostasis; renal and hepatic function; and selected exogenous toxins such as tricyclic antidepressants, organophosphates, cyanide, and mercury may have a direct damaging effect on neural tissue.[24]

Brain edema is often a common response to mechanical, ischemic, and the other aforementioned mechanisms of injury. It is a common element of secondary injury, and even without elevation of ICP may cause irreversible cellular damage. As our imaging techniques improve, the frequency and response to therapy for cerebral edema will be better understood. Considering the problems of the timely availability of these adjuncts, empiric treatment of cerebral edema will remain a mainstay of brain resuscitation.

Ischemia is a common cause of initial and subsequent brain injury. As noted earlier, since cerebral perfusion pressure and vascular resistance are the basic measurements of cellular circulation, ischemia can occur without hypotension. For example, intracerebral hemorrhage may cause both increased ICP and intense vascular spasm resulting in tissue ischemia without hypotension. Therefore, though commonly combined, systemic shock and brain ischemia do not always occur together. Even perfusion pressure may not have as close a relation to brain ischemia as previously thought. The "luxury perfusion syndrome" describes damaged and dying cells with normal or heightened regional perfusion thought to be caused by local adenine release from injured cells.[25] Our understanding of ischemia in the brain is made more difficult by limitation of measurement devices, animal differences, regional and cellular differences of flow and range, and tolerance for hypoperfusion.

Tertiary injury, elevated ICP, is often the end result of any combination of the secondary mechanisms. It has been shown to increase both morbidity and mortality in a variety of insults to the brain.[26-28] It is often the common denominator of death and disability in brain tissue; although as noted in global ischemia studies (cardiac arrest), tremendous damage may be inflicted without ICP elevation. Present measurement devices may be too insensitive to pick up subtle compensatory changes in the brain, e.g., CSF shifts, which may cause damage before a pressure rise is noted.[28,29] The evolution of bedside technology for regional brain perfusion monitoring[30,31] may significantly enhance the sensitivity of our ICP monitoring in detection of early deleterious changes in brain homeostasis.

BRAIN RESPONSE TO INJURY AND REPERFUSION

Understanding brain response to injury is complicated by the complexity of the normally functioning organ and the finding that each specific mechanism of injury has its own pathology, which can overlap with those of other injuries. Much of the information we have is based on animal research, which varies in design as well as in applicability to humans. Despite these difficulties, the response of the brain to no-flow, low-flow, and reperfusion states has been better defined in the last decade.

Hypoxia

It is important to differentiate brain response to ischemia from the response to hypoxia. Hypoxia may be caused by anemia or inadequate hemoglobin oxygenation, e.g., drowning. It represents a decrease in available oxygen in relation to metabolic demands. Ischemia is a critical decrease in cerebral perfusion. Though it may result in hypoxia, it also involves other substrates, blood rheology, and cellular waste disposal.

The brain tolerates Pa_{O_2} greater than 50 mm Hg reasonably well. With oxygen concentration below this level, functional changes may occur, but energy metabolism is maintained. At a Pa_{O_2} of 20 mm Hg, the autoregulatory response increases CBF up to fivefold, ATP remains normal, and intracellular lactic acid levels increase slightly. Functional changes at this level may be related to alterations in levels and effectiveness of chemical transmitters.[5,32] In severe hypoxia, irreversible neuronal damage can occur, but ischemia from myocardial insufficiency or arrest has usually occurred first.[33]

Ischemia

Ischemia must be considered as either a global or regional (focal) circulatory problem. Though focal damage may be precipitated, shock states result primarily in incomplete or complete global injury. Most shock states represent an incomplete global ischemic insult to the brain. Cardiac arrest is the prototype for complete global ischemia. The brain response to incomplete ischemia is less well studied, and is dependent on the factors listed in Table 5-2, particularly the amount of residual blood flow. Comparisons of literature studies are difficult, because the flow is variably reported as percentage of cardiac output, blood pressure, cerebral blood flow, or cerebral perfusion pressure. Also, cerebral ischemia causes metabolic changes that vary greatly in different regions of the brain.[34] Clinically, CNS depression still correlates best with CPP.[35]

After autoregulatory compensation is exhausted at MAP of 50 to 60 mm Hg, oxygen extraction increases. Tissue energy metabolism changes below 40% of normal CBF,[36] and energy changes similar to complete ischemia occur at less than 5%.[37,38] Increased lactate levels are seen with continued supply of glucose. This "trickle flow" state of less than 10% cerebral blood flow is believed to be more damaging than complete global ischemia because of the elevation in intracellular lactic acid level[39,40] and decreased tissue washout.[41,42] Low oxygen delivery may also allow increased free radical production,[43] and resultant membrane injury.[44]

The impact of "low-flow" states (10 to 20% of CBF) are presently the topic of considerable debate. This is the flow produced by standard closed-chest CPR, and its value in sustaining neuron integrity is under assessment.[40,45,46] In monkeys, CBFs of 12 ml/100 g/mm (approximately 20% CBF) for 60 min have been maintained with complete return of neurologic function.[47] CBFs over 20 to 30% seem to be satisfactory for maintaining cellular function without significant compromise.[48,49] This remains an unstable flow range, and prolonged ischemia at this level may lead to irreversible damage.[50] Open chest CPR and experimental "new" CPRs, e.g., simultaneous ventilation-compression (SVC) and interposed abdominal compression (IAC), have been shown to maintain CBF above this level, and are being evaluated for clinical suitability.[46,51-55] Augmentation of CBF and coronary blood flow during closed-chest CPR with epinephrine has also been promising in

Table 5-2. Factors Influencing Brain Response to Ischemia.

Age of patient
Status cerebral circulation
Preischemic metabolic rate
Previous injury
Degree of ischemia
Nature of shock state, i.e. hemorrhage, septic, cardiogenic
Duration of ischemia
Cerebral perfusion pressure (MAP-ICP)
Pa_{CO_2} influence on vascular resistance

the canine model and is under study.[56] Effect on coronary perfusion pressure and ICP must always be included in the evaluation of artificial perfusion techniques.[53,57,58]

Neurons are more susceptible to similar degrees of ischemia than glial or vascular tissue. Neurons in different areas have differing responses, and there is little predictability of distribution.[34] Without reperfusion, complete ischemia evolves, and neurons show similar patterns of injury.[59,60] The heterogenous nature of brain response to ischemia is manifested only with reperfusion. Much of the work to date describes the effect of transient global ischemia with reperfusion. Clinically, this represents a severe shock state, i.e., cardiopulmonary arrest, followed by resuscitation of varying effectiveness. There are projected corollaries between brain response in this model and hemorrhagic or septic shock, but little work has been done in these specific areas.

With transient global ischemia and reperfusion, a cascade of events at the cellular level is begun by an abrupt decrease in energy metabolites and depletion of high energy phosphates, particularly in arterial border zones.[61] These are areas of marginal blood supply most susceptible to hypotension. Glucose availability declines, ATP level decreases, and lactic acid level increases, causing a breakdown in homeostatic metabolism.[41] This condition undermines the cell's ability to maintain ionic gradients. Cells and mitochondria absorb water and swell, as ion shifts (K^+,Na^+,Ca^{++}) occur with equilibration between intra- and extracellular compartments.[62-64]

Ca^{++} influx occurs through a variety of mechanisms.[65,66] It activates destructive proteases and phospholipases, and is shifted between mitochondrial and cytosol compartments.[67,68] Free fatty acids (FFA), especially arachidonic acid, are released by phospholipases and act as detergents and injure cell membranes, allowing persistent ion decompartmentalization.[69-72] All these changes are potentially reversible with adequate reperfusion and re-establishment of energy metabolism. Unfortunately, reperfusion may accelerate oxidative injury mechanisms after ischemia and result in irreversible cell injury.

Reperfusion

Postischemic cells are particularly vulnerable because of altered membrane stability and energy metabolism. It is presently thought that the injury initiated during ischemia matures during reperfusion.[73] Continued swelling and Ca^{++} influx during reperfusion cause substantial increases in total tissue calcium content, and affect a number of different areas, possibly leading to cell death.[74] Calcium accumulates in mitochondria, with uncoupling of oxidative phosphorylation.[75,76] Ca^{++} overload in vascular smooth muscle causes constriction and cerebral vasospasm.[74,77] This vasospasm is at least partially responsible for the prolonged reduction in cortical CBF found after experimental global ischemia, and is decreased by the use of calcium channel blockers.[46,78-81] Ca^{++} is also believed to influence negatively platelet function and blood viscosity in the postreperfusion state.[74,82,83]

With reperfusion, the extra arachidonic acid is oxidatively metabolized to a number of potentially cytotoxic substances, including endoperoxides, prostaglandins, thromboxane, and leukotrienes.[43] Thromboxane is highly vasospastic,[84] and a potent platelet-activating substance.[85] The arachidonic acid cascade may also contribute to free radical production, which experimentally leads to increased cell injury by degrading membranes, protein, and DNA,[74,86] The clinical role of oxygen radicals remains unclear, however.[43] Other cations, particularly Mg^{++} are currently under investigation as to their role in vasospasm.[87,88]

Cerebral Edema

Elevated ICP is a late sequela of ischemia, occurring 48 to 72 hours after injury. Cellular edema at levels not influencing ICP is an important component of the process begun by ischemia. Cytotoxic or cellular edema is an early response to ATP and energy loss. Fluid accumulates primarily in the astrocytes and capillary endothelium,[89] theoretically from failure of the ATP-dependent Na-K pump.[33,90,91] Tissue changes can be seen in 5 to 7 min. This form of edema is more associated with altered neuronal dysfunction than its common counterpart, vasogenic edema. Vasogenic edema is associated with trauma,[92,93] infection, and prolonged ischemia. The blood brain barrier is altered, allowing water and protein to enter the interstitial space. The theoretic origins of this alteration include opening of cytoplasmic channels, loosening of endothelial tight junctions, and membrane injury from free radicals, fatty acids, and lysosomal enzymes.[94] Once begun, a pressure gradient spreads the edema into the interstitium, which resides primarily in the more compliant white matter.[95] Therefore, both intracellular and extracellular responses to ischemia of varying degree set in motion a series of changes that may be advanced by reperfusion at certain levels. Though cerebral edema (cytotoxic) participates in the mechanism of postischemic injury, elevated ICP does not play a major role.

Late sequelae at 36 to 72 hours have been found in animals that survived the initial neuronal insult after treatment with Ca^{++} blockers.[96] These included late-developing seizures, episthotonos, and deterioration of the level of consciousness. Such late deterioration is difficult to explain biochemically, and thus biochemical injuries whose functional maturation may be slow have been invoked. These include DNA injury by OH radical or perferryl radical-mediated lipid peroxidation in the membranes. These reactions require a transitional metal (one with two stable ionic states) to catalyze the reactions. Iron is such a metal, and the brain has rich iron stores. Recent experiments have been conducted to examine the brain for iron delocalization during ischemia. Data from White[96] and McCabe (in progress) indicate marked increases in CSF iron content during laboratory resuscitation by closed chest CPR methods. Moreover, the brain tissue content of low molecular weight chelate, nonprotein-bound iron has tripled 2 hours after a 15-min cardiac arrest and resuscitation. This increase in decompartmentalized iron is accompanied by a 50% increase in tissue malondialdehyde (MDA) levels. (MDA is a terminal product of membrane injury by lipid peroxidation.) Both the "free" iron and malondialdehyde levels are corrected by early postischemic treatment with the iron chelator deferoxamine. These data suggest that the postischemic reperfusion injury is mediated by perferryl radical species derived from decompartmentalized brain iron, and that this biochemical injury can be ameliorated by making the iron chemically inert and removing it in the ferrioxamine complex.[73] Outcome studies are now underway to examine the combination of calcium antagonists and iron chelators for further improvement in pharmacologic protection of the postischemic brain.

NONPHARMACOLOGIC THERAPEUTIC INTERVENTION

Volume replacement is the mainstay of therapy in shock. Infusion of sufficient crystalloid or blood to maintain a mean arterial pressure (MAP) of 90 to 100 mm Hg is a present-day standard of brain-oriented treatment of shock. The effectiveness of therapeutic intervention in cerebral injury from shock is still being evaluated.[35]

Most non-drug therapies are used after volume has been restored, and are used to control intracranial pressure and restore cerebral blood flow (CBF).[97] These measures include hyperventilation, patient positioning, hemodilution, drainage of cerebral spinal fluid, hypothermia, and hyperbaric oxygen.

Hyperventilation

Although the relationship between Pa_{CO_2} and CBF had been known for sometime, one of the first clinical applications occurred in the late 1950s, when Furness demonstrated that reduced Pa_{CO_2} improved intracranial operating conditions.[98] Beneficial effects have been found in head injury[99-101] and cerebral edema.[102] They are related to a decrease in CBF, which, to a degree, favorably influences cerebral perfusion pressure.

Blood vessel response is controlled by pH at the arteriolar-CSF interface.[103] The pH is determined by the ratio of Pa_{CO_2} and CSF bicarbonate.[7] Since the CO_2 rapidly diffuses across the blood-brain barrier, it has a more immediate effect on the pH. The precise relationship between pH and arteriolar tone in the brain is unclear, but a 1 mm Hg decrease in Pa_{CO_2} decreases CBF 1 to 2 ml/min/100 g of brain tissue.[7,104] Bicarbonate correction within the CSF is 50% at six hours, causing the vascular response to hyperventilation, in normal cerebral tissue, to decrease over time.[105] Also, the response may be blunted by a vasomotor paralysis associated with severe head injury and cerebral ischemia.[15,106] Hyperventilation may serve another role in brain protection by its action on restoring autoregulation.[107]

Hyperventilation is not without potential hazard. At Pa_{CO_2} levels of less than 20 mm Hg, cerebral hypoxia and increase in CSF lactate level have been reported, particularly when associated with hypotension.[108-110] This hypoxia has been experimentally linked to regional hypoperfusion, left shift of the oxygen-hemoglobin dissociation curve, and altered glucose metabolism.[111,112] These findings were not confirmed in normal brains of cats by all laboratories.[113]

After global ischemic injury, hyperventilation improved outcome only if ICP elevation was present. Soloway, et al. found a reduction in regional infarct size experimentally when hyperventilation was begun shortly after the occlusion.[114] Evaluation in humans after one hour of occlusion showed no benefit.[106]

Presently, maintaining Pa_{CO_2} between 25 to 30 mm Hg is recommended for patients with elevated ICP on monitoring, and in unresponsive patients with injuries causing early ICP rise. Despite the lack of favorable evidence, it is also recommended as part of the resuscitative effort in comatose patients after shock.[115]

Patient Positioning

Head, neck, and back elevation to a 20 to 30° angle decreases ICP secondary to CBF and central venous pressure changes.[116] Elevation should not be considered before cervical spine evaluation and blood pressure stabilization. There is little to recommend its use in the postglobally ischemic patient.[117] Head-down positions or ones of neck extension, flexion, or rotation are to be avoided.

Hemodilution

Fluid shifts in cerebral tissue after injury from shock may increase blood viscosity.[118] This increased viscosity and associated sludging was believed to be one of the reasons for the early difficulty in establishing cerebral perfusion after ischemia, deemed the "no-reflow" phenomenon by Ames, et al. in 1968.[119] Hemodilution has been shown to improve cerebral blood flow in experimental animals because of the effect of lowered viscosity on resistance.[120,121] Jurkiewicz has also found an inhibitory effect on the elevation of ICP during induced cerebral edema in cats.[122]

Safar has advocated hemodilution to a hematocrit of 25 to 30% combined with mild hypertension as a modality in both focal and global ischemia.[117] Better experimental support is available for focal ischemia.[123] Presently, it should be considered experimental in the postshock patient. Oxygen-carrying solutions may have some use as diluents.[124]

Cerebrospinal Fluid Drainage

CSF drainage to control elevated ICP is used only under monitored conditions. Most of the work has been in posttrauma or near-drowning patients.[125,126] Withdrawal of small amounts have significant, but short-lived effects on ICP. A theoretic benefit is an improvement of transit of extracellular fluid from the edematous area to the ventricular CSF.[127] Continuous CSF drainage is reserved for selected use in neurosurgical intensive care units. Presently it has no use in the treatment of postischemic brain injury.

Hypothermia

There is a linear relationship between the cerebral metabolic rate of O_2 (CMR-O_2) and body temperature. Experimentally, a 50% decrease in CMR-O_2 occurs at 28 to 30°C, and a 40% decrease in ATP depletion at 30°C.[128,129] These findings were the basis for studies that found a reduction of cerebral edema or ICP with hypothermia.[130,131] In global ischemia, early studies found hypothermia beneficial both for protection and resuscitation from circulatory arrest.[132−134] Safar wrote that without elevated ICP, hypothermia does not improve outcome.[115] Experimentally, hypothermia has reduced infarct size in focal ischemia only if begun within 30 min.[135]

Hypothermia has its major benefit as a second or third line therapy for ICP reduction, with monitored cooling to 30 to 32°C. Recent data cause one to question the decreased CMR-O_2 benefit below 34°C.[136] It is a complex process, necessitating sedation, shivering control including paralysis, respiratory control, temperature control, and close monitoring of neurologic, cardiac, and metabolic status. It is used for near-drownings, after head injury, and other elevated ICP states.[115,126] Complications include arrhythmia and increased blood viscosity.[117,137] The latter may be benefited by hemodilution.

Hyperbaric Oxygen

Hyperbaric oxygen lowers ICP by decreasing CBF and may effect ischemic tissue by increasing the oxygen content of blood.[138,139] This effect has been found to occur only during barotreatment and has not been sustained in either animal or human studies.[138,140] Though theoretically useful, hyperbaric therapy for brain resuscitation in the shock model is still experimental.

A number of other nonpharmacologic interventions are under evaluation. Cantodore, et al. have reported cardiopulmonary bypass effective in controlling pressure, flow, composition, and temperature of blood after 20 min of normothermic and 90 min of hypothermic cardiac arrest in dogs.[141] It may be useful for resuscitation after prolonged arrest times. Negovsky, et al. found that detoxification through hemoperfusion in the early postresuscitative period improved metabolism and ameliorated hemodynamic disorders, including impaired tissue perfusion and oxygenation.[142] Both of these modalities need further testing.

PHARMACOLOGIC THERAPEUTIC INTERVENTIONS

The drug therapy for ischemic brain injury is directed at preventing secondary damage to brain tissue. Though protective effects of medications have been demonstrated in brain injury,[143] the drug therapy of the brain "in shock" is essentially "after shock" or resuscitative therapy. The present status of corticosteroids, osmotic and diuretic agents, barbiturates, and calcium channel blockers will be reviewed in the context of global ischemia.

Corticosteroids

The mechanism of action of corticosteroids is still controversial. Preserved membrane integrity, reduced vascular permeability, radical scavenging activity, lysosome stabilization, improved intracranial compliance, and metabolic changes have all been considered.[144–147] Each may have a role in the pharmacodynamics of this complex drug.

The basis for steroid use in brain resuscitation is its effectiveness in reducing peritumoral edema.[148–150] It has become a standard therapy in this area.[151,152] Attempts to extrapolate the benefit to other forms of cytotoxic or vasogenic edema have been exhaustive and disappointing. Research has been muddled and prolonged by controversy regarding the "correct" dose and dosage, the "right" drug, and the "no harm done" arguments surrounding short-term steroid use. The cytotoxic edema associated with global ischemia is poorly responsive to steroids.[91] No studies have demonstrated steroid effectiveness in this setting. In shock states, steroid use is confined to early septic shock, and this remains a controversial subject.[153]

Animal and human studies in focal ischemia have found that steroids offer little or no improvement when given after injury.[154–156] Increased gastrointestinal complications from short-course steroids have been found in stroke patients.[157] Last, several well controlled studies of high and low dose steroids in head trauma have demonstrated no improvement in outcome, but have found serious complications, including gastrointestinal bleeding and infection.[158–161] Until new data are available, the empiric use of steroids in postischemic cerebral resuscitation is discouraged.

Osmotic/Diuretic Agents

These drugs are used primarily for rapid reduction of intracranial pressure. Mannitol and furosemide are the most commonly used agents in these two categories.

MANNITOL

Mannitol is a metabolically inert sugar that removes water from the brain by creating an osmotic gradient between the intravascular and extravascular compartments, using the blood-brain barrier as a semipermeable membrane.[162] Mannitol is also the best hydroxyl radical scavenger known. Other benefits include improved microcirculation through increased CBF and hemodilution,[163] and increased oxygen consumption.[164] The latter change may be detrimental in a compromised oxygen supply. Serial studies have shown reduced ICP after mannitol administration[91,165] It is used in the patient with acute or anticipated manifestations of ICP elevation, and may be given as a bolus (0.25 to 1.0 g/kg) or continuously in a monitored setting. Marshall, et al. found a low-dose regimen of 0.25 to 0.50 g/kg maintained a pressure reduction for 2 to 3 hours and was associated with fewer complications.[165] Despite its benefits, mannitol has potential hazards. Osmotic rebound with pressures exceeding those being treated is a known problem. Continuous administration and combination therapy have been found to decrease the rebound of ICP that occurs in approximately 30% of patients treated with bolus therapy. Its osmotic effect is exerted on normal, undamaged tissue. This effect may allow expansion of the damaged area and shifts in intracranial contents.[91,166] The increase in intravascular fluid could theoretically raise blood pressure and increase ICP.[167,168] Finally, the generalized hyperemic response to head injury in children precludes the use of mannitol because increased cerebral circulation may be more harmful than beneficial.[91,166]

The long-term effectiveness of mannitol is difficult to ascertain because it is usually not used alone in treating rises in ICP. It is a useful drug in attenuating the damage of elevated ICP from mass lesions or after near-drowning, but has little use in early therapy for postshock brain injury.

FUROSEMIDE

Furosemide is a loop diuretic that inhibits chloride anion transport and causes a naturesis and associated diuresis. The gradient created by this diuresis favors diffusion from the brain to the intravascular space, decreases brain water, and decreases ICP.[169] It also has effects on decreasing CSF by carbonic anhydrase inhibition,[170] decreasing sodium uptake by the brain,[171] and possibly decreasing cell swelling from cytotoxic edema.[172] Uniquely, its removal of brain water selectively affects injured brain tissue, and does not alter cerebral blood volume or flow.[173] Both human and animal studies have emphasized the post-traumatic setting, in which it effectively decreases ICP without significant rebound.[170,174] A standard intravenous regimen is 1 mg/kg initially followed by 0.3 to 0.5 mg/kg every 4 to 6 hours as necessary. Studies in other forms of cerebral edema are few,[175] and specific use in postshock states is, as with mannitol, primarily as part of combination therapy directed at lowering ICP.[125,176-178] In this setting, both mannitol and furosemide have proved effective, but continued research, particularly related to neurologic outcome in humans, is necessary.

Barbiturates

Barbiturates have long been known to have a depressant effect on CMR-O_2, and a protective benefit in cerebral ischemia.[179-181] They have also been considered as beneficial in postischemic resuscitation. Although the mechanism of action is incompletely understood, barbiturates are known to decrease CMR-O$_2$ in proportion to CBF, by depressing neural function,[182,183] and not by slowing ATP depletion.[38,184,185] This effect is different from that of hypothermia,[186] and the two have demonstrated an additive effect.[187] Studies by Steen, Nemoto, and others point to a barbiturate benefit in assisting cerebral metabolism recovery after ischemic insult.[184,185,188] Other theories under exploration include improvement of regional reperfusion, possibly from a calcium channel blocking effect,[187,189–191] membrane protection against free radicals,[192–194] and direct anesthetic effect.[195]

Barbiturates also have an effect on decreasing ICP,[196] and blunting changes from ICU stimulation.[197] Most of the benefit from ICP control has been noted in head trauma[197] and Reye's syndrome.[198] At present, refractory ICP elevation is the only indication for high-dose barbiturate therapy.

In global ischemia, early work demonstrated significant neurologic recovery in rabbits and monkeys[143,199] but inconclusive results in canine and human pilot studies.[200,201] Data from the Brain Resuscitation Clinical Trials I, conducted by Abramson, et al. from 1979 to 1983 found no significant benefit from high-dose barbiturates in global ischemia except when arrest was prolonged before CPR institution.[202] In focal ischemia, barbiturates have shown some benefit in animals,[181,203,204] but some adverse cardiovascular effects in high doses.[202,205] Additional studies are necessary.

Barbiturates have use as an anesthetic and for seizure control in the postischemic brain-injured patient. There is little evidence to support use of high-dose barbiturates after global ischemia unless monitored refractory ICP elevation complicates the clinical course.

Calcium Channel Blockers

As outlined, calcium has multiple roles in the postischemic reperfusion syndrome. Calcium antagonists may favorably modify these activities and thereby influence neurologic outcome. Potential benefits include decreased platelet activation, maintenance of microvascular perfusion, decreased free radical production, and limiting vasospasm.[206] There are numerous calcium "antagonists," and as the pathophysiology of postischemic brain injury has become better understood, selected drugs have come to the forefront as being of potential benefit.[206–208] These include nimodipine, lidoflazine, and flunarizine.

Canine studies by White, et al.[46,206,209,210] and others[211–213] have demonstrated improvement in CBF and CMR-O$_2$ when Ca^{++} antagonists are given in postglobally ischemic settings. Additional studies have demonstrated an improvement in neurologic outcome in other animal models.[81] A recent report by Schwartz, using verapamil, found improvement in humans.[214] Because of the strong evidence supporting the favorable influence of calcium channel blockers given after global ischemia, the Brain Resuscitation Clinical Trials II, designed by Safar, et al. have been established. The study compares therapy with or without lidoflazine on neurologic outcome in post-cardiac arrest patients meeting selected criteria. The study should be completed in 1986.

Additional drugs under evaluation in postshock brain injury include dimethyl sulfoxide,[215] phenytoin,[216,217] naloxone,[218] deferoxamine,[96] vasopressors,[219] fructose-diphosphate,[220] ATP-MG^{++} complex,[221] indomethacin,[222] magnesium,[191] and others.[223]

ASSESSMENT, STABILIZATION, AND MANAGEMENT

Assessment and stabilization cover the care of the brain-injured patient in the prehospital and emergency department setting. Information gathering and intervention must proceed expectantly and quickly. It often is difficult to differentiate between reversible and irreversible injury in this short time frame. With the exception of the brain-dead patient, every effort must be made to preserve functional neural capacity. Always consider the potential of presentation-modifying drugs, particularly alcohol, in the initial evaluation. The brief management discussion is directed toward intensive care.

Assessment

Patient assessment usually consists of a history, a physical examination, and laboratory tests, which are integrated into a diagnostic and therapeutic approach. In the patient with ischemic brain injury, these precepts continue, but the task is made difficult by the frequent combination of poor history, lack of cooperation or response in the physical examination, and no readily available laboratory measurement of cerebral function. Still, considerable information can be gained from an organized assessment. Although discussed in traditional order, the assessment, stabilization, diagnosis, and treatment usually occur simultaneously, but can be divided into two stages (Table 5–3).[224]

Pertinent history is listed in Table 5–4. All sources must be explored. Discussion with prehospital personnel, search of the patient's belongings, sending the police to the scene of the injury, and retrieval of medication are all part of locating that person or clue that will assist in the patient's care.

PHYSICAL EXAMINATION

After "ABC" assessment and interpretation of vital signs, the patient must have a rapid physical examination with neurologic emphasis. Particular attention must be given to protection and early roentgengraphic evaluation of the cervical spine.

Using the guidelines of Plum and Posner,[24] a protocol for rapid and repetitive neurologic examination can be developed, which will provide preliminary injury

Table 5–3.   Stages in Treatment of the Injured Patient.

Stage I. Assessment and stabilization of life-threatening insults
    Airway, breathing, circulation
    Cervical spine
    Screening physical and neurologic examination
    Consideration of secondary causes of injury, including substrate support, metabolic support,
        endogenous toxin reversal, correction of ischemia, possible mass lesion, and edema potential
    Initiation basic ICP management (tertiary injury)
Stage II. Diagnosis and management
    Detailed history
    Complete physical evaluation
    Repeat neurologic evaluation
    Laboratory evaluation
    Bladder and stomach drainage
    Tetanus or antibiotic prophylaxis
    Imaging/roentgenographic evaluation

Table 5-4.   History Pertinent to the Brain-Injured Patient.

General	
Name	Next of kin
Address	Physician
Age	
Medical Background	
Medications (available?)	Allergies
Operations	Family History
Medical problems (particularly renal, hepatic, cardiac, CNS)	Psychiatric status
	Previous neurologic status
Last hospitalization	
Incident Specifics	

  Approximate timing (when last seen, onset of incident, time until initial therapy, travel time)
  Mechanism(s) of injury (if trauma, amount and direction of forces involved, potential for cervical spine injury)
  Status at scene (both patient condition and setting)
  Intervention and response to therapy outside hospital
  Witnesses available
  Potential of exo/endogenous toxin

localization and good information on progression of neurologic status. This protocol emphasizes five major areas of examination: 1. Level of consciousness, 2. respiratory pattern, 3. extraocular movements, 4. pupil position and light response, and 5. posturing.

Coma is defined as unarousable unconsciousness. This state is caused by either diffuse *bilateral* hemispheric injury, or injury to the central core of grey matter in the brain stem at the level of the caudal pons, the reticular activating system (RAS).

Major altered respiratory patterns include Cheyne-Stokes respiration, which generally corresponds to bilateral insult in the internal capsule, or occasionally metabolic abnormalities such as uremia. Grossly irregular respiratory patterns and apnea correspond to insult to the respiratory centers in the medulla.

Altered extraocular movements include loss of the corneal reflexes and fixed ocular deviation in lateral gaze. Loss of corneal reflexes is a particularly critical sign in the head trauma patient with other signs of an acute intracranial mass lesion. In this environment, the loss of corneal reflexes frequently indicates that the process of brain stem herniation is occurring, and loss of the corneal reflexes is often quickly followed by respiratory arrest. There is rarely good neurologic outcome following respiratory arrest in the milieu of progressing neurologic signs following head trauma, because at that point the secondary injury to the brain stem from hemorrhagic-ischemic process (resulting from compromise of perfusion branches of the basilar artery) has irreversibly injured the RAS. Three major etiologic possibilities with fixed ocular deviation include: 1. A seizure with the irritative focus in the contralateral cortex from the direction of ocular deviation; 2. A massive ischemic infarction of the cortex on one side with the eyes deviated toward the side of the injury and away from the paralysis; or 3. An injury to the nucleus of cranial nerve VI on one side, which is frequently seen with hypertensive intracranial hemorrhage in the pons. In this case, the eyes are deviated toward the paralyzed side and away from the lesion because the pyramidal tracts have not yet crossed at the level of the pons.

Spontaneous conjugate eye movements reflect an intact brainstem. Oculomotor reflexes are preferentially tested by the oculovestibular pathway and cold caloric irrigation. It is more sensitive than oculocephalic testing and does not require special motion. The test is done by establishing tympanic membrane integrity in each ear, elevating head to 30° after cervical spine clearance, irrigating the ear with 50 to 200 ml ice water, and waiting up to two minutes for a response. The brainstem between cranial nerves III and VIII moves the eye tonically toward the infusion, and the cerebrum rapidly corrects to the midline. Therefore, both components of consciousness are tested. In the awake patient, the response is usually over-ridden by higher centers, but nystagmus vomiting and vertigo can be precipitated. A variety of patterns may occur, dependent on cranial nerve and cerebral function. The most common response after shock is tonic deviation without correction, representing an intact brainstem and dysfunctional cerebrum.[24,225] Asymmetric and dysconjugate eye movements may occur in drug coma or structured damage of efferent pathways. Loss of oculovestibular reflexes may represent severe brainstem damage, drug coma, or severe hypothermia. A fundoscopic examination should conclude the eye evaluation, because signs of acute or underlying disease may be present. Subhyloid (preretinal) hemorrhage and elevated ICP signs are uncommon but valuable when discovered.

Bilateral pupillary dilation may occur with administration of adrenergic agonists, administration of cholinergic antagonists, brain death, or rarely, bilateral transtentorial herniation of the uncus secondary to central mass lesions. Bilateral pupillary constriction may occur with interruption of the downflowing sympathetic tracts; this is again often seen with pontine hemorrhage. Bilateral pupillary constriction may also be observed with ocular administration of miotic agents used in the treatment of glaucoma. Unilateral pupillary dilation is frequently seen in association with unilateral transtentorial herniation of the uncus resulting in direct pressure being applied to cranial nerve III on the ipsilateral side.

Two types of altered posturing include decorticate and decerebrate posturing. Decorticate posturing is characterized by flexion posturing of the upper extremities and is associated with interruption of the normal downflowing motor tone at the level of the rostral pons. This is again often seen with pontine hemorrhage. Decerebrate posturing is characterized by hyperextension of the elbows and flexion of the wrists and is associated with compromise of the upper medulla.

The cerebral manifestations of shock range from confusion and delerium to drowsiness and coma. Alterations of cerebrum are more common and affect content more than arousal. The examination must localize and quantify the injury in the context of these varied presentations. A neurologic examination scheme linked to the aforementioned structural correlates and the Glasgow Coma Scale (GCS) is outlined in Table 5–5.[24,225,226]

The GCS has demonstrated usefulness in predicting outcome from a variety of brain injuries, including ischemia. It may also be used to replace the clumsy descriptions lethargic, obtunded, and stuporous. A score of seven or less correlates with coma, three being brain dead. The scale has two important qualifiers. First, concomitant exogenous toxins such as alcohol must be ruled out. Second, the noxious stimulus is standardized as either thumbnail pressure with a pencil or supraorbital nerve pressure.[24]

Severe injury to the cortex with an intact brainstem may be found after severe shock or arrest. The cortex is more susceptible to anoxic-ischemic damage. These

Table 5-5. Neurologic Examination of Brain-Injured Patient, Linking Structural Correlates and the Glasgow Coma Scale.

Glasgow Coma Scale (GCS)	Neurologic Examination Correlates
Eye opening	Wakefulness (represents ascending reticular activating system)
Spontaneous (4)	
Mild stimulus (3)	
Noxious stimulus (2)	
Absent (1)	
Language	(Content represents cerebral hemispheres)
Appropriate (5)	
Confused (4)	
Audible words (3)	
Unintelligible sounds (2)	
Absent (1)	
	Pupils (size, shape, symmetry, reactivity)
	Oculomotor reflexes (spontaneous movement, oculocephalis, oculovestibular)
Motor response	Motor activity (spontaneous/stimulated, symmetry, decerebrate/decorticate posturing)
Obeys commands (6)	
Localizes noxious stimulus (5)	
Withdraws from noxious stimulus (4)	
Decorticate posturing (3)	
Decerebrate posturing (2)	
Flaccid (1)	
	Respiratory pattern (of least value since often altered by medications, intubation, or ventilation)

(Numbers in parentheses indicate points assessed using the GCS.)

awake but unaware patients are termed to be in a "vegetative" state. The prognosis is poor.[227]

LABORATORY AND OTHER EVALUATION

The laboratory evaluation for brain-injured patients is relatively standardized (Table 5–6). An important bedside test is measurement of serum blood glucose

Table 5-6. Laboratory Evaluation of Brain-Injured Patient.

Chemistry
  Electrolytes (Na, K, Cl, HCO_3)
  Creatinine, BUN
  Calcium, Magnesium*
  SGOT*, SGPT*, LDH*, Bilirubin
  CPK with isoenzymes
Hematology
  CBC
  Platelets
  PT*/PTT*
Urinalysis
Toxicology Screen
Electrocardiology
Radiology
  Chest roentgenogram
  Skull roentgenogram
  CT scan

(*Indicates evaluations in selected situations)

level by test stick (Dextro-stix, Chem-stix). The importance of this test before glucose is routinely given is emphasized by the finding that both low and high glucose levels before and after ischemia have a detrimental impact on outcome.[21]

Roentgenograms of the skull can be selected if history or suspicion war-
rants.[227,228] CT scanning is most useful in the acute onset of altered sensorium and
when suspicion of a mass lesion is high.[230,231] Toxicologic screening is chosen on
the basis of history, clinical findings, or high suspicion. One must not allow a
positive toxicologic screen, particularly for alcohol, to preclude a thorough search
for other mechanisms of brain injury. One must also not be deceived by the diagnostic lull created by the unconscious "known alcoholic" or patient with the
breath odor of an alcoholic beverage.

DIFFERENTIAL DIAGNOSIS

As assessment and stabilization evolve, a differential diagnosis of the ischemic
state is being considered. Response to stabilization is often useful in determining
causation. The differential of shock states is discussed in Chapter 1 and must
include myocardial infarction, hemorrhage, sepsis, and drug overdose. A well
known acronym for reviewing the differential of coma is listed in Table 5–7.[232]
Careful consideration of each of the letters is necessary, because multiple factors
may cause or complicate ischemic injury. An early diagnostic mind-set is a path
to disaster.

Stabilization

Safar and others have stressed the importance and impact of "brain-oriented"
therapy in the salvage of patients.[233,234] Table 5–8 is derived from the research and
clinical experience of the last decade and offers specific recommendations for preventing secondary injury. These may be disappointing in their present limits, particularly in relation to calcium channel blockers. At the same time, these guidelines
save quality lives and should not be discounted. It is hoped that the currently
"underaggressive" material on treatment will be substantially resolved in the next
few years.

Management

Intensive care of brain-injured patients consists primarily of monitoring and
maintenance of cerebral homeostasis. Table 5–9 lists the areas that should be considered for monitoring. They can be categorized into anatomic assessment, func-

Table 5–7.   Causes of Coma—Two Useful Acronyms.

A-E-I-O-U	T-I-P-S
Alcohol	Trauma
Encephalopathy (hypertensive, hepatic)	Infection (CNS, sepsis, pulmonary)
Endocrinopathy (adrenal, thyroid)	Psychogenic effects
Electrolytes (hyper/hypo-Na, K, Ca, Mg)	Shock, stroke, seizure, subarachnoid bleed
Insulin	
Overdose (medications, poison)	
Uremia	

Table 5–8. Guidelines for "Brain-Oriented" Stabilization and Prevention of Secondary Injury.

Substrate Deficiency

Maintain PaO_2 over 80 mm Hg. Avoid PEEP if possible; it raises ICP.

Check blood glucose level at bedside. If it is less than 100 mg% give 25 ml of 50% glucose (see below), and recheck in 15 to 30 min. If it is greater than 250 mg%, use 0.5% NaCl and consider use of insulin for control.

Give thiamine, 50 mg IV and 50 mg IM, in advance of glucose in suspected instances of chronic alcoholism or unknown status.

Hematoma/Mass Formation

Use high index of suspicion. Use CT scan liberally. Use selected cerebral angiography if CT is unavailable or unclear.

Perform early surgical decompression or removal of accessible lesions.

Altered Metabolism

Monitor temperature; maintain normothermia.

Prevent or control seizures. Barbiturates: short-acting (thiopental, pentobarbital for rapid control); long-acting (phenobarbital for sustained control, prevention, and sedation). Phenytoin: for prevention and control.

Provide sedation and immobilization. For patients with restlessness and straining, use sedating doses of barbiturates and low-dose neuromuscular blockade.

Maintain pH between 7.3 and 7.6, and Pa_{CO_2} between 30 and 40 mm Hg unless hyperventilating for elevated ICP.

Toxins

Consider exogenous toxins. Use toxicologic screening liberally, particularly alcohol. Routinely administer an initial dose of 2 to 4 ampules (0.4 mg/ml) of naloxone in suspected cases. Use 8 to 10 ampules if propoxyphene is present or there is a partial response to the initial dose, then reassess.[240]

Perform laboratory evaluation of renal, hepatic, and electrolyte status. Correct if necessary.

Ischemia

In shock states, use replacement therapy of crystalloid and blood products, as necessary, to maintain MAP between 90 and 100 mm Hg.

May use vasopressors to augment perfusion after volume repletion.

Perform invasive monitoring in unstable states after initial resuscitation.

Maintain adequate oxygen-carrying levels of hemoglobin, 10 to 12 mg%.

Reserve calcium channel blockers for approved experimental protocols.

Edema

Use the following measures empirically to control anticipated cerebral edema and elevated ICP. They should be considered routinely in patients with GCS less than 8.

Check plasma colloid osmotic pressure. Maintain over 15 mm Hg (or albumin level of 3 g/dl). Once stabilized, give maintenance fluid D5/0.2 to 0.5% NaCl. Maintain MAP; monitor input and output closely.

Hyperventilate to bring arterial P_{CO_2} between 25 and 30 mm Hg.

Use the following optional therapy in the stabilization phase for the patient with a deteriorating course and high suspicion of ICP rise. Although ICP monitoring is preferred, it is unlikely it will be available at this stage of care.

Give furosemide 1 mg/kg IV

Give mannitol 0.25 to 0.5 g/kg IV, usually as 20% solution over 5 to 10 min, then reassess. May repeat 0.3 g/kg/hr IV, short term.

Perform skull trephination, but only in catastrophic situations demonstrating focal findings.[241]

---

tional condition, and metabolic and circulatory measurements.[235] The frequency of these measurements depends on the setting and clinical circumstance, but a regular schedule should be followed by both nurses and physicians. Early discovery of improvement or deterioration correlated with cessation or institution of therapy is a primary goal of ICU management.

A problem unique to the management of the postischemic brain-injured patient involves ICP monitoring. The measurements reflect the total pressure generated by the dynamic interplay of the intracranial contents. It has had demonstrated

Table 5-9. Guidelines for Monitoring the Brain-Injured Patient.

Serial vital signs
Serial neurologic assessment
    —trained nurses
    —comprehensive quantitative coma scale,[225] including higher cortical functions
    —standardized recording form[242]
Laboratory surveillance
Serum and urine
    —electrolytes, particularly sodium in context of osmolar balance
    —serum osmolality, in suspicion of diabetes insipidus or syndrome of inappropriate antidiuretic
       hormone production (SIADH)
    —hemoglobin/hematocrit, reflecting adequate oxygen-carrying capacity and stabilized hemato-
       logic status.
    —arterial blood gases, assessing acid base and potential secondary damage from hypoxia/
       hypercarbia.
Hemodynamic monitoring (invasive)
    —pulmonary artery catheterization to assess volume status and cardiac function in the postshock
       patient
Intracranial pressure monitoring (invasive)
    —in high-risk circumstances, to avoid empiric therapy and to assess response to treatment, to
       avoid tertiary injury by other therapeutic modalities such as ventilation and fluid challenges
Radiologic imaging techniques
    —serial chest roentgenograms
    —computerized tomography[230]
Electrophysiologic monitoring
    EEG, as "compressed special array"[243]
    Evoked potentials[244-246]

usefulness and safety since Lundberg's description in 1960.[29] Its benefits to date are primarily in head injury,[27,28] drowning,[126] and Reye's syndrome.[236] Monitoring is performed through a ventricular catheter, subarachnoid screw, or epidural transducer.[29,237,238] The choice is often based in the experience of the treating physician. Because elevated ICP is a late and unpredictable problem in shock, little investigative work has been done. The pathophysiology of global ischemia reveals one of the problems in ICP monitoring; that is, considerable damage may occur without manifesting a change in ICP. Assessing intracranial compliance by measuring the response to a volume impulse may enhance the sensitivity of ICP monitoring.[235] Nonetheless, invasive ICP monitoring should be considered in the postischemic patient who has shown either deterioration or lack of recovery in the first 24 to 48 hours. These patients have a poor prognosis, but to avoid aggressive assessment at this early stage is an error.

Monitoring of spontaneous (EEG) or stimulated (evoked potential) brain electrical activity has demonstrated benefit in intensive care monitoring. Although discussed in the section on predictors, it should also be mentioned here as a useful method to monitor the effects of drug therapy and announce secondary insults.[235,239]

Table 5–10 outlines the present maneuvers available to maintain ICP equal to or less than 15 mm Hg beyond the initial measures given in Table 5–8. Uncontrolled ICP above 25 mm Hg in patients with head injury is associated with greater than 70% mortality.[27,28] At present, data are unavailable in the postshock patient. It can be assumed when elevated ICP is a complication, the potential for increased morbidity and mortality exists.

Table 5–10. Maneuvers for ICP Control in the ICP-Monitored Patient.

1. Hyperventilation between 20 to 25 mm Hg
2. Mannitol 0.25 to 0.50 g/hg IV
3. Furosemide 0.5 to 1.0 mg/hg IV
4. Sedation with pentobarbital 2 to 5 mg/hg IV; use of high-dose (30 mg/kg) barbiturates under protocol only
5. Hypothermia, 30 to 32°C, with controlled ventilation, anesthesia, muscle relaxant
6. CSF removal

PREDICTORS IN POSTISCHEMIC BRAIN INJURY

Forecasting a patient's outcome is always difficult but is necessary to prepare family, adjust treatment plans, and appropriately use expensive and limited resources. Its use is particularly important in the postischemic patient, since CPR, coma, and shock are the three most predictive variables for ICU mortality.[247] It is the salvageable subset of these patients that must be located.[247] In recent years, a number of predictive criteria have been developed for head trauma and coma.[248,250] There is little on the postshock patient; therefore the discussion will emphasize predictors in postglobally ischemic brain injury. They range from a single physical finding to complex integrated scales. Each attempts to alleviate the mystery of the future.

When using and evaluating these indicators, it is important to understand the timing of measurement, the influence of extracranial factors—drugs, hypotension, patient variation within the measurement period—and to have a clear definition of outcome. Problems in standardizing this definition have precluded accurate comparisons, though the Glasgow Outcome Scale has offered some uniformity using five disability categories measured six months after injury.[251,252] The categories are: 1. brain dead, 2. vegetative state, 3. severe disability, 4. moderate disability, and 5. good recovery. Though crude, it has demonstrated reproducibility in a variety of brain injuries, and a number of prognosticators measured at less than 48 hours have been linked to it.

History

Both patient age and duration of ischemia have been used as prognostic tools. Children do recover with less morbidity than adults with similar injuries. A separate category for children is usually considered in developing predictive criteria, and most studies do not involve a mix of adults and children.[253,254] One study has found ischemic time above and below 5 min was not associated with major differences in outcome;[255] but the length of coma continues to be a negative prognostic sign.[256,257] Levy, et al.[256] found a relationship with diagnosis in 500 patients with nontraumatic coma. Patients with structural lesions were 50% more likely not to recover or remain in a vegetative state than those with metabolic or diffuse disease. Of the 210 patients with hypoxia-ischemia as the cause of coma, 10% had severe disability, 20% were in a vegetative state, and 58% had died at one year. Ten percent made a good recovery.[256]

Physical Examination

Beyond the poor prognosis associated with flaccidity, isolated evaluation of motor and respiratory patterns have no demonstrated predictive significance.[252,257]

Brain-stem reflexes have been evaluated by Snyder, et al.[258] in patients who have had a cardiac arrest. In reviewing eye movement, pupil size, pupillary light reflex, corneal reflex, and oculocephalic/vestibular reflexes, it was noted that all survivors had normal reflexes at 48 hours. None of the survivors had three or more abnormalities; any abnormality after six hours was associated with poor outcome. This correlation was supported in a recent study on nontraumatic coma.[256]

Teasdale and Jennett introduced the Glasgow Coma Scale for outcome prediction linked to GCS in head trauma in 1974.[254] This scale gives a number to a response level in three categories covering wakefulness (eye opening), anatomically based in the ARAS, and two components of awareness, based in the cerebral hemispheres—content of consciousness (verbal response), and purposeful motor response. The best score is 15, 3 is brain death, and 7 or less connotes coma. Though modified by others,[259] this score has proved useful in predicting survival and disability in head trauma and after global and focal ischemia, and near-drowning. The GCS has received good acceptance, and finally offers a reproducible scale for comparison of data. Work by Gennarelli, et al. has shown that different lesions with the same GCS score have different outcomes; therefore comparison should be between similar injuries.[260]

Isolated motor responses, deep tendon reflexes, and respiratory pattern have not demonstrated predictive value to date. The use of multiple signs has greatly strengthened the accuracy of prognosis.

Laboratory Evaluation and Special Equipment

Mullie, et al. evaluated a number of CSF substances in an attempt to quantify and predict outcome in postischemic encephalopathy. No marker of initial insult was found, but patterns of GOT, LDH, and CPK were found to be similar to those of myocardial infarction.[261]

Longstreth, et al. used measurements of serum and CSF creatinine kinase-BB fraction (CKBB) taken six hours after global ischemia to predict survival.[262] Both qualitative and quantitative measurements had some predictive capability. In serum, CKBB was present in 100% of nonsurvivors and 4% of survivors with good recovery (GOS 5). All those who recovered had less than 2 units/L in their CSF; those with greater than 10 units/L had severe impairment or death. Other studies have measured CSF adenylate kinase at 24 hours and found it correlative with coma scoring and with an index of intellectual function postoperatively.[263,264]

Electroencephalographic (EEG) studies have found it to be a good predictor of who will not survive,[251,265] and of mixed benefit in predicting neurologic outcomes.[266] The latter is best linked to a detailed grading system.[267,268] Certain patterns in a 16-hour "compressed spectral array" EEG tracing have shown use in predicting survivors.[243] Additional correlation is necessary.

Evoked potential (EP) is a test of neural pathway integrity. Auditory, visual, or somatosensory stimuli are given peripherally, and "averaged" cortical responses are made. It may be better correlated with prognosis than with diagnosis.[239,245] Somatosensory testing in patients with head injuries has been prognostically useful in dividing patients into two groups of GOS 1,2,3 and GOS 4,5 combinations.[239,244] This testing is more sensitive in assessing lesions of the cerebral hemispheres than are auditory EPs, which originate at or below the midbrain.[239] Auditory testing has shown prognostic usefulness in deeply comatose children.

All patients with normal auditory nerve brain response lived, regardless of cause or depth of coma.[269] Unfortunately, adult studies have not supported this relationship.[239]

Experimentally, brain tissue viability has been evaluated by measuring high energy phosphate concentrations and the oxidation reduction state after ischemic injury.[36,270] Since both are noninvasively measured by magnetic resonance imaging (MRI) the predictive possibility is real. Unfortunately, these substances return to normal under conditions incompatible with functional recovery. As yet, they are not useful indicators for prognosis.[271,272]

Though the prognosticators discussed in this section have advanced our ability to forecast outcome, it is literally only a beginning. A minimal observation time must be found, predictive computer programs must be designed, noninvasive tests must be developed and evaluated, and better discrimination between outcome groups must be established.

BRAIN DEATH

Despite our best efforts, a number of postischemic brain-injured patients will remain comatose.[249,273] The difficult medical, legal, and ethical issues of resource conservation and life support termination eventually confront all who care for the critically ill.

Unfortunately an easily applicable and legally acceptable definition of brain death does not exist. Not all states have legislation, and those that do vary from accepting "cessation of circulatory systems and function" to the "irreversible cessation of all functions of the entire brain," as the basis for defining death.[274] In addition to the state models, a number of other professional groups have developed their own definitions, including the American Medical Association and the American Bar Association. The topic has reached such scope that the National Library of Medicine has published an extensive bibliographic reference list to aid researchers in this field.[275]

Recently, the Medical Consultants on the Diagnosis of Death reported to the President's Commission for the Study of Ethical Problems in Medicine and Biomedical and Behavioral Research.[276] This report, entitled "Guidelines for the Determination of Death," outlines criteria for physicians to use in reliably recognizing that death has occurred. Its purpose was to supply the "accepted medical standards" as stated in the Uniform Determination of Death Act model statute.[276] The standards are divided into the clinical situations of irreversible cessation of respiration and circulation and the artificial maintenance of cardiopulmonary functions. These standards are adaptable and, importantly, allow a determination of death to be made without unreasonable delay. A summary of the outline is given in Table 5–11.

The standards come with a number of qualifiers. The most important is that any physician referring to the guidelines be thoroughly familiar with the entire document, including explanatory notes on complicating conditions. The complicating conditions include drug and metabolic intoxicants, hypothermia, children, and shock states.[276] As has been discussed, neurologic criteria in patients in a state of shock may be inaccurate because decreased cerebral perfusion can change the accuracy of clinical and laboratory examinations.

Table 5-11. The Criteria for Determination of Death.

An individual presenting the findings in either Section A (cardiopulmonary) or Section B (neurologic) is dead. In either section, a diagnosis of death requires that both cessation of functions, as set forth in Subsection 1, and irreversibility, as set forth in Subsection 2, be demonstrated.

A. An individual with irreversible cessation of circulation and respiration is dead.
　1. Cessation is recognized by an appropriate clinical examination.
　2. Irreversibility is recognized by persistent cessation of functions during an appropriate period of observation and/or trial of therapy.
B. An individual with irreversible cessation of all functions of the entire brain, including the brainstem, is dead.
　1. Cessation is recognized when evaluation discloses findings of a and b:
　　a. Cerebral functions are absent, and
　　b. Brainstem functions are absent.
　2. Irreversibility is recognized when evaluation discloses findings of a, b, and c:
　　a. The cause of coma is established and any brain function is excluded, and
　　b. The possibility of recovery of any brain function is excluded, and
　　c. The cessation of all brain functions persists for an appropriate period of observation and/or trial of therapy.

REFERENCES

1. Rappaport, S.I.: The Blood-Brain Barrier in Physiology and Medicine. New York, Raven Press, 1976.
2. Lee, J.C.: Anatomy of the blood-brain barrier under normal and pathological conditions. *In* Histology and Histopathology of the Nervous System. Edited by R.D. Haymaker Ward Adams. Springfield, Charles C Thomas, 1982.
3. Garoutte, B.: Survey of functional neuroanatomy. Greenbrae, CA, Jones Medical Publications, 1981.
4. Rappaport, Z.H., Ransohoff, J., and Hass, W.K.: Cerebral metabolism in head injury. *In* Craniocerebral Trauma: Progress in Neurological Survey. Vol. 10. Basel, Karger, 1981.
5. Rehncrona, S., and Siesjo, B.K.: Metabolic and physiologic changes in acute brain failure. *In* Brain Failure and Resuscitation. Clinics in Critical Care Medicine. Edited by A. Grenvik, and P. Safar. New York, Churchill Livingstone, 1981.
6. Inqvas, D.H., et al.: Normal value of cerebral blood flow in man including flow and weight estimates of grey and white matter. Acta Neurol. Scand., *41(14)*:72, 1967.
7. Lassen, N.A., and Christensen, M.S.: Physiology of cerebral blood flow. Br. J. Anaesth., *48*:719, 1976.
8. Wilkinson, I.M.S., et al.: Regional blood flow in the normal cerebral hemisphere. J. Neurol. Neurosurg. Psychiatry, *32*:367, 1969.
9. Miller, J.D.: Volume and pressure in the craniospinal axis. Clin. Neurosurg., *22*:76, 1976.
10. Betz, E.: Cerebral blood flow: its measurement and regulation. Physiol. Rev., *52(3)*:595, 1972.
11. Newfield, P., and Cotrell, J.E.: Neurologic-pharmacologic considerations of brain, protection and resuscitation. *In* Brain Failure and Resuscitation. Clinics in Critical Care Medicine. Edited by A. Grenvik, and P. Safar. New York, Churchill Livingstone, 1981.
12. Todd, M.M., Shapiro, H.M., and Obrist, W.D.: Cerebral blood flow measurement in the critically ill patient. *In* Brain Failure and Resuscitation. Clinics in Critical Care Medicine. Edited by A. Grenvik, and P. Safar. New York, Churchill Livingstone, 1981.
13. Fitch, W., et al.: Autoregulation of cerebral blood flow during controlled hypotension in baboons. J. Neurol., *39*:1014, 1976.
14. Grubb, R., et al.: Regional cerebral blood flow and cerebral oxygen utilization in superficial temporal-middle cerebral artery anastomosis patients. Acta Neurol. Scand., *60(Suppl. 72)*:502, 1979.
15. Koch, K.A., et al.: Total cerebral ischemia: effect of alterations in arterial P_{CO_2} on cerebral microcirculation. J. Cereb. Blood Flow Metab., *4*: 343, 1984.
16. Langfitt, T.W., and Obrist, W.D.: Cerebral blood flow and metabolism after intracranial trauma. Prog. Neurol. Surg., *10*:14, 1981.
17. Rose, M.W.: Avoidable factors contributing to death after head injury. Br. Med. J., *2*:615, 1977.
18. Agardh, C.D., Folbergrova, J., and Siesjo, B.K.: Cerebral metabolic changes in profound, insulin-induced hypoglycemia, and in the recovery period following glucose administration. J. Neurochem., *34*:1135, 1978.
19. Ginsberg, M.D., Welsh, F.A., Budd, W.W., and Reider, W.: Deleterious effect of glucose pre-

treatment on recovery from diffuse cerebral ischemia in the cat: I. Local cerebral blood flow and glucose utilization. II. Regional metabolite levels. Stroke, *11*:347, 1980.

20. Pulsinelli, W.A., et al.: Moderate hyperglycemia augments ischemic brain damage: a neuropathologic study in the rat. Neurology, *32*:1239, 1982.

21. Gardiner, M., et al.: Influence of blood glucose concentration on brain lactate accumulation during severe hypoxia and subsequent recovery of brain energy metabolism. J. Cereb. Blood Flow Metab., *2*:429, 1982.

22. Seelig, J.M., et al.: Traumatic acute subdural hematoma, major mortality reduction in comatose patients treated under 4 hours. N. Engl. J. Med., *304*:1511, 1981.

23. Bowers, S.A., and Marshall, L.F.: Outcome in 200 consecutive cases of severe head injury treated in San Diego County. Neurosurgery, 6:237, 1980.

24. Plum, F., and Posner, J.B.: The Diagnosis of Stupor and Coma, 3rd Ed. Philadelphia, F.A. Davis Co., 1980.

25. Lassen, N.A.: The luxury perfusion syndrome and its possible correlation to acute metabolic acidosis localized within the brain. Lancet, *2*:1113, 1966.

26. Mickell, J.J., et al.: Intracranial pressure: monitoring and normalization therapy in children. Pediatrics, *59*:606, 1977.

27. Miller, J.D., et al.: Significance of intracranial hypertension in severe head injury. J. Neurosurg., *47*:503, 1977.

28. Saul, T.G., Ducker, T.B.: Effect of intracranial pressure monitoring and aggressive treatment on mortality in severe head injury. J. Neurosurg., *56*:498, 1982.

29. Lundberg, N.: Continuous recording and control of ventricular fluid in neurosurgical practice. Acta Neurol. Psychiatr. Scand. *36*:1, 1960.

30. Weirnsperger, N., Sylvia, A.L., and Jobsis, F.F.: Incomplete transient ischemia: a non-destructive evaluation of in vivo cerebral metabolism and hemodynamics in rat brain. Stroke, *12*:864, 1981.

31. Colazino, J.M., Grubb, B., and Jobsis, F.F.: Infra-red technique for cerebral blood flow: comparison with 133-xenon clearance. Neurol. Res., *3*:17, 1981.

32. Siesjo, B.K., and Ljunggren, B.: Cerebral energy reserves after prolonged hypoxia and ischemia. Arch. Neurol., *29*:400, 1973.

33. Garcia, J.H., et al.: Post-ischemic brain edema: quantitation and evolution. *In* Brain Edema— Pathology, Diagnosis, and Therapy. Advances in Neurology, Vol. 28. Edited by J. Cervos-Navarro, and R. Ferszt. New York, Raven Press, 1980.

34. Welsh, F.A.: Regional evaluation of ischemic metabolic alterations. J. Cereb. Blood Flow Metab. *4*:309, 1984.

35. Kovach, A.G.B., and Sandor, P.: Cerebral blood flow and brain function during hypotension and shock. Ann. Rev. Physiol., *38*:571, 1976.

36. Marshall, L.F., et al.: Experimental cerebral oligemia and ischemia produced by intracranial hypertension. Part 3: Brain energy metabolism. J. Neurosurg., *43*:323, 1975.

37. Nordstrom, C.-H., and Rehncrona, S.: Postischemic central blood flow and oxygen utilization rate in rats anaesthetized with nitrous oxide or phenobarbital. Acta Physiol. Scand., *101*:230, 1977.

38. Nordstrom, C.-H., and Siesjo, B.K.: Effects of phenobarbital in cerebral ischemia. Part 1: Cerebral energy metabolism during pronounced incomplete ischemia. Stroke, *9*:327, 1978.

39. Myers, R.E.: A unitary theory of causation of anoxic and hypoxic brain pathology. *In* Advances in Neurology. Vol. 26. Edited by S. Fahn, J.N. Davis, L.P. Rowland. New York, Raven Press, 1974.

40. Steen, P.A., Michenfelder, J.D., and Milde, J.H.: Incomplete versus complete cerebral ischemia: improved outcome with a minimal blood flow. Ann. Neurol., 6:389, 1979.

41. Hossman, K.A., and Kleihues, P.: Reversibility of ischemic brain damage. Arch. Neurol., *29*:375, 1973.

42. Rehncrona, S., Rosen, I., and Siesjo, B.K.: Brain lactic acidosis and cell damage: biochemistry and neurophysiology. J. Cereb. Blood Flow Metab., *1*:297, 1981.

43. Siesjo, B.K.: Cell damage in the brain: a speculative synthesis. J. Cereb. Blood Flow Metab., *1*:155, 1981.

44. Demopoulos, H.B.: The basis of free radical pathology. Fed. Proc., *32(8)*:1859, 1973.

45. Rogers, M.C., Weistfeldt, M.L., and Traystan, R.J.: Cerebral blood flow during CPR. Anesth. Analg., *60*:73, 1981.

46. White, B.C., et al.: Cerebral cortical perfusion during and following resuscation from cardiac arrest in dogs. Am. J. Emerg. Med., *1*:128, 1983.

47. Morawetz, R.B., et al.: Cerebral blood-flow determined by hydrogen clearance during middle cerebral-artery occlusion in unanesthetized monkey. Stroke, *9*:143, 1978.

48. Hossman, K.A.: Neuronal survival and revival during and after cerebral ischemia. Am. J. Emerg. Med., *1*:191, 1983.

49. Paschen, W., et al.: Regional blood flow and regional distribution of biochemical substrates in experimental stroke of gerbils. J. Cereb. Blood Flow Metab., *1(Suppl)*:174, 1981.

50. Jennings, R.B., Ganote, C.E., and Reimer, K.A.: Ischemic tissue injury. Am. J. Pathol., *81*:179, 1975.

51. Kohler, R.C., et al.: Augmentation of cerebral perfusion by simultaneous chest compression and lung inflation with abdominal binding following cardiac arrest in dogs. Circulation, *67*:266, 1983.

52. Bircher, N., Safar, P., and Stewart, R.: A comparison of standard, MAST-augmented and open-chest CPR in dogs. A preliminary investigation. Crit. Care Med., *8*:147, 1980.

53. Bircher, N., and Safar, P.: Comparison of standard and "new" closed-chest CPR and open-chest CPR in dogs. Crit. Care Med., *9*:5, 1981.

54. Sanders, A.B., et al.: Improved resuscitation from cardiac arrest with open-chest massage. Ann. Emerg. Med., *13(9)*:672, 1984.

55. Bircher, N., and Safar, P.: Preserving the brain during cardiopulmonary resuscitation in dogs. Crit. Care Med., *12(3)*:251, 1984.

56. Jackson, R.E., et al.: Blood flow in the cerebral cortex during cardiac resusciation in dogs. Ann. Emerg. Med., *13(9)*:657, 1984.

57. Alifimoff, J.K., et al.: Cardiac resuscitability after closed-chest, MAST-augmented and open-chest cardiopulmonary resuscitation (CPR). Anesthesiology, *53*:S151, 1980.

58. Niemann, J.T., et al.: Coronary perfusion pressure during experimental CPR. Ann. Emerg. Med., *11*:127, 1982.

59. Jenkins, L.W., et al.: Complete cerebral ischemia. An ultrastructural study. Acta Neuropathol. *48*:113, 1979.

60. Kalimo, H., Garcia, J.H., and Kamijyo, Y.: Cellular and subcellular alterations of human CNS: Studies utilizing in situ perfusion fixation at immediate autopsy. Arch. Pathol., *97*:352, 1974.

61. Romanul, F.C.A., and Abramowicz, A.: Changes in brain and pial vessels in arterial border zones. A study of 13 cases. Arch. Neurol., *11*:40, 1964.

62. Baue, A.E., Chaudry, I.H., and Wurth, M.A.: Cellular alterations with shock and ischemia. Angiology, *25*:31, 1974.

63. Hossmann, K.A.: Development and resolution of ischemic brain swelling. *In* Dynamics of Brain Edema. Edited by H. Pappius, and W. Feindel. New York, Springer Verlag, 1976.

64. Robbins, S.L., and Cotran, R.S.: Cell injury and cell death. *In* Pathologic Basis of Disease. 2nd Ed. Phildelphia, W.B. Saunders, 1979.

65. Grinwald, P.M., and Nayler, W.G.: Calcium entry in the calcium paradox. J. Mol. Cell Cardiol. *13*:867, 1981.

66. Harris, R.J., et al.: Changes in extracellular calcium activity in cerebral ischemia. J. Cereb. Blood Flow Metab., *1*:203, 1981.

67. Weglicki, W.B., et al.: Hydrolysis of myocardial lipids during acidosis and ischemia. *In* Recent Advances of Studies on Cardiac Structure and Metabolism. Edited by N.S. Dhalla. Baltimore, University Park Press, 1972.

68. Fiskum, G.: Involvement of mitochondria in ischemic cell injury and in regulation of intracellular calcium. Am. J. Emerg. Med., *2*:147, 1983.

69. Yatsu, F.M., and Moss, S.A.: Brain lipid changes following hypoxia. Stroke, *2*:587, 1971.

70. Chan, P.H., and Fishman, R.A.: Brain edema: induction in cortical slices by polyunsaturated fatty acids. Science, *201*:358, 1978.

71. Katz, A.M., and Messineo, F.C.: Lipid-membrane interactions and the pathogenesis of ischemic damage in the myocardium. Circ. Res., *48*:1, 1981.

72. Messineo, F.C.: The possible role of endogenous amphiphiles in the membrane abnormalities of ischemic and reperfused myocardium. Am. J. Emerg. Med. *1*:162, 1983.

73. White, B.C., Krause, G.S., Aust, S.F., and Eyster, G.E.: Post-ischemic tissue injury by iron-mediated free radical lipid peroxidation. Ann. Emerg. Med. (in press).

74. Winegar, C.D., and White, B.C.: Physiology of resuscitation. Emerg. Med. Clin. North Am., *1(3)*:479, 1983.

75. Borgers, M., et al.: The role of calcium in cellular dysfunction. Am. J. Emerg. Med., *1*:154, 1983.

76. White, B.C., Hoehner, P.J., and Wilson, R.F.: Mitochondrial O_2 use and ATP synthesis: kinetic effect of Ca^{2+} and HPO_{42}—modulated by glucocorticoids. Ann. Emerg. Med., *9*:396, 1980.

77. Braunwald, E.: Mechanism of action of calcium channel blocking agents. N. Engl. J. Med., *307*:1618, 1982.

78. Gadzinski, D.S., et al.: Alterations in canine cerebral cortical blood flow and vascular resistance post-cardiac arrest. Ann. Emerg. Med., *99*:58, 1982.

79. Rehncrona, S., Abdul-Rahman, A., and Siesjo, B.K.: Local cerebral blood flow in the post ischemic period. Acta Neurol. Scand., *60(Suppl. 72)*:294, 1979.

80. Winegar, C.D., et al.: Prolonged hypoperfusion in the cerebral cortex following cardiac arrest and resuscitation in dogs. Ann. Emerg. Med., *12*:414, 1983.

81. Hoffmeister, F., Kazda, S., and Krause, J.P.: Influence of nimodipine on the postischemic changes of brain function. Acta Neurol. Scand., *60(Suppl. 72)*:358, 1979.

82. De Cree, J., et al.: The rheological effects of cinnarizine and flunarizine in normal and pathological conditions. Angiology, 30:505, 1979.
83. Hossmann, V., Hossmann, K.A., and Takagi, N.: Effect of intravascular platelet aggregation on blood recirculation following prolonged ischemia of the cat brain. J. Neurol., 222:159, 1980.
84. Towart, R., and Perzborn, E.: Nimodipine inhibitis carboxcyclic thromboxane-induced contractions of cerebral arteries. Eur. J. Pharmacol., 69:213, 1981.
85. Muller, R., and Lehrach, F.: Haemorheological role of platelet aggregation and hypercoagulability in microcirculation: Therapeutic approach of pentoxifylline. Pharamatherapeutica, 2:372, 1980.
86. Hammond, B., Kontos, H.A., and Hess, M.L.: Oxygen radicals in the adult respiratory distress syndrome in myocardial ischemia and reperfusion injury, and in cerebral vascular damage. Can. J. Physiol. Pharmacol., 63:173, 1985.
87. Altura, B.M., and Altura, B.T.: Cerebral and peripheral vascular actions of magnesium ions: role in resuscitation and cerebrovasospasm. Am. J. Emerg. Med., 2(4):347, 1984.
88. Widener, L.L., and Mela-Riker, L.M.: Verapamil pretreatment preserves mitochondrial function and tissue magnesium in the ischemic kidney. Circ. Shock, 13:27, 1984.
89. Klatzo, I.: Neuropathological aspects of brain edema. J. Neuropathol. Exp. Neurol., 26:1, 1976.
90. Brierlye, J.B., Meldrum, B.S., and Brown, A.W.: The threshold and neuropathology of cerebral "anoxic-ischemic" cell change. Arch. Neurol., 29:367, 1973.
91. Fishman, R.A.: Brain edema. N. Engl. J. Med., 293:706, 1975.
92. Vigouroux, R.P., and Guillermain, P.: Post-traumatic hemispheric contusion and laceration. In Craniocerebral Trauma. Progress in Neurological Surgery, Vol. 10. Edited by H. Krayenbuehl, et al. Basel, S. Karger, 1981.
93. Fishman, R.A., and Chan, P.A.: Metabolic basis of brain edema. In Brain Edema—Pathology, Diagnosis, and Therapy. Advances in Neurology, Vol. 28. Edited by J. Cervos-Navarro, and R. Ferszt. New York, Raven Press, 1980.
94. O'Brien, M.D.: Ischemic cerebral edema: a review. Stroke, 10:623, 1979.
95. Marmarou, A., Takagi, H., and Shulman, K.: Biomechanics of brain edema and effects on local cerebral blood flow. In Brain Edema—Pathology, Diagnosis, and Therapy. Advances in Neurology, Vol. 28. Edited by J. Cervos-Navarro, and R. Ferszt. New York, Raven Press, 1980.
96. White, B.C., et al.: Brain injury by ischemic anoxia: hypothesis extension—a tale of two ions? Ann. Emerg. Med., 12:862, 1984.
97. Mullie, A. et al.: Cerebral resuscitation: a review. Acta Anaesthesiol. Belg. 31(2):147, 1980.
98. Furness, D.N.: Controlled respiration in neurosurgery. Br. J. Anaesth., 29:415, 1957.
99. Crockard, H.A., Coppel, D.L., and Morrow, W.F.K.: Evaluation of hyperventilation in treatment of head injuries. Br. Med. J., 4:634, 1973.
100. Rowed, D.W., et al.: Hypocapnia and intracranial volume-pressure relationship. Arch. Neurol., 32:369, 1975.
101. Gordon, E.: Controlled respiration in the management of patients with traumatic brain injuries. Acta Anaesthesiol. Scand., 15:193, 1971.
102. Rossanda, M., et al.: Oxygen supply to the brain and respirator treatment in severe comatose status. Acta Anaesthesiol. Scand., 3(Suppl.23):766, 1966.
103. Richle, M.E., and Plum, F.: Hyperventilation and cerebral blood flow. Stroke, 3:566, 1972.
104. Reivich, M.: Arterial Pco_2 and cerebral hemodynamics. Am. J. Physiol., 206:25, 1964.
105. Christensen, M.S., et al.: Cerebral apoplexy (stroke) treated with or without prolonged artificial hyperventilation. 2. Cerebrospinal fluid acid-base balance and intracranial pressure. Stroke, 4:620, 1973.
106. Langfitt, T.W.: Increased intracranial pressure and the cerebral circulation. In Neurological Surgery. 2nd Ed. Vol. 2. Edited by J.R. Youmans. Philadelphia, W.B. Saunders Co., 1982.
107. Paulson, O.B., Olesen, J., and Christensen, M.S.: Restoration of autoregulation of cerebral blood flow by hypocapnia. Neurology, 22:286, 1972.
108. Carlsson, C., Nilsson, L., and Siesjo, B.K.: Cerebral metabolic changes in arterial hypocapnia of short duration. Acta Anaesthesiol. Scand., 18:104, 1974.
109. Plum, F., Posner, J.B., and Smith, W.W.: Effect of hyperbaric-hypoxic hyperventilation on blood, brain, and CSF lactate. Am. J. Physiol., 215:1240, 1968.
110. Harp, J.R., and Wollman, H.: Cerebral metabolic effects of hyperventilation and deliberate hypotension. Br. J. Anaesth., 45:256, 1973.
111. Gotoh, F., Meyer, J.S., and Takagi, Y.: Cerebral effects of hyperventilation in man. Arch. Neurol., 12:410, 1965.
112. Kogure, K., et al.: Effect of hyperventilation on dynamics of cerebral energy metabolism. Am. J. Physiol., 228:1862, 1975.
113. Gibbons, P.A., et al.: Extreme hypocapnia does not cause cerebral ischemia in normal cat brain. Crit. Care Med., 12(3):229, 1984.

114. Soloway, M., et al.: The effect of hyperventilation on subsequent cerebral infarction. Anesthesiology, *29*:975, 1968.
115. Safar, P., Bleyaert, A., and Nemoto, E.M.: Resuscitation after global brain ischemia-anoxia. Crit. Care Med., *6*:215, 1978.
116. Cuypers, J., Matakas, F., and Potolicchio, S.J.: Effect of central venous pressure on brain tissue pressure and brain volume. J. Neurosurg., *45*:89, 1976.
117. Safar, P.: Resuscitation after brain ischemia. Clin. Crit. Care Med., *2*:155, 1981.
118. Wells, R.E.: Rheology of blood in the microvasculature. N. Engl. J. Med., *270*:832,889, 1964.
119. Ames, A., et al.: Cerebral ischemia II. The no-reflow phenomenon. Am. J. Pathol., *52*:437, 1968.
120. Gottshein, U., Held, K., and Seldmeyer, J.: Cerebral and peripheral blood flow as affected by induced hemodilution. *In* Haemodilution: Theoretical Basis and Clinical Application. Edited by K. Messmer, and H. Schmidt-Schonbing. Basel, S. Karger, 1972.
121. Jurkiewicz, J., and Kozniewska, E.: Effect of haemodilution on the cerebral blood flow and blood brain barrier in experimental cerebral edema in cats. Resuscitation, *6*:227, 1978.
122. Jurkiewicz, J.: The effect of haemodilution on experimental cerebral edema in cats. Resuscitation, *6*:197, 1978.
123. Sundt, R., Naltz, A.G., and Sayre, G.P.: Experimental cerebral infarction: modification of treatment with hemodiluting, hemoconcentrating and dehydrating agents. J. Neurosurg., *26*:46, 1967.
124. DeVenuto, F.: Hemoglobin solutions as oxygen-carrying resuscitation solutions. Crit. Care Med., *10*:238, 1982.
125. James, H.E., et al.: Treatment of intracranial hypertension. Acta Neurochir., *36*:189, 1977.
126. Conn, A.W., Edmonds, J.F., and Barlow, G.A.: Cerebral resuscitation in near drowning. Pediatr. Clin. North Am., *26*:691, 1979.
127. Reulen, H.J., et al.: The role of tissue pressure and bulk flow in the formation and resolution of cold induced edema. *In* Dynamics of Brain Edema. Edited by H.M. Pappius, and W. Feindel. Berlin, Springer Verlag, 1976.
128. Rosomoff, H.L., and Holaday, D.A.: Cerebral blood flow and cerebral oxygen consumption during hypothermia. Am. J. Physiol., *179*:85, 1954.
129. Michenfelder, J.D., and Theye, R.A.: The effects of anesthesia and hypothermia on canine cerebral ATP and lactate during anoxia produced by decapitation. Anesthesiology, *33*:430, 1970.
130. Clasen, R.A., et al.: Hypothermia and hypotension in experimental cerebral edema. Arch. Neurol., *19*:472, 1968.
131. Shapiro, H.M., Wyte, S.R., and Loeser, J.: Barbiturate augmented hypothermia for reduction of persistent intracranial hypertension. J. Neurosurg., *40*:90, 1974.
132. White, R.J., et al.: Differential extracorporeal hypothermic perfusion of the circulatory arrest to the human brain. Med. Res. Eng., *6*:18, 1967.
133. Rainey Williams, G., and Spencer, R.D.: The clinical use of hypothermia following cardiac arrest. Ann. Surg., *148*:462, 1958.
134. Benson, D.W., et al.: The use of hypothermia after cardiac arrest. Anesth. Analg., *38*:423, 1958.
135. Rosomoff, H.L.: Hypothermia and cerebral vascular lesions. Arch. Neurol. Psychiatry, *78*:454, 1957.
136. Frewen, T., et al.: Cerebral blood flow and cross brain oxygen consumption during hyperventilation and hypothermia. Crit. Care Med., *12(3)*:275, 1984.
137. Michenfelder, J.D., and Milde, J.H.: Failure of prolonged hypocapnia, hypothermia, or hypertension to favorably alter acute stroke in primates. Stroke, *8*:87, 1977.
138. Miller, J.D., and Ledingham, I.M.: Reduction of increased intracranial pressure: comparison between hyperbaric oxygen and hyperventilation. Arch. Neurol., *24*:210, 1971.
139. Sukoff, M.H., et al.: The protective effect of hyperbaric oxygenation in experimental cerebral edema. J. Neurosurg., *29*:236, 1968.
140. Mogami, H., et al.: Clinical applications of hyperbaric oxygenation in the treatment of acute cerebral damage. J. Neurosurg., *31*:636, 1969.
141. Cantadore, R., et al.: Cardiopulmonary bypass for emergency resuscitation after prolonged cardiac arrest. Am. J. Emerg. Med., *2(4)*:348, 1984.
142. Negovsky, V.A., Zaks, I.O., and Shapiro, V.M.: Extracorporeal hemosorption in the post-resuscitation period in experiment. Resuscitation, *7*:145, 1979.
143. Yatsu, F.M., et al.: Experimental brain ischemia; protection from irreversible damage with a rapid-acting barbiturate (methohexital). Stroke, *3*:726, 1972.
144. Miller, J.D., and Leed, P.: Effects of mannitol and steroid therapy on intracranial volume-pressure relationships in patients. J. Neurosurg., *42*:274, 1975.
145. Anderson, D.K., and Means, E.D.: Lipid peroxidation in spinal cord: $FeCl_2$ induction and antioxidants. Neurochem. Pathol., *1*:249, 1983.
146. Long, D.M., et al.: Multiple therapeutic approaches in the treatment of brain edema induced by

a standard cold lesion. *In* Steroids and Brain Edema. Edited by H.J. Reulen, and K. Schurmann. Berlin, Springer Verlag, 1972.

147. Demopoulos, H.V., et al.: Molecular aspects of membrane structure and cerebral edema. *In* Steroids and Brain Edema. Edited by H.J. Reulen, and K. Schurmann. New York, Springer Verlag, 1972.

148. Kofman, S., et al.: Treatment of cerebral metastasis from breast cancer with prednisolone. J.A.M.A., *163*:1473, 1957.

149. Weinstein, J.D., et al.: The effect of dexamethasone on brain edema in patients with metastatic brain tumors. Neurology, *23(1)*:121, 1973.

150. Reulen, H.J., Hadjumos, A., and Schurmann, K.: The effect of dexamethasone or water and electrolyte content on +CBF in perifocal brain edema in man. *In* Steroids and Brain Edema. Edited by J.H. Reulen, and K. Schurmann. Berlin, Springer Verlag, 1972.

151. Ignelzi, R.J.: Cerebral edema: present perspectives. Neurosurgery, *4/4/*:338, 1979.

152. Harbaugh, R.D., et al.: Acute therapeutic modalities for experimental vasogenic edema. Neurosurgery, *5(6)*:656, 1979.

153. Houston, M.C., Thompson, W.L., and Robertson, D.: Shock: diagnosis and management, Arch. Intern. Med., *144*:1433, 1984.

154. Anderson, P.C., and Cranford, R.E.: Corticosteroids in ischemic stroke. Stroke, *10(1)*:68, 1978.

155. Bauer, R.B., and Telleg, H.: Dexamethasone as treatment in cerebrovascular disease: a controlled study in acute cerebral infarction. Stroke, *4*:547, 1973.

156. Norris, J.W.: Steroid therapy in acute cerebral infarction. Arch. Neurol., *33*:67, 1976.

157. Ottonello, G.A., and Primavera, A.: Gastrointestinal complications of high-dose corticosteroid therapy in acute cerebrovascular patients. Stroke, *10*:208, 1970.

158. Gudeman, F.K., Miller, J.D., and Becker, D.P.: Failure of high-dose steroid therapy to influence intracranial pressure in patients with severe head injury. J. Neurosurg. *51*:301, 1979.

159. Cooper, P.R. et al.: Dexamethasone and severe head injury: a prospective double-blind study. J. Neurosurg., *51*:307, 1979.

160. Sal, T.G., et al.: Steroids in severe head injury: a prospective randomized clinical trial. J. Neurosurg., *54*:596, 1981.

161. Pitts, L.H., and Kaktis, J.V.: Effect of megadose steroids in ICP in traumatic coma. *In* Intracranial Pressure IV. Edited by K. Shulman, et al. Berlin, Springer Verlag, 1980.

162. Warren, S.E.: Mannitol. Arch. Intern. Med., *141*:493, 1981.

163. Little, J.R.: Modification of acute focal ischemia by treatment with mannitol. Stroke, *9*:4, 1978.

164. Galuboff, B., Shenkin, H.A., and Haft, H.: The effects of mannitol and urea on cerebral hemodynamics and cerebral spinal fluid pressure. Neurology, *14*:891, 1964.

165. Marshall, L.F., Shapiro, H.M., and Rauscher, A.L.: Mannitol dose requirements in brain-injured patients. J. Neurosurg., *48*:169, 1978.

166. Bruce, D.A., Gennarelli, T.A., and Langfitt, T.W.: Resuscitation from coma due to head injury. Crit. Care Med., *6*:254, 1978.

167. Shenkin, H.A., and Bouzarth, W.F.: Medical progress: clinical methods of reducing intracranial pressure. Role of cerebral circulation. N. Engl. J. Med., *282*:1465, 1970.

168. Raulen, H.D., et al.: Role of pressure gradients and bulk flow in dynamics of vasogenic brain edema. J. Neurosurg. *46*:24, 1977.

169. Reulen, H.J., et al.: Clearance of edema fluid into cerebrospinal fluid: a mechanism for resolution of vasogenic brain edema. J. Neurosurg., *48*:754, 1978.

170. Tornheim, P.A., McLaurin, R.L., and Sawaya, R.: Effect of furosemide on experimental traumatic cerebral edema. Neurosurgery, *4(1)*:48, 1979.

171. Burhley, L.E., and Reed, D.J.: The effect of furosemide on sodium-22 uptake into cerebrospinal fluid and brain. Exp. Brain Res., *14*:503, 1972.

172. Bourke, R.S., et al.: Studies on the formation of astroglial swelling and its inhibition by chemically useful agents. *In* Seminars in Neurological Surgery. Edited by A.J. Popp, et al. New York, Raven Press, 1979.

173. Cottrell, J.E., et al.: Furosemide and mannitol induced changes in intracranial pressure and serum osmolality and electrolytes. Anesthesiology, *47*:27, 1977.

174. Cottrell, J.E., and Marlin, A.E.: Furosemide and human head injury. J. Trauma, *21(9)*:805, 1981.

175. Gaab, M., et al.: Effect of furosemide (Lasix) on acute severe experimental cerebral edema. J. Neurol., *220*:185, 1979.

176. James, H.E.: Combination therapy in brain edema. *In* Brain Edema—Pathology, Diagnosis, and Therapy. Advances in Neurology, Vol. 28. Edited by J. Cervos-Navarro, and R. Ferszt. New York, Raven Press, 1980.

177. Bremer, A.M., Yamada, K., and West, C.R.: Ischemic cerebral edema in primates: effects of acetazolamine, phenytoin, sorbitol, dexamethasone and methylprednisolone on brain water and electrolytes. Neurosurgery, *6*:149, 1980.

178. Meinig, G., et al.: Clinical, chemical, and CT evaluation of short-term and long-term antiedema therapy with dexamethasone and diuretics. In Brain Edema—Pathology, Diagnosis, and Therapy. Advances in Neurology, Vol. 28. Edited by J. Cervos-Navarro, and R. Ferszt. New York, Raven Press, 1980.

179. Wechsler, R.L., Dripps, R.D., and Kety, S.S.: Blood flow and oxygen consumption of the human brain during anesthesia produced by thiopental. Anesthesiology, 12:308, 1951.

180. Michenfelder, J.D., and Theye, R.A.: Cerebral protection by thiopental during hypoxia. Anesthesiology, 39:510, 1973.

181. Michenfelder, J.D., Milde, J.H., and Sundt, I.M.: Cerebral protection by barbiturate anesthesia. Arch. Neurol., 33:345, 1976.

182. Nilsson, L., and Siesjo, B.K.: The effect of phenobarbitone anesthesia on blood flow and oxygen consumption in the rat brain. Acta Anaesthesiol. Scand., 57(Suppl 57):18, 1975.

183. Michenfelder, J.D.: The interdependency of cerebral functional and metabolic effects following massive doses of thiopental in the dog. Anesthesiology, 41:231, 1974.

184. Steen, P.A., Milde, J.H., and Michenfelder, J.D.: Cerebral metabolic vascular effects of barbiturate therapy following complete global ischemia. J. Neurol., 31:1317, 1978.

185. Nordstrom, C.-H., Rehncrona, S., and Siesjo, B.K.: Effects of phenobarbital in cerebral ischemia. Part II: Restitution of cerebral energy state, glycolytic metabolites, citric acid cycle intermediates and associated amino acids after pronounced incomplete ischemia. Stroke, 9:335, 1978.

186. Steen, P.A., and Michenfelder, J.D.: Barbiturate protection in tolerant and nontolerant hypoxic mice. Anesthesiology, 50:404, 1979.

187. Nemoto, E.M., et al.: Impaired reperfusion: effect of barbiturate therapy after total cerebral ischemia in monkeys. Crit. Care Med., 9:183, 1981.

188. Nemoto, E.M., et al.: Studies on the pathogenesis of ischemic brain damage and the mechanism of its ameliorization by thiopental. Acta Neurol. Scand. 56(Suppl 64):142, 1977.

189. Branston, N.M., Hope, D.T., and Simon, L.: Barbiturates in focal ischemia of primate cortex: effects on blood flow distribution, evoked potential and extracellular potassium. Stroke, 10:647, 1979.

190. Altura, B.T., Turlapaty, P.D., and Altura, B.M.: Pentobarbital sodium inhibits calcium uptake in vascular smooth muscle. Biochem. Biophys. Acta, 595:309, 1980.

191. Altura, B.M., and Altura, B.T.: Pharmacologic inhibition of cerebral vasospasm in ischemia, hallucinogen ingestion, and hypomagnesemia: barbiturates, calcium antagonists, and magnesium. Am. J. Emerg. Med., 2:180, 1983.

192. Siesjo, B.K., et al.: Brain metabolism in the critically ill. Crit. Care Med., 4:283, 1976.

193. Flamm, E.S., et al.: Barbiturates and free radicals. In Neural Trauma. Edited by A.G. Popp, et al. New York, Raven Press, 1979.

194. Smith, D.S., et al.: Lipid peroxidation in brain tissue in vitro: antioxidant effects of barbiturates. Acta Physiol. Scand. 105:527, 1979.

195. Steen, P.A., and Michenfelder, J.D.: Cerebral protection with barbiturates: relation to anesthetic effect. Stroke, 9:140, 1978.

196. Rockeff, M.A., Marshall, L.F., and Shapiro H.M.: High dose barbiturate therapy in humans: a clinical review of 60 patients. Ann. Neurol., 6:194, 1979.

197. Marshall, L.F., Smith, R.W., and Shapiro, H.M.: The outcome with aggressive treatment in severe head injuries. Part II: Acute and chronic barbiturate administration in the management of head injury. J. Neurosurg., 50:26, 1979.

198. Marshall, L.F., et al.: Pentobarbital therapy for intracranial hypertension in metabolic coma: Reye's syndrome. Crit. Care Med., 6:1, 1978.

199. Bleyaert, A.L., et al.: Thiopental ameliorization of brain damage after global ischemia in monkeys. Anesthesiology, 49:390, 1978.

200. Steen, P.A., Milde, J.H., and Michenfelder, J.D.: No barbiturate protection in a dog model of complete cerebral ischemia. Ann. Neurol., 5:343, 1979.

201. Snyder, B.D., et al.: Failure of thiopental to modify global anoxic injury. Stroke, 10:135, 1979.

202. Abramson, N.A., et al.: Thiopental loading in cardiopulmonary resuscitation survivors. The brain resuscitation clinical trial (BRCT) I study group. Crit. Care Med. 12(3):227, 1984.

203. Smith, A.L., et al.: Cerebral protection in acute focal cerebral ischemia. Stroke, 5:1, 1974.

204. Selman, W.R., Spetzler, R.F., and Roski, R.A.: Barbiturate resuscitation from focal cerebral ischemia—a review. Rescue, 9:189, 1981.

205. Astrup, J.: Barbiturate protection in focal cerebral ischemia (editorial). Scand. J. Clin. Lab. Invest. 40:201, 1980.

206. White, B.C., et al.: Possible role of calcium blockers in cerebral resuscitation: a review of the literature and synthesis for future studies. Crit. Care Med., 11(3):202, 1983.

207. Fleckenstein, A.: Specific pharmacology of calcium in myocardium, cardiac pacemakers, and vascular smooth muscle. Ann. Rev. Pharmacol. Toxicol., 17:149, 1977.

208. Young, G.P.: Calcium channel blockers in emergency medicine. Ann. Emerg. Med., *13(Part 1)*:712, 1984.
209. White, B.C., et al.: Effect of flunarizine on canine cerebral cortical blood flow and vascular resistance post cardiac arrest. Ann. Emerg. Med., *11(3)*:119, 1982.
210. Winegar, C.D., et al.: Early amelioration of neurologic deficit by lidoflazine after fifteen minutes of cardiopulmonary arrest in dogs. Ann. Emerg. Med., *12*:471, 1983.
211. Wauguier, A., et al.: Flunarizine in the treatment of experimental canine cardiac arrest. Am. J. Emerg. Med., *2(4)*:361, 1984.
212. Vaagenes, P., et al.: The effect of lidoflazine and verapamil on neurological outcome after 10 minutes ventricular fibrillation cardiac arrest in dogs. Crit. Care Med., *12(3)*:228, 1984.
213. Steen, P.A., et al.: Nimodipine improves cerebral blood flow and neurologic recovery after complete cerebral ischemia in the dog. J. Cereb. Blood Flow Metab. *3*:38, 1983.
214. Schwartz, A.C.: Calcium blockers: status post cardiac arrest. Ann. Emerg. Med., *12*:10, A-137, 1983.
215. De la Torre, J.C., et al.: Dimethyl sulfoxide in central nervous system trauma. Ann N.Y. Acad. Sci., *243*:362, 1975.
216. Cullen, J.P., et al.: Protective action of phenytoin in cerebral ischemia. Anesth. Analg., *58(3)*:165, 1979.
217. Aldrete, J.A., et al.: Phenytoin for brain resuscitation after cardiac arrest: an uncontrolled clinical trial. Crit. Care Med., *9(6)*:474, 1981.
218. Handal, K.A., Schauben, J.L., and Salamone, F.R.: Naloxone. Ann. Emerg. Med., *12*:438, 1983.
219. Jackson, R.E., et al.: Blood flow in the cerebral cortex during cardiac resuscitation in dogs. Ann. Emerg. Med., *13* (9 pt. 1):657, 1984.
220. Markov, A.K., et al.: Irreversible hemorrhagic shock: treatment and cardiac pathophysiology. Circ. Shock, *8*:9, 1981.
221. Chaudry, I.H., Mohammed, S., and Baue, A.E.: Effect of adenosine triphosphate-magnesium chloride administration in shock. Surgery, *75*:220, 1974.
222. Hallenbeck, J.M., and Furlow, T.W.: Prostaglandin I_2 and indomethacin prevent impairment of post-ischemic brain reperfusion in the dog. Stroke, *10*:629, 1970.
223. Safar, P.: Cerebral resuscitation after cardiac arrest: summaries and suggestions. Am. J. Emerg. Med., *2*:108, 1983.
224. Epstein, F.B., and Hamilton, G.C.: Initial approach to the brain injured patient. Crit. Care Quart. *5(4)*:13, 1983.
225. Jennett, B., and Teasdale, G.: Assessment of coma and impaired consciousness. A practical scale. Lancet, *2*:81, 1974.
226. Sigsbee, B., and Plum, F.: The unresponsive patient—diagnosis and early management. Med. Clin. North Am., *63(4)*:813, 1979.
227. Caronna, J.J.: Diagnosis, prognosis, and treatment of hypoxic coma. Edited by S. Fahn, J.H. Davis, and E.P. Rowland. *In* Advances in Neurology. Vol. 26. Raven Press, New York, 1979.
228. Bell, R.S., and Loop, J.W.: The utility and futility of radiographic skull examination from trauma. N. Engl. J. Med., *284(5)*:236, 1971.
229. Jennett, B.: Skull X-rays after recent head injury. Clin. Radiol. *31*:463, 1980.
230. Saul, T.G., and Ducker, T.B.: The role of computer tomography in acute head injury. J. Comp. Tomog., *4(4)*:296, 1980.
231. James, H.E., et al.: Priorities and indications of computerized tomography in clinical practice. Acta Neurochir., *36*:1, 1977.
232. Duffy, T.P.: Coma and altered mental states. *In* The Principles and Practice of Medicine. 19th ed. Edited by A.M. Harvey, et al. New York, Appleton Century Crofts, 1976.
233. Safar, P.: Brain resuscitation. Crit. Care Med., *6*:199, 1978.
234. Abramson, N., et al.: Long term follow-up of cardiac arrest survivors. Crit. Care Med., *10*:215, 1982.
235. Greenberg, R.P., et al.: Advanced monitoring of the brain. *In* Brain Failure and Resuscitation. Edited by A. Grenvik and P. Safar. New York, Churchill Livingstone, 1981.
236. Mickell, J.J., et al.: ICP monitoring in Reye-Johnson syndrome. Crit. Care Med., *4*:1, 1976.
237. Vries, J.K., Becker, D.P., and Young, H.F.: A subarachnoid screw for monitoring intracranial pressure. J. Neurosurg., *39*:416, 1973.
238. Gjerris, F., Borgesen, S.E., and Sorensen, S.C.: Clinical evaluation of a new epidural pressure transducer. *In* Intracranial Pressure IV. Edited by K. Shulman, et al. Berlin, Springer Verlag, 1980.
239. Chiappa, K.H., and Ropper, A.H.: Evoked potentials in clinical medicine, N. Engl. J. Med., *306*:1140,1205, 1982.
240. Martin, W.R.: Naloxone. Ann. Intern. Med., *85*:765, 1976.
241. Mahoney, B.D., et al.: Emergency twist drill trephination. Neurosurgery, *8(5)*:551, 1981.

242. Bouzarth, W.F., and Lindermuth, J.R.: Head injury watch sheet modified for a digital scale. J. Trauma, *19*:571, 1978.
243. Karnaze, D.S., Marshall, L.F., and Bickford, R.G.: Part I:EEG monitoring of clinical coma: the compressed spectral array. Neurology, *32*:289, 1982.
244. Greenberg, R.P., et al.: Evaluation of brain function in severe human head injury with multimodality evoked potentials. Part I: Evoked brain injury potentials, methods, and analyses. J. Neurosurg., *47*:150, 1977.
245. Greenberg, R.P., et al.: Evaluation of brain function in severe human head trauma with multimodality evoked potentials. Part II: Localization of brain dysfunction and correlation with posttraumatic neurological conditions. J. Neurosurg., *47*:163, 1977.
246. Salcman, M., Schepp, R.S., and Ducker, T.B.: Calculated recovery rates in severe head trauma. Neurosurgery, *8(3)*:301, 1981.
247. Teres, D., Brown, R.B., and Lemeshow, S.: Predicting mortality of intensive care unit patients: the importance of coma. Crit. Care Med., *10*:86, 1982.
248. Bates, D., et al: A prospective study of non-traumatic coma: methods and results in 310 patients with severe head injury. Ann. Neurol., *2*:211, 1977.
249. Jennett, B., et al.: Prognosis of patients with severe head injury. Neurosurgery, *4*:283, 1979.
250. Plum, F., and Ferry, D.: Predicting prognosis in coma. Am. J. Med., *65*:224, 1978.
251. Teasdale, G., and Galbraith, S.: Head trauma and intracranial hemorrhage. *In* Brain Failure and Resuscitation. Clinics in Critical Care Medicine. Edited by A. Grenvik, and P. Safar. New York, Churchill Livingstone, 1981.
252. Jennett, B.: Predictors of recovery in evaluation of patients in coma. Adv. Neurol., *22*:129, 1979.
253. Bruce, D.A., et al.: Pathophysiology, treatment and outcome following severe head injury in children. Child. Brain, *5*:174, 1979.
254. Teasdale, G., and Jennett, B.: Assessment of coma and impaired conscousness. Lancet, *2*:81, 1974.
255. Hesse, B., Jensen, G., and Sigurd, B.: Emergency-room patients with cardiac arrest. Dan. Med. Bull., *20(1)*:30, 1973.
256. Levy, D.E., et al. Prognosis in nontraumatic coma. Ann. Int. Med., *94*:293, 1981.
257. Snyder, B.D., Ramirez-Lassepas, M., and Lippert, D.M.: Neurologic status and prognosis after cardiopulmonary arrest. I. A retrospective study. Neurology, *27*:807, 1977.
258. Snyder, B.D., et al.: Neurologic prognosis after cardiopulmonary arrest. IV. Brain-stem reflexes. Neurology, *31*:1092, 1981.
259. Safar, P.: Resuscitation after Brain Ischemia. *In* Brain Failure and Resuscitation. Clinics in Critical Care Medicine. Edited by A. Grenvik, and P. Safar. New York, Churchill Livingstone, 1981.
260. Gennarelli, T.A., et al.: Influence of the type of intracranial lesion on outcome from severe head injury. J. Neurosurg., *56*:26, 1981.
261. Mullie, A., et al.: Monitoring of cerebrospinal fluid enyzme levels in postischemic encephalopathy after cardiac arrest. Crit. Care Med., *9(5)*:399, 1981.
262. Longstreth, W.T., Jr., Clayson, K.J., and Sumi, S.M.: Cerebrospinal fluid and serum creatine kinase BB activity after out-of-hospital cardiac arrest. Neurology, *31*:455, 1981.
263. Edgren, E., Terent, A., Hedstrand, U., and Ronquist, G.: Cerebrospinal fluid markers in relation to outcome in patients with global cerebral ischemia. Crit. Care Med., *11*:4, 1983.
264. Aberg, T., Ronquist, G., and Tyden, H.: Release of adenylate kinase into cerebrospinal fluid during open-heart surgery and its relation to postoperative intellectual function. Lancet, *2*:1139, 1982.
265. Binnie, C.D., Prior, P.F., and Lloyd, D.S.L.: Electroencephalogram prediction of fatal anoxic brain damage after resuscitation from cardiac arrest. Br. Med. J., *4*:265, 1970.
266. Wagner, I., and Greenbaum, D.: Cerebral function monitoring in deeply comatose patients. Crit. Care Med., *9(4)*:305, 1981.
267. Moller, M., et al.: Electroencephalographic predictions of anoxic brain damage after resuscitation from cardiac arrest in patients with acute myocardial infarction. Acta Med. Scand., *203*:31, 1978.
268. Lemmi, H., Hubbert, C.H., and Faris, A.A.: The electroencephalogram after resuscitation of cardiopulmonary arrest. J. Neurosurg. Psychiatry, *36*:997, 1973.
269. Goitein, K.J., et al.: Diagnostic and prognostic value of auditory nerve brainstem evoked responses in comatose children. Crit. Care Med., *11*:91, 1983.
270. Welsh, F.A., Ginsberg, M.D., Rieder, W., and Budd, W.W.: Diffuse cerebral ischemia in the cat: II. Regional metabolites during severe ischemia and recirculation. Ann. Neurol., *3*:493, 1978.
271. Yatsu, F.M., Lee, L.-W., and Liac, C.-L.: Energy metabolism during brain ischemia. Stroke, *6*:678, 1975.
272. Garcia, J.H., and Conger, K.A.: Ischemic brain injuries: structural and biochemical effects. *In* Brain Failure and Resuscitation. Clinics in Critical Care Medicine. Edited by A. Grenvik, and P. Safar. New York, Churchill Livingstone, 1981.

273. Levy, D.E., Knill-Jones, R.P., and Plum, F.: The vegetative state and its prognosis following non-traumatic coma. Ann. N.Y. Acad. Sci., *315*:293, 1978.
274. Wallace-Barnhill, G., et al.: Medical, legal, and ethical issues in critical care. Crit. Care Med., *10(1)*:57, 1982.
275. Kenton, C.: Brain death criteria. Literature search 82-2, National Library of Medicine, January 1977 through April 1982.
276. Guidelines for the determination of death. Report of the medical consultants on the diagnosis of death to the President's commission for the study of ethical problems in medicine and biomedical and behavioral research. Crit. Care Med., *10(1)*:62, 1982.

Chapter 6
HEART IN SHOCK

Wolfgang Johannes Mergner • Louis Marzella

The Heart in Hemorrhagic Shock

The heart is one of the best protected organs in shock.[1] If it becomes affected in shock, the heart may be a crucial determinant of survival or death.[2] The natural course of shock is progressive. If in the progression of clinical shock the heart's function suffers, the patient enters a downward spiral, which enhances underperfusion and depressed cellular metabolism and may cause lethal organ failure. Lefer,[3] who believes that the heart is the target of several local and systemic factors in shock,[4] stressed that although impairment of heart function is an important event in shock it occurs relatively late.

Definitions and Time Course of Shock

An essential feature of shock then is the critical reduction of nutrient flow. In considering the effects of hemorrhagic shock on the heart, a review of the phases of shock contributes to an understanding of the sequence of events. In response to a falling blood pressure, regulatory responses of the negative feedback control system are activated. The baroreceptors found in the aortic arch and carotid sinus relay the information to the cardiovascular center in the medulla oblongata that in turn adjusts the blood pressure through the effector organs—the heart and blood vessels. These organs maintain blood pressure during the compensatory phase of hemorrhagic shock at set point. The cardiac output is altered by changing the heart rate and myocardial contractility. The arterioles and venules also constrict. Most compensating vasoconstriction occurs in splanchnic and dermal arterioles, but kidney, liver, and skeletal muscle contribute as well. In cases of severe blood pressure reduction, the neurons of the cardiovascular center are directly affected, resulting in the intense sympathetic stimulation in an emergency attempt to raise the blood pressure. This is known as the central nervous system ischemic response. If therapeutic measures are timely and effective at this point, blood pressure and microcirculatory flow may be restored. Tissues, including the heart, return to normal functional status (Fig. 6–1). In tissues damaged by hypoxia, adequate flow will allow regeneration and repair. The clinical situation is called nonprogressive shock. The siginicant factor in progressive shock is the damage to the circulatory structures themselves. This leads to further circulatory damage (Figs. 6–2 and 6–3). The essential component of this progressive shock is depression of cardiac function by the reduction of the coronary circulation. Prolonged ischemia to the cardiovascular center of the CNS may reduce the auto-

Supported in part by grant 1R01-22281-01, by the University of Maryland Foundation, and by funds from MIEMSS. This is publication UM #1890 from the Cellular Pathobiology Laboratory at the University of Maryland, Department of Pathology.

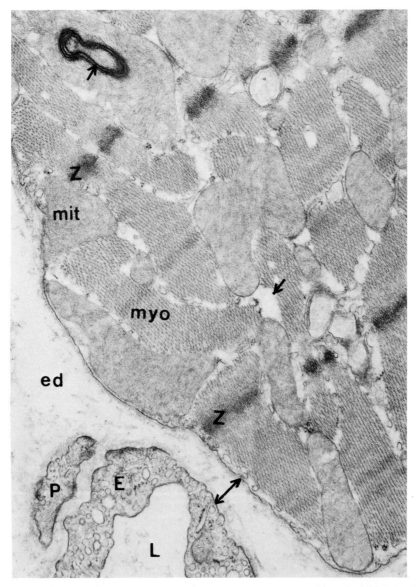

Fig.6-1. An electron micrograph of the myocardium of a dog. Shock was produced by bleeding to maintain the oxygen deficit at a predetermined level. The dog had hemorrhagic shock for 1 hour then underwent reinfusion, first with plasmanate and then with whole blood. The photograph shows inter-stitial edema (double-headed arrow) and the beginning of cellular edema. The mitochondria show a mild degree of swelling. Original magnification × 15,000 (ed = edema; mit= mitochondria; Z = z-band; E = endothelial cell; P = pericyte; myo = myofilaments; arrow = myelin body).

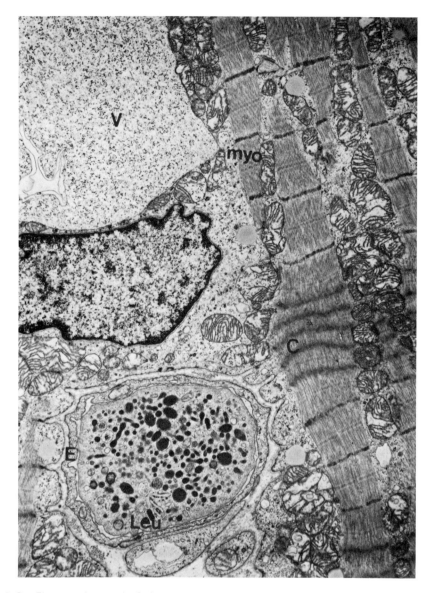

Fig. 6-2.   Electron micrograph of a human heart obtained during an autopsy immediately after death, showing myocyte with contraction band. A capillary with a leukocyte is adjacent to it. There is a limited degree of cellular swelling and mitochondrial alteration. V = cytoplasmic bleb; myo = myofilaments; C = contraction bands; Leu = leukocyte; E = endothelial cell. (Reprinted with permission from Trump, B.F., et al.: The application of electron microscopy and cellular biochemistry to autopsy. Observation on cellular changes in human shock. Human Pathol., 6:499, 1975.)

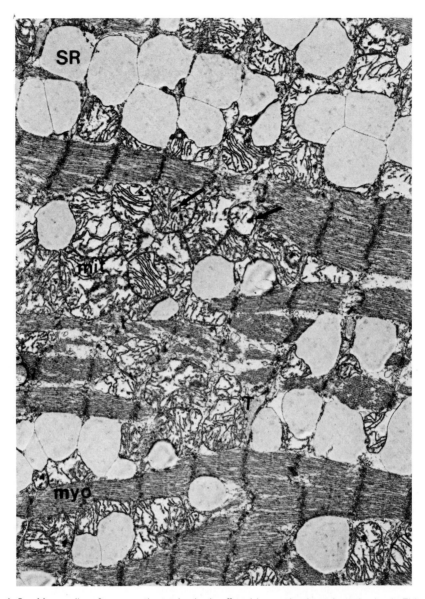

Fig. 6-3. Myocardium from a patient who had suffered hemorrhagic and septic shock. This is an example of severe alteration of myocardium. Note the swollen mitochondria and the very swollen sarcoplasmic reticulum system. SR = sarcoplasmic reticulum; T = T tubule; myo = myofilaments; mit = mitochondria. (Reprinted with permission from Trump, B.F., et al.: The application of electron microscopy and cellular biochemistry to autopsy. Observation on cellular changes in human shock. Human Pathol., 6:499, 1975.)

nomic output to the heart, thus releasing the heart from the counterregulatory effort. Vasoconstrictive failure results in peripheral pooling of blood, reduced venous return, and reduced filling of the heart.[5-9] In many clinical situations the true stage of shock is not known at the initiation of resuscitation. It would be desirable, however, to assess exactly the state of shock and to be able to measure predictive cardiovascular parameters in order to be guided by them toward purposeful therapy.

GENERAL CONSIDERATIONS

Morbid Anatomy

The postmortem pathologic condition of the heart in hemorrhagic shock is quite distinct, as reported by Hackel, et al.[10] and Ratliff,[11] causing the so-called "zonal lesions"[12] and "endocardial and epicardial hemorrhages." McGovern[13] has stressed that one of the most important features in hemorrhagic shock with lethal outcome is the high incidence of cardiac lesions. Of 207 postmortem examinations as a result of hemorrhage, 120 necropsy reports of individuals dying of hemorrhagic shock showed histologic manifestations of shock. The heart was involved in 39.2%, next in frequency to the lung, with 50%. Grossly there were hemorrhages into the epicardium posteriorly and into the endocardium in the interventricular septum. Microscopically there was frank necrosis, particularly endocardial and septal lesions affecting scattered fibers and single groups of fibers in a pattern not seen in other conditions; large areas of infarction were also noted. Banding of hypercontraction was frequently seen, as were "wavy fibers" of Bouchardy and Majno.[14] Ratliff and Unger[15] reported severe deformities of the intercalated discs in persons and cats subjected to hemorrhagic shock. These deformities were considered a manifestation of cell swelling of myocytes and thus were reversible. In general, a good correlation was found between structure and function on an ultrastructural level (Fig. 6–4).[16,17]

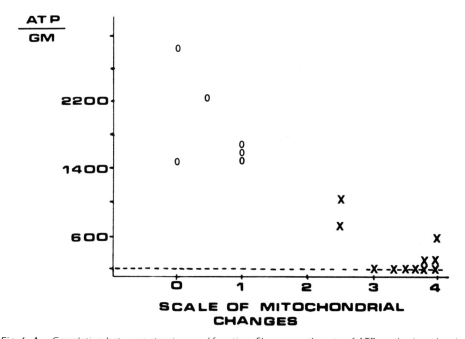

Fig. 6–4. Correlation between structure and function. Shown are the rate of ATP synthesis and scale of change in mitochondrial structure in human autopsy specimens. o = control patients with head trauma; x = trauma patients with hemrrohagic shock. ATP synthesis is measured in μmol/min. (Reprinted with permission from Mergner, W.J., et al.: Cells in shock: The effects of ischemia, microprobe, morphological and biochemical studies. *In* International Symposia on Emergency Medical Service System Development, Traumatology and Trauma Nursing. Edited by R.A. Cowley. Baltimore, Williams & Wilkins, 1979.)

Pathophysiology

The mechanical myocardial dysfunction of hemorrhagic shock has been considered to be a major contributing factor leading to irreversible myocardial injury. Because myocardial oxygen consumption is great even under physiologic conditions, modest diminution of coronary perfusion may be critical. Recent studies on the relationship of mitochondrial ATP synthesis to ischemic tolerance have stressed the low tolerance of cardiac myocytes and myocyte mitochondria to total ischemia of 25 to 30 min.[18,19] Once myocardial viability has been compromised, even treatment of the primary cause such as restoration of severe blood loss may not restore depressed ventricular function.[20] Such depression has been measured by reduced stroke work, [21,22] positive dp/dt_{max}, negative dp/dt_{max}, and cardiac output.[23,24] The effects of hemorrhagic shock have been reproduced in experimental animal models. Hackel, et al.[10] postulated at least three general mechanisms responsible for shock-induced cardiac failure: 1. decreased coronary blood flow, 2. increased heart rate, and 3. flooding the coronary circulation with toxins such as the myocardial depressant factor or endotoxins.[25] Hormones may also affect the heart. In the studies by Hackel, et al.[10] high levels of serum catecholamines have been associated with two distinct cardiac lesions, "zonal lesions" and "subendocardial ischemia," suggesting that hormonal counterregulation to hypovolemia enhances cardiac injury. Both lesions may, as suggested by the authors, be directly associated with cardiac failure. Boutet, et al.[26] defined catecholamine-induced injury. Similar mechanisms have been described in humans by Trump, et al., [16] who demonstrated cardiac lesions in trauma victims even if the trauma did not directly affect the heart. Although the events are complex, a certain time sequence and a certain order of reaction prevails. The cardiovascular adjustments in the initial phase of shock seem to be induced mainly by circulating hormones. Neurogenic vasoconstrictor discharge is accelerated, and skeletal muscle, skin, and splanchnic bed are the main targets for these vasomotor reflexes. As a result, the proportion of cardiac output reaching the vital organs, such as heart and brain, is increased, but absolute blood flow is still subnormal, more to the kidney and liver than to the heart and brain.[20] The late reactions to persistent shock may involve significant organ damage, possibly caused by hypoxia, hormonal agents, or peptides generated during severe underperfusion of the splanchnic bed.[27]

Role of Hypoxia

Hypovolemic shock causes inadequate tissue oxygenation.[28] This knowledge has been used by Guyton, et al.,[6] Crowell and Smith,[29] Crowell and Guyton,[2] Dunham, et al.,[30] and Linberg et al.[31] to quantify the severity of shock. The measurement of total body oxygen deficit over a period of time corresponded closely with other criteria used to indicate the severity of shock, such as mixed venous oxygen, blood lactate, systolic pressure, transcutaneous oxygen, or muscle interstitial pH. The same criteria also correspond to the organ damage in kidney or liver. The heart is not one of the early target organs. Therefore, these criteria do not, in general, reflect the degree of injury to the heart. Total body hypoxia, thus, is uneven during the compensatory phase of shock. This does not mean that the heart is entirely spared (Fig. 6-2).

The sensitivity of heart cells to hypoxia depends on the work performed. Mild degrees of underperfusion can be tolerated by the heart cells. Heart cells in a resting stage have been said to tolerate hypoxia up to 50% of normal.[32] Many physiologic reactions, however, keep hypoxia low and favor coronary circulation. The heart cells, though, are very dependent on the intact microcirculation. If in the late phases of shock coronary and microvascular perfusion is significantly reduced, the low tolerance of myocytes to hypoxia becomes apparent and dominates the clinical situation. Then a sequence of cellular reactions is seen, which will, in the end, affect the contractile machinery of the heart or its electrophysiologic behavior and lead to arrythmia or heart failure and death of the individual (Fig.6–3).

EFFECT OF SHOCK ON THE MYOCYTE

Excitation-Contraction Coupling

Goldfarb[33] pointed out that alteration of the mechanical performance of the heart is central to cardiovascular reaction to shock and can only be detected by refined methods such as the end systolic pressure-diameter relationship. The excitation-contraction coupling during the last postinfusion state following hemorrhagic shock was studied by Warner, el al.,[34] who focused on the integrity of the sarcoplasmic reticulum and myofibrils. Hemorrhagic shock was induced for 90 min and monitored by systolic blood pressure depression. Blood was then reinfused. Thirty minutes after reinfusion no change occurred in peak developed left ventricular pressure, positive dp/dt_{max}, stroke work, mean arterial pressure, coronary flow, or total peripheral resistance. However, at 90 min after reinfusion, all these parameters were significantly depressed, whereas coronary flow had returned to the same level as before shock was induced. This decrease in mechanical performance was linked to a severe depression of calcium uptake by the sarcoplasmic reticulum (SR),[35] uncoupling of ATP hydrolysis from calcium transport in the SR, and depression of myofibrillar ATPase activity characterized by a decreased enzyme affinity for calcium. It was concluded that the late postinfusion phase of hemorrhagic shock is characterized by an intrinsic decrease in myocardial contractility. The depression in contractility is associated with a depression in excitation-coupling and in an altered affinity of the myofibrillar ATPase for calcium. These observations clearly imply direct myocardial damage in the late postinfusion phase.

Role of Depressed Metabolism

General Considerations

The effect of shock on myocyte metabolism is complex, and it is not possible to decide on a hierarchy of events. Shock is a state of hypoperfusion, i.e., partial, not total ischemia. The effect of partial ischemia is different from that of total ischemia, as has been worked out by Opie, et al.[36] or Garfinkel and Adis,[37] and Kohn and Garfinkel.[38] Shock and hypoxia affect the overall cell metabolism by partially limiting the suppy of oxygen and substrate and by metabolic inhibition (acidosis). The foremost target in shock on myocyte metabolism seems to be the energy metabolism. Energy metabolism of the heart is largely dependent on ATP generation by mitochondria. Anaerobic glycolysis cannot replace oxidative phosphorylation under physiologic and pathologic conditions. At least for a while, however, under anaerobic conditions, myocardial viability seems to depend in part on glycolysis. Thus, perfusion with glucose does improve ventricular function in hypoperfusion syndromes.[39] Yet this beneficial effect is only partially realized since anaerobic glycolysis is further inhibited by the rate-limiting influence of developing cellular acidosis. Schumer[40,41] stressed that a common denominator exists at the cellular and molecular level. Since energy metabolism is severely depressed, the individual cells within hypoxic and underperfused tissue have less substrate available and are also less able to metabolize substrate to its full energy content. The cells are starving for oxygen and substrate. Substrate use in the heart is severely retarded.[42,43] For example, fatty acids are preferentially incorporated into triglycerides in hypoxic states, increasing the neutral lipid content of myocytes. The accumulation of triglycerides is readily visible microscopically as small fat globules. Hypoperfusion states may also lead to loss of purine nucleotides because nucleotide biosynthesis is not maintained effectively in myocytes.[36,44] Hypoperfusion syndromes cause structural and functional alteration to cell organelles, some reversible, some irreversible.

SARCOPLASMIC RETICULUM

Ratliff[11] demonstrated the disruption of the sarcoplasmic reticulum contained within the aforementioned zonal lesions in the late phase of hemorrhagic shock. After 30 min of ischemia, isolated sarcoplasmic reticulum showed depressed calcium accumulation, a deficiency that affects excitation-contraction coupling as described earlier.[45] A defect at this site causes reduced speed of accumulation of calcium by the reticulum and impaired regulation of calcium-dependent cell functions, such as contraction. Thus such a defect in the function of the sarcoplasmic reticulum leads to heart failure.[35] The altered calcium metabolism is reflected by the reduced response of the myocardium to calcium during endotoxic shock[46] and possibly other forms of shock as well.[45] Also, loss of regulation of cytosolic calcium levels may have deleterious stimulating effects on the catabolism of the cytoplasm or of membranes and on cytoskeletal function. In this way such defects of calcium sequestration could lead to cell injury. Although the primary target of low-flow ischemia is the energy metabolism, the contribution to cell decay by other organelles is overshadowing. Chaudry, et al.[47–49] maintain that if energized substrate could be supplied to cells in low flow states survival periods could be prolonged.

PLASMA MEMBRANE

Another organelle affected severely in prolonged low-flow ischemia is the plasma membrane. Hess and Krause[45] argue that the plasma membrane (plasmalemma) is structurally and functionally preserved even after relatively prolonged periods of shock. Yet catecholamine effects may induce selected cell necrosis and scattered or localized changes in the permeability of cells. In late phases of prolonged hypoperfusion states the plasmalemma is altered. The damaged cell then loses its control over volume regulation and the interior milieu. This plasmalemmal cell damage is expressed by leakage of potassium and of molecules such as lactate dehydrogenase.[50] Elevations in the lactate dehydrogenase level may be detected in cardiac lymph and serum after anoxia and shock. Hypoperfusion, as described earlier, does affect a specialized region in the plasmalemma—the nexus. The nexus thus altered was examined by serial sections by Ratliff and Unger.[15] The evidence supported the hypothesis that swelling on these special slides may be the cause of the contraction band lesions, possibly as the result of specific calcium accumulation.

MYOFILAMENTS

There is good evidence of myofibrillar changes in heart failure induced by shock or hypoperfusion. Such myofibrillar changes may be visible in the subendocardial hemorrhagic lesions.[11] Kleinman, et al.[51] and Ratliff[11] distinguished between two myofibrillar lesions.[52] One was present in the zonal lesions and showed sarcomere disruption, and the other one was called myofibrillar degeneration and revealed focal dissolution of myofilaments. The lesions are similar to those induced experimentally by Dhalla[53] with oxidized isoproterenol or those induced by catecholamine overdose by Boutet, et al.[26] Shock-induced acidosis may be an element that greatly depresses myofibrillar function.[42,54] This effect is perhaps in part explained by the competition between calcium and protons.[55]

MITOCHONDRIA

Parenchymal tissue mitochondria isolated immediately after death from tissues of persons who died of shock showed severe depression of ATP synthesis.[56] The tissues with the most severe alteration of oxidative phosphorylation were kidney and liver. In these individuals heart mitochondria were relative unaffected, reflecting the afore-described phase difference of organ involvement between the heart and the remainder of the organ systems. In late phases of hemorrhagic shock and in situations in which the individual has experienced prolonged decompensation, the heart mitochondria also show vulnerability. It may be that the vulnerability of heart mitochondria is similar in situations of oxygen deprivation of ischemia and during late phases of shock. Costa, et al.[18] described the limit of ischemic tolerance of heart myocyte mitochondria to be between 25 and 30 min of total ischemia. Jennings, et al.[57] reported similar data for in vivo ischemia of dog myocardium. Thus fast and severe or prolonged shock states are able to affect the energy metabolism of the heart and can contribute to the circulatory decompensation. The result of alteration of heart mitochondria is loss of the ability to generate ATP.[18,58]

Progression of Cardiac Lesions

Gutovitz, et al.[59] described the progressive nature of myocardial injury in cardiogenic shock and compared it with hypovolemic shock. In hypovolemic shock serum MB creatine kinase level was lower and less sustained than in cardiogenic shock. It was argued that patients with cardiogenic shock entered a vicious circle of myocardial destruction. This is different in hypovolemic conditions in which cardiac alteration appears less distinct and later in the course of the reactions to shock. Still a number of distinct cellular alterations may be related to the observed depression of cardiac function

It is postulated that the late effects of hypovolemic shock on the heart are 1. pathophysiologic, related to cardiac filling, reduced cardiac output, and reduced coronary perfusion; 2. microcirculatory, related to the effect of myocardial depressant factor, platelets, leukocytes, and viscosity changes of red blood cells, and thus affecting oxygenation and perfusion; 3. endocrine, related to dysregulation of calcium metabolism, possibly stimulated by factors such as catecholamines; 4. metabolic, related to acidosis, oxygen, and substrate depletion; 5. toxic, related to peroxidation, endothelial injury, and edema. Other substances may also be toxic.

PATHOGENESIS OF LESIONS IN SHOCK

The pathogenesis of lesions in shock is still uncertain, although the search has focused on a variety of distinct mechanisms. Some authors stress that the organ manifestations of shock are the result of interrelated factors until the process reaches a stage from which it is self-perpetuating.

The Mediators

Because many of the manifestations of shock seem to occur at some distance from any potential injury site, it seems reasonable to assume that cell injury in target organs is mediated by factors that are responsible for the manifestations of organ lesions. As much as certain mediators seem established, it certainly seems that several mediators act in concert in the pathogenesis of organ lesions. This may be particularly true for the heart during late stages of decompensation.

FREE RADICALS

The question has been raised about how tissue damage is mediated. The generation of free radicals, particularly oxygen free radicals, plays an essential damage-mediating role in the microvasculature and parenchymal cells in shock and ischemia. Parks, et al.,[60] demonstrated that oxygen free radicals create increased microvascular permeability in small venules. In shock states oxygen radicals are formed by xanthine oxidase if and when the intravascular volume is restored. Taylor, et al.[61] suspected that oxygen radicals also affect capillary permeability and lead to pulmonary edema. Lefer, et al.,[62] showed that there is a beneficial effect of free radical scavengers MK-447 in traumatic shock and myocardial ischemia. The agent partially restored normal contractility in hearts perfused at low perfusion rates, partially prevented edema in low-perfusion ischemia of the isolated heart, and prolonged survival in traumatic shock. The effects could be enhanced by the cyclo-oxygenase inhibitor meclofenamate.

BLOOD CONSTITUENTS

The microcirculation is a central problem in the general pathology and pathologic anatomy of shock.[63] It is affected by activated blood constituents and by hormonal regulation. Among the blood constituents are the red blood cells, the platelets, and the leukocytes. Altered viscosity of the blood is also a factor that has found considerable attention in previous research efforts. Such change may be caused in part by loss of water and in part by a change of the corpuscular elements by hypoxia.

RED BLOOD CELLS

It is reported that red blood cells have a decrease in filterability and crenelation in vivo as morphologic evidence of increased red blood cell viscosity in low-flow states. The relationship of altered flow characteristics in low-flow states has been described by Chien.[64] Red blood cells become less pliable, possibly as a consequence of the altered ion regulation in hypoperfused tissues caused by energy deficiency.[65,66] The same alteration may induce endothelial cells to form luminal blebs, thus creating a mechanical obstacle to regional perfusion and reperfusion.

PLATELETS

Blood coagulation, including fibrin formation and platelet-induced coagulation, is abnormal in shock.[67] Platelet-activating factor causes circulatory collapse.[68] In fact, Matthias and Lasch[69] described the role of disseminated intravascular coagulation as an important and clinically frequently undetected event in the progression of circulatory shock.

LEUKOCYTES

In shock, the leukocytes, if activated, may affect the circulation, including the coronary microcirculation[70] The effect of the leukocytes may be twofold. It may affect the release of lytic enzymes, although it has not yet been shown that this event plays any general and contributing role, or it may affect peroxidation. In a number of models invasion by leukocytes induced local peroxidation injury. One of the targets of local peroxidation injury is the endothelial cell with consequent tissue edema. Leukocyte activation predominantly occurs through complement, although other activators such as cardiolipin have been postulated.

LYSOSOMES

Although the contribution to myocardial injury by lysosomal enzymes derived from leukocytes has not been proved, Glenn and Lefer[71] have postulated a role for lysosomes from the splanchnic bed tissues in the progression of shock and in generation of the depressed cardiac function. The depression of cardiac funtion was shown in cats after ligation and release of the splanchnic artery. Similar characteristic cardiac depression has been shown by Lee, et al.[72] in acute pancreatitis. Characteristic morphologic alterations of the lysosomes occur in many types of cell injury, including ischemia.[73,74] In particular, an accumulation of degradative vacuoles called autophagic vacuoles is seen in cells. The autophagic vacuoles are an important site for the normal process of degradation of cellular proteins and lipids[75] and are functionally a part of the lysosomal system. These lysosomal changes seen in injury are thought to reflect primarily altered turnover of cellular constituents.[75]

Hormonal Substances, Peptides, and Receptors

HORMONES AND ENDOGENOUS PEPTIDES

Said[76] postulated a crucial role for a number of recently discovered vasoactive peptides. Because of their effect on smooth muscle, these peptides are known to influence local blood flow, in particular to the heart and lung. Bradykinin, opioid peptides, vasopressin, and vasoactive intestinal peptides (VIP) have been implicated in all forms of shock.

Recently VIP, neurotensin, and substance P have been identified in nerves of the heart, including nerves of the sinoatrial node, the specialized conduction tissue, and atrial and ventricular myocardium, as well as in the walls of coronary vesicles. VIP and substance P have dilatory effects on coronary vessels.[76]

BRADYKININ

Bradykinin is a potent systemic vascular dilator. Bradykinin also increases systemic, not pulmonary vascular, permeability.[77] Bradykinin seems intensely involved in all inflammatory reactions with reactivation of corpuscular elements of the blood.

OPIOID PEPTIDES

The opioid peptides, endorphins and enkephalins, have important effects on cardiovascular function. When given intravenously opioid peptides cause vascular dilation and a decrease in systemic blood pressure. The central nervous system effects differ. The implication of the role of opioid peptides in shock is derived from 1. the beneficial effect of antagonists on morbidity and mortality that can be observed with different types of shock, and 2. the discovery that endotoxin and probably also severe hemorrhage stimulate release of opioid peptides.[78-85]

VASOPRESSIN

Vasopressin is secreted by the neurohypophysis. It is a potent vasoconstrictive agent. It also has antidiuretic functions. The chief evidence of the effects of vasopressin is derived from experiments with Brattleboro rats, a genetically deficient species of rat that does not secrete vasopressin and is vulnerable to severe hemorrhage.[86,87]

VASOACTIVE INTESTINAL PEPTIDES

Vasoactive intestinal peptides (VIP) have also been found in brain and peripheral nervous tissue. They are potent vasodilators for certain organs—the heart, the brain, and the splanchnic bed. VIP cause systemic hypotension. It could be shown that VIP are secreted into the circulation during shock and hemorrhage. It is postulated that these peptides increase flow to the heart, brain, and the splanchnic bed during the reaction to shock.[84]

CATECHOLAMINES

The heart is the target of the body's counteroffensive and counter-regulation. Elevated catecholamine levels have been linked to the pathogenesis of posterior epicardial hemorrhage, septal subendocardial hemorrhage, and the zonal lesions described by Hackel and Ratliff and Ratliff.[10,11] It has been postulated that these vasoactive amines are related to an uncontrolled and damaging influx of calcium into myocytes.[26,88]

DOPAMINE

Dopamine is a therapeutic cardiovascular active amine. The effects of dopamine may be both positive and negative. The effects of dopamine on hemodynamics and myocardial metabolism in cardiogenic shock following myocardial infarction might be significantly different from normal reactions of the heart. Dopamine may improve cardiac performace at the expense of cardiac oxygenation.[89] Therefore, dopamine adminstration may be of questionable benefit when the heart is damaged. Hirsch and Rone,[90] however, pointed out that mesenteric blood flow response to dopamine infusion may have a beneficial effect during myocardial infarction and possibly also during other forms of shock that cause prolonged hypotension.

HISTAMINES

Histamine shock encountered in anaphylactic reactions and immune reactions also causes ultrastructural cardiac lesions. Hegewald, et al.[91] described the cardiac effects of histamine on the rabbit myocardium. Mitochondria and sarcoplasmic reticulum showed swelling 15 min after injection of polymyxin-B-sulphate, a substance that releases histamine. The sarcolemma revealed blister-like protrusions, and cytoplasmic components were found in the interstitium. There was also pericapillary edema. Altura[92] described the role of histamine release in shock and trauma with the focus on the microcirculation.

The Microcirculation

The microcirculation in the heart is highly refined. The myocytes are surrounded by a network of capillaries which form numerous Y- and H-shaped connections. Whether these are the basis for a countercurrent system is not known.[93]

How can we imagine that the injury to the microvasculature is transmitted and progresses? The flow behavior of blood depends on the geometry of the vasculature and on the flow properties of the blood.[64] We may first focus on the blood itself. The properties that change are called the rheologic properties. The blood viscosity changes in low-flow situations.[64] It also changes in hypoxia.[66] The main factor at the capillary level is increased stiffness of red blood cells. But white blood cell stickiness and the formation of microthrombi may also augment such sluggishness of the blood. Blood flow on the other hand is increased and viscosity reduced if the hematocrit decreases. Thus in the compromised circulation of shock a shift of the hematocrit from 45 to 25% is beneficial to flow particularly in the coronary circulation.[64,94-96]

Another factor is the perfusion pressure. Goldfarb[33] pointed out that the mechanism for coronary hypoperfusion could easily reduce coronary perfusion pressure. The argument is based on experiments by Downey, et al.,[97] who prepared external circuits to perfuse coronary arteries during systemic hypotension. In these experiments significant myocardial ischemia appeared during systemic hypotension below 40 mm Hg and this reduction was linked to reduced contractility. Experiments by Hinshaw, et al.,[24] on the isolated perfused heart preparation corroborated these results.

The second category of changes are those that affect the vessel wall. Loss of endothelium enhances microthrombi. Loss of endothelium or damage to endothelium also enhances interstitial edema. The latter could increase the outside pressure on the vessels in critically restricted microvascular beds. This situation can exist in the heart even during diastole. Endothelial denudation also increases the exposure of constrictive vessels to vasoactive agents. This has been shown with reactions to thromboxanes. Because great portions of the body's reactions use the microvasculature as an effector organ, the exposure of the cells of the microcirculation may have both beneficial and detrimental effects. The beneficial effects may dominate during the compensated phase of shock and are indeed critical to survival, as shown by Altura[87] using Brattleboro rats, which lack vasopressin. Among the damaging mediators of the shock reaction, the renin-angiotensin system, the prostacyclin-thromboxane system, and the hydrolases have acquired particular concern.

Another factor that may enhance organ damage in shock is redistribution of blood away from vital organs or from critical organ regions, such as the endocardium.[3,51,98] Hirota and Seki[99] proposed also that shock may affect the alpha and beta receptors of the coronary circulation.

Myocardial Depressant Factor

One of the "amines" released during shock is the myocardial depressant factor (MDF). The molecular mass of MDF is about 500 daltons.[100] MDF forms in the plasma during shock and reaches toxic levels approximately 2 to 7 hrs after the shock.[101]

Evidence for myocardial depression following ischemia, anoxia, or disease of the splanchnic bed region, in particular of the pancreas, has come from many studies, Lee, et al.,[72] for example examined 24 patients with acute pancreatitis using systolic time intervals and found that during the acute phase PEP/LVET ratio was significantly prolonged. MDF has a number of biologic functions, which are 1. negative inotropic action, observed in papillary muscle, the isolated perfused heart, and the intact animal; 2. splanchnic constriction, seen in isolated vessel strips and the isolated perfused pancreas; and 3. depression of phagocytosis mainly in fixed macrophages, sparing the circulating leukocytes. Lefer[102] has postulated that a positive feedback loop exists between secretion of the MDF and these three effects. Shock enters a vicious circle. It could be shown that intravenous injection of MDF causes progressive impairment of left ventricular function within 60 min, and a state of shock ensues.[71,103] If MDF can be convincingly identified as a lethal systemic shock factor, then therapeutic efforts have to be directed toward detoxification of such a factor or toward interruption of the positive feedback loop. This has been explored by Lefer and co-workers.[104]

Intracellular degradation of secretory granules by the lysosomes serves to regulate the intracellular levels of secretory proteins. In pancreatic acinar cells the lysosomes are a potential site for the activation of zymogen enzyme and the induction of pancreatic injury.[105] Such tissue injury may result in the generation of toxic factors.

Healing and Recovery

Cardiac function remains depressed during recovery from acute pancreatitis, a situation of massive release of MDF.[72] Downing and Lee[106] reported that after two hours of hemorrhagic shock in the newborn lamb, subsequent blood pressure elevation to 100 mm Hg could not improve the depressed cardiac function. The cardiac output remained around 45% of control. However, if the shock period lasted only for 30 minutes, cardiac function returned to normal. At that short interval, the cardiac depression was fully reversed with elevation of the coronary perfusion pressure. These data demonstrate that myocardial lesions can and do heal after short periods of hypoxemia, but prolonged hypoperfusion will reduce the chances of partial or complete recovery. At a given point the shock effects on the heart may become lethal. Death of shock may occur from severe heart failure, leading to an accentuated hypoperfusion syndrome or arrhythmia.[107]

When cardiovascular depression is noted in the course of hemorrhagic shock, the patient has entered a late and critical phase for survival. Not only for research but also for therapy it is important to identify the numerous systemic and local factors that promote, accelerate, and determine the fatal outcome of hemorrhagic shock.

Hinshaw, et al.[108] proposed the following scheme for alterations of the heart:

1. Hypoperfusion leads to increased coronary capillary permeability and increased myocardial cell permeability.

2. Increased coronary capillary permeability is related to myocardial interstitial edema and intracellular edema.

3. Increased interstitial edema alters postcapillary resistance (increased) and depresses ventricular relaxation and compliance.

4. Increased filling pressure results from depressed ventricular contractility (the result of electrolyte disturbance and alteration of bioenergetic mechanisms as well as depressed ventricular response to stimuli).

5. The outcome is myocardial dysfunction and enhancement of shock.

Research and therapy designed to salvage the victim of severe shock will have to focus on the following:

1. Monitoring. Better information should be available to define the status of the heart and vessels as guide to therapy. Currently used techniques might not be sensitive enough.

2. Preserving the fluidity of blood. This has been the goal of emergency treatment, but its full impact is incompletely understood.

3. Preserving the coronary perfusion pressure. This may be the most efficient countermeasure.

4. Preserving the microvasculature. This may involve two linked items, preservation of cells and function. This may be the target of the beneficial effects of peptide receptor antagonists.

5. Preserving the heart cell and the contractile ability of the heart. The heart cell may be another target of hormones and peptides; in particular, disturbance of the cellular calcium metabolism may be detrimental.

The underlying mechanisms of cell injury are similar in ischemia and hypoxia. The final determining factor will be the status of the plasma membrane, the excessive leak of calcium from storage sites, and the status of the bioenergetic system—mitochondria and anaerobic glycolysis.

REFERENCES

1. Siegel, H.W., and Downings, S.E.: Reduction of left ventricular contractility during acute hemorrhagic shock. Am. J. Physiol., *218*:772, 1970.
2. Crowell, J.W., and Guyton, A.C.: Evidence favoring a cardiac mechanism in irreversible hemorrhagic shock. Am. J. Physiol, *201*:893, 1961.
3. Lefer, A.M.: Positive feedback actions of a myocardial depressant factor in circulatory shock. Texas Rep. Biol. Med., *39*:200, 1979.
4. Dole, W.P., and O'Rourke, R.A.: Hypotension and cardiogenic shock. *In* Internal Medicine. Edited by J. H. Stein Boston, Little Brown and Co., 1983.
5. Emes, J.H., and Nowak, T.J.: Introduction to Pathophysiology. Baltimore, University Park Press, 1983.
6. Guyton, A.C.: Textbook of Medical Physiology. 3rd Ed. Philadelphia, W.B. Saunders, 1971.

7. Bell, G.H., Emslie-Smith, D., and Paterson, C.P.: Textbook of Physiology. New York, Churchill Livingstone, 1980.
8. DeSanctis, R.W.: Shock. Sci. Am. Med., *2*:1, 1981.
9. Walter, J.B.: An Introduction to the Principles of Disease. Philadelphia, W.B. Saunders, 1977.
10. Hackel, D.B., Ratliff, N.B., and Mikat, E.: The heart in shock. Circ. Res., *35*:805, 1974.
11. Ratliff, N.B.: Ultrastructural comparison of myocardial zonal lesions and myofibrillar degeneration in cats subjected to hemorrhagic shock. Circ. Shock, *2*:221, 1975.
12. Ratliff, N.B., Hackel, D.B., and Mikat, E.: Myocardial zonal lesions. Circ. Shock, *3*:77, 1976.
13. McGovern, V.J.: Hypovolemic shock with particular reference to cardiac and pulmonary lesions. Pathology, *12*:63, 1980.
14. Bouchardy, B., and Majno, G.: Histopathology of early myocardial infarcts. A new approach. Am. J. Pathol., *74*:301, 1974.
15. Ratliff, N.B., and Unger, S.W.: The nexus in serial cross-sections of myocardium from cats subjected to hypovolemic shock: A three-dimensional interpretation. Lab. Invest., *41*:193, 1979.
16. Trump, B.F., et al.: The application of electron microscopy and cellular biochemistry to autopsy. Observation on cellular changes in human shock. Human Pathol., *6*:499, 1975.
17. Galankina, I.E., and Permiakov, N.K.: Myocardial pathomorphology in exotoxic shock. Arkh. Patol. *43*:47, 1981.
18. Costa, M., Shute, B., and Mergner, W.J.: Direct measurement of ATP synthesis and development of flocculent densities in mitochondria isolated from ischemic rat, heart, and liver. Virch. Arch. Pathol. (Accepted for publication).
19. Stevens, R., and Mergner, W.J.: Studies on mitochondrial ATPase and proton gradient in global ischemia of the rat heart (in preparation).
20. Haljamäe, H., et al.: Pathophysiology of shock. Pathol. Res. Pract., *165*:200, 1979.
21. Goldstein, M.A., et al.: Ultrastructural and contractile characteristics of isolated papillary muscle exposed to acute hypoxia. J. Mol. Cell. Cardiol., *9*:285, 1977.
22. Winslow, E.J., et al.: Hemodynamic studies and results of therapy in patients with bacteremic shock. Am. J. Med., *54*:421, 1973.
23. Kelman, G.R.: Cardiac output in shock. In. Anesthesiol. Clin., *7*:739, 1969.
24. Hinshaw, L.B., et al.: Myocardial function in shock. Am. J. Physiol., *226*:357, 1974.
25. Sarnoff, S.F., Case, R.B., Waithe, P.E., and Isaacs, J.P.: Insufficient coronary flow and myocardial failure as complicating factors in later hemorrhagic shock. Am. J. Physiol., *176*:439, 1954.
26. Boutet, M., Huttner, I., and Rona, G.: Permeability alterations of sarcolemmal membrane in catecholamine induced cardiac muscle injury. Lab. Invest., *34*:482, 1976.
27. Saunders, C.R., and Doty, D.B.: Myocardial contusion. Surg. Gynecol. Obstet., *144*:595, 1977.
28. Ninikoski, J.: Tissue oxygenation in hypovolemic shock. Ann. Clin. Res., *9*:1977.
29. Crowell, J.W., and Smith, E.E.: Oxygen deficit and irreversible hemorrhagic shock. Am. J. Physiol., *206*:313, 1964.
30. Dunham, C.M., Linberg, S.E., Mergner, W.J., and Marzella, L.L.: Oxygen consumption as a useful determinant of outcome in human and experimental hemorrhagic shock. Surg. Forum, Oct. 1984.
31. Linberg, S.E., Dunham, C.M., Mergner, W.J., and Marzella, L.L.: The development of a clinically applicable hemorrhagic shock model. Circ. Shock (In preparation).
32. Schaper, W.: Experimental coronary artery occlusion III. The determinants of collateral blood flow in acute coronary occlusion. Basic Res. Cardiol., *73*:584, 1978.
33. Goldfarb, R.D.: Cardiac mechanical performance in circulatory shock: A critical review of methods and results. Circ. Shock, *9*:633, 1982.
34. Warner, M., et al.: The excitation-contraction coupling system of the myocardium in canine hemorrhagic shock. Circ. Shock, *8*:563, 1981.
35. Estes, J.E., Farley, P.E., and Goldfarb, R.D.: Effect of shock on calcium accumulation by cardiac sarcoplasmic reticulum. Adv. Shock Res., *3*:229, 1980.
36. Opie, L.H.: Effects of regional ischemia on metabolism of glucose and fatty acids: Relative rates of aerobic and anaerobic energy modulation during myocardial infarction and comparison with effects on anoxia. Cir. Res., *38*(Suppl. 1):152, 1976.
37. Garfinkel, D., and Adis, M.I.: Metabolism of totally ischemic excised dog heart. II. Interpretation of a computer model. Am. J. Physiol., *237*:R327, 1979.
38. Kohn, M.C., and Garfinkel, D.: Computer simulation of ischemic rat heart purine metabolism. II. Model behavior. Am. J. Physiol., *232*:H386, 1977.
39. Hinshaw, L.B., Archer, L.T., Benjamin, B., and Bridges, C.: Effects of glucose or insulin on myocardial performance in endotoxin shock. P.S.E.M.B., *152*:529, 1976.
40. Schumer, W.: The effects of shock on the energy pathways of the cell. *In* The Cell in Shock. Kalamazoo, Upjohn Co., 1975.
41. Schumer, W.: Overall cell metabolism. Prog. Clin. Biol. Res., *111*:1, 1983.

42. Spitzer, J.J.: Myocardial metabolism during acute shock induced by hemorrhage, endotoxin, or physiostigmine infusion. Rec. Adv. Stud. Cardiac Struct. Metab., *3*:161, 1973.

43. Spitzer, J.J., Greenfield, L.J., and Hinshaw, L.B.: Effect of prolonged coronary hypotension on myocardial substrate utilisation. Rec. Adv. Stud. Cardiac Struct. Metab., *10*:235, 1975.

44. Kuttner, R.E., Apantaku, F.O., and Schumer, W.: Glycolytic intermediates in rat heart after endotoxin treatment. Circ. Schock, *7*:405, 1980.

45. Hess, M.L., and Krause, S.M.: Myocardial subcellular function in shock. Tex. Rep. Biol. Med., *30*:193, 1979.

46. McCaig, D.J., and Parratt, J.R.: Reduced myocardial response to calcium during endotoxin shock in the cat. Circ. Shock, *7*:23, 1980.

47. Chaudry, I.H.: Cellular mechanisms in shock and ischemia and their correction. Am. J. Physiol., *245*:R117, 1983.

48. Chaudry, I.H., and Baue, A.E.: Overview of hemorrhagic shock. *In* Pathophysiology of Shock, Anoxia, and Ischemia. Edited by R.A. Cowley, and B.F. Trump. Baltimore, Williams & Wilkins, 1982.

49. Chaudry, I.H., Ohkawa, M., Clemens, M.G., and Baue, A.E.: Alteration in electron transport and cellular metabolism with shock and trauma. Prog. Clin. Biol. Res., *111*:67, 1983.

50. Szabo, G., Vandor, E., and Anda, E.: The lymphatic transport of lactate dehydrogenase. Effect of tissue anoxia and shock. Res. Exp. Med. (Berl.), *161*:39, 1973.

51. Kleinman, W.M., Krause, S.M., and Hess, M.L.: Cardiogenic endotoxin shock: Role of coronary flow and subendocardial ischemia. Circ. Shock, *6*:197, 1979.

52. Stone, M.J., Willerson, J.T., and Waterman, M.R.: Radioimmunoassay of myoglobin. Meth. Enzymol., *84*:172, 1982.

53. Dhalla, N.S., Yates, J.C., Lee, S.L., and Singh, A.: Functional and subcellular changes in the isolated rat heart perfused with oxidized isoproterenol. J. Mol. Cell. Cardiol, *10*:31, 1978.

54. Fabiato, A., and Fabiato, F.: Effect of pH on the myofilaments and sarcoplasmic reticulum of skinned cells from cardiac and skeletal muscles. J. Physiol, *276*:233, 1978.

55. Katz, A.M.: Effects of ischemia on the contractile processes of heart muscle. Am. J. Cardiol., *32*:456, 1973.

56. Mergner, W.J., et al.: Structural and functional changes in human kidney and liver mitochondria in acute cell injury after shock and trauma. Am. J. Pathol., *66*:36a, 1972.

57. Jennings, R.B., and Ganote, C.E.: Structural changes in myocardium during acute ischemia. Circ. Res., *34(Suppl.III)*:156, 1974.

58. Mergner, W.J., and Schaper, J.: Cellular and subcellular changes in myocardial infarction. *In* Pathophysiology of Shock, Anoxia, and Ischemia. Edited by R.A. Cowley, and B.F. Trump, Baltimore, Williams & Wilkins, 1982.

59. Gutovitz, A.L., Sobel, B.E., and Roberts, R.: Progressive nature of myocardial injury in selected patients with cardiogenic shock. Am. J. Cardiol., *41*:469, 1978.

60. Parks, D.A., Bulkley, G.B., and Granger, D.N.: Role of oxygen free radicals in shock, ischemia and organ preservation. Surgery, *94*:428, 1983.

61. Taylor, A.E., Martin, D., and Parker, J.C.: The effects of oxygen radicals in pulmonary edema formation. Surgery, *94*:433, 1983.

62. Lefer, A.M., Araki, H., and Ikamatsu, S.: Beneficial actions of a free radical scavenger in traumatic shock and myocardial ischemia. Circ. Shock *8*:273, 1981.

63. Permiakov, N.K.: Central problems in the general pathology and pathologic anatomy of shock, Arch. Patol., *45*:3, 1983.

64. Chien, S.: Rheology in the microcirculation in normal and low flow states. Adv. Shock. Res. *8*:71, 1982.

65. Poraicu, D., Sandore, S., and Menessy, I.: Decrease of red blood cell filterability seen in intensive care. II. Red blood cell crenelation "in-vivo" as morphological evidence of increased red blood cell viscosity in low flow states. Resuscitation, *10*:305, 1983.

66. Weed, R.I., La Celle, P.L., and Merrill, E.W.: Metabolic dependence of red cell deformability. J. Clin. Invest., *48*:793, 1969.

67. Saldeen, T.: Blood coagulation and shock. Pathol. Res. Pract., *165*:221, 1979.

68. Bessin, P., et al.: Acute circulatory collapse caused by platelet-activating factor. Eur. J. Pharmacol. *88*:403, 1983.

69. Matthias, F.R., and Lasch, H.G.: Disseminated intravascular coagulation and circulatory shock. Kardiologiia, *22*:39, 1982.

70. Bagge, U.: Leukocytes and capillary perfusion in shock. Kroc. Found. Ser., *16*:285, 1984.

71. Glenn, T.M., and Lefer, A.M.: The role of lysosomes in the pathogenesis of spanchnic ischemic shock in cats. Circ. Res., *27*:783, 1970.

72. Lee, W.K., et al.: Depression of myocardial function during acute pancreatitis. Circ. Shock, *8*:369, 1981.

73. Marzella, L., and Glaumann, H.: Effects of *in vivo* liver ischemia on microsomes and lysosomes. Virch. Arch. Cell. Pathol., *36*:1, 1981.

74. Marzella, L., Ahlberg, J., and Glaumann, H.: Isolation of autophagic vacuoles from rat liver. Morphological and biochemical characterization. J. Cell Biol., *93*:144, 1982.

75. Glaumann, H., Ericsson, J.L.E., and Marzella, L.: Mechanisms of intralysosomal degradation with special reference to autophagocytosis and heterophagocytosis of cell organelles. Intern. Rev. Cytol., *73*:149, 1981.

76. Said, S.I.: Vasoactive peptides: state of the art review. Hypertension, *5*:117, 1983.

77. Erdös, E.G.: Bradykinin, kallidin and kallikrein. *In* Handbook of Experimental Pharmacology. Edited by E.G. Erdös. New York, Springer Verlag, 1979.

78. Curtis, M.T., and Lefer, A.M.: Actions of opiate antagonists with selective receptor interactions in hemorrhagic shock. Circ. Shock, *10*:131, 1983.

79. Vargish, T., et al.: Naloxone reversal of hypovolemic shock in dogs. Circ. Shock, *7*:31, 1980.

80. Reynolds, G.D., et al.: Blockade of opiate survival and cardiac performance in canine endotoxin shock. Circ. Shock, *7*:39, 1980.

81. Janssen, H.F., and Lutherer, J.O.: Ventriculocisternal administration of naloxone protects against severe hypotension during endotoxin shock. Brain Res., *194*: 608, 1980.

82. Faden, A.I., and Holaday, J.W.: Experimental endotoxin shock: The pathophysiologic function of endorphins and treatment with opiate antagonists. J. Infect. Dis., *142*: 229, 1980.

83. Peters, W.P., Johnson, M.W., Friedman, P.A., and Mitch, W.E.: Pressure effect of naloxone in septic shock. Lancet, *1*:529, 1980.

84. Bone, R.C., et al.: Endorphins in endotoxin shock. Microcirculation, *1*:285, 1981.

85. Gahhos, F.N., Chiu, R.C.J., Hinchey, E.J., and Richards, G.K.: Endorphins in septic shock: Hemodynamic and endocrine effects of an opiate receptor antagonist and agonist. Arch. Surg., *117*:1053, 1982.

86. Zerbe, R.L., Bayorh, M.A., and Feuerstein, G.: Vasopressin: An essential pressure factor for blood pressure recovery following hemorrhage. Peptides, *3*:509, 1982.

87. Altura, B.M.: Microcirculatory and vascular smooth muscle behavior in the Brattleboro rat: Relationship to the reticuloendothelial system function and resistance to shock and trauma. Ann. N.Y. Acad. Sci., *394*:375, 1982b.

88. Chekareva, G.A., et al.: Catecholamine lesions of the myocardium as a model of cardiac pathology in shock. Vrach. Delo., *3*:36–39, 1984.

89. Mueller, H.S., Evans, R., and Ayers, S.H.: Effect of dopamine on hemodynamics and myocardial metabolism in shock following acute myocardial infarction in man. Circulation, *57*:361, 1978.

90. Hirsch, L.J., and Rone, A.S.: Mesenteric blood flow response to dopamine infusion during myocardial infarction in the awake dog. Circ. Shock, *10*:173, 1983.

91. Hegewald, G., Nikulin, A., Bärenwald, G., and Schwanengel, H.: Ultrastructure of rabbit myocardium in experimental histamine shock. Zentralbl. Allg. Pathol., *126*:487, 1982.

92. Altura, B.M.: Reticuloendothelial system function and histamine release in shock and trauma; Relationship to microcirculation. Klin. Wochenschr., *60*:882, 1982a.

93. Stoiko, M.A., Pendergrass, R.B., and Mergner, W.J.: Aspects of three dimensional structure of cardiac microcirculation in the dog. J. Mol. Cell. Cardiol., *15*:40, 1983.

94. Jan, K.M., Heldman, J., and Chien, S.: Coronary hemodynamics and oxygen utilization after hematocrit variations in hemorrhage. Am. J. Physiol., *239*:H326, 1980.

95. Heine, H., Trenkel, K., Arbogast, J., and Eisenbach, J.: Functional morphology of the terminal vascular bed and transit space: Problems caused by shock. Med. Welt., *31*:558, 1980.

96. Neuhof, H., Mittermayer, C., and Freudenberg, N.: Macro and microcirculation in shock. Verh. Dsch. Ges. Pathol. *62*:80, 1978.

97. Downey, J.M., et al.: Adequacy of coronary blood flow during hypertension. Circ. Shock, *13*:83, 1976.

98. Harden, W.R., III, Barlow, C.H., Simson, M.B., and Harken, A.H.: Heterogeneity of the coronary microcirculation during low flow ischemia: A model for the heart in shock. Adv. Shock Res., *3*:239, 1980.

99. Hirota, A., and Seki, K.: Shock and microcirculation, including the question of alpha, beta receptors in microcirculation, Nippon Rinsho., *38*:1825, 1980.

100. Lefer, A.M., and Martin, P.: Role of a myocardial depressant factor in the pathogenesis of circulatory shock. Fed. Proc., *29*:1836, 1970.

101. Lefer, A.M.: Blood borne humoral factors in the pathophysiology of circulatory shock. Circ. Res. *32*:129, 1973.

102. Lefer, A.M.: The heart in shock. Tex. Rep. Biol. Med., *39*:155, 1979.

103. Pagni, E.: The role of the myocardial depressant factor in the pathogenesis of shock. Minerv. Anestesiol., *46*: 1001, 1981.

104. Lefer, A.M.: Vascular mediators in ischemia and shock. *In* Pathophysiology of Shock, Anoxia and Ischemia. Edited by R.A. Cowley, and B.F. Trump. Baltimore, Williams & Wilkins, 1982.
105. Resau, J.H., Marzella, L., Trump, B.F., and Jones, R.T.: Degradation of zymogen granules by lysosomes in cultured pancreatic explants. Am. J. Pathol., *115*:39, 1984.
106. Downing, S.E., and Lee, J.C.: Cardiac function and metabolism following hemorrhage in the newborn lamb. Ann. Surg., *184*:743, 1977.
107. Zapriageaev, V.V.: Reparative regenaration of the myocardium after focal injury following orthostatic collapse. Arkh. Anat. Gistol. Embriol., *60*:74, 1971.
108. Hinshaw, L.B., Benjamin, B., Archer, L.T., and Peyton, M.D.: The heart and endotoxin shock. Texas Rep. Biol. Med., *39*:173, 1979.

Chapter 7
KIDNEY IN SHOCK

William M. Stahl

The kidney is a composite organ made up of nephron units, which provide two types of vital function. Filtration of the circulating plasma by the glomerular capillary network allows passage of all small ions and water into the proximal renal tubule while retaining large molecules such as proteins and blood cells within the circulation. In a healthy adult, the total plasma volume of approximately 3 to 3.5 liters is filtered more than 40 times daily, with the production of 140 liters of proximal tubular filtrate. This massive laundering of plasma is an efficient way to remove those chemical moieties that can be filtered through the glomerular capillary membrane. It is the only way to remove those ions produced by cell metabolism that cannot be converted into a gaseous state and removed by respiration. The primary ions of this type are nitrogen, sulfate, phosphate, potassium, sodium, and chloride. It is clear that if the level of filtration falls below a critical level, these ions will not be adequately removed from the circulating plasma, and renal insufficiency will exist. It is also clear that excretion of this massive amount of fluid could not take place without rapid dehydration of the organism. To this end, the renal tubule, with its ability to resorb most of the isotonic filtrate in its proximal portion and to regulate the composition of the filtrate in the long loop and distal collecting ducts, plays a vital role. Tubular cells modify the filtrate and regulate body water balance, serum osmolality, and specific ion concentrations. These interrelated mechanisms function to maintain homeostasis in the individual. However, these same mechanisms make the kidney exquisitely sensitive to changes in total body fluids, cardiac index, and excessive loss of electrolytes.

THE EFFECT OF SHOCK

Shock states can conveniently be considered in two categories. The first, transport failure, is caused by a decrease in cardiac index as a result of loss of fluid, volume shock, or deficiency of myocardial function, pump shock. The second is the complex state known as septic shock. In shock caused by transport deficiency the primary injury is cellular ischemia. This occurs because of overall decrease in blood flow and because the overriding principle of the cardiovascular system is to maintain blood pressure. When cardiac index falls, peripheral resistance is increased to maintain a normal perfusion pressure to the brain and heart. Organ systems of lesser immediate need are deprived of blood to permit this survival mechanism. Homer Smith demonstrated in 1936 that small decreases in cardiac index cause large decreases in renal blood flow and glomerular filtration rate.[1] On the other hand, the primary insult in septic shock is the presence of damaging molecular species or toxins that cause direct cellular injury. It is therefore important to determine what changes occur in the kidney because of ischemia and because of toxins.

Ischemic Injury

Renal ischemia is produced when blood flow to the kidney decreases as the result of a severe fall in perfusion pressure or from intense vasoconstriction. Such vasoconstriction is usually part of a general increase in total peripheral resistance as a response to a decrease in cardiac output. Alterations in systemic and intra-renal blood flow distribution occur in states of hepatic failure and sepsis diverting flow from the renal cortex. Direct interruption of renal arterial flow with supra-renal aortic or renal artery clamping and removal of the kidney during renal trans-plantation produce total ischemia.

The cellular response to acute ischemia has been extensively studied. Oxygen deprivation appears predominantly to affect structures in the renal cortex, includ-ing glomerular capillary cells and the pars recta of the proximal renal tubule. Var-ious segments of the nephron may be injured more easily than others, but clearly an interruption of one vital portion of the nephron unit may cause failure of the entire nephron. Renal cell energetics seem to be affected more rapidly than those in cells of other organs, such as liver or heart, and renal tissue ATP levels fall to 22% of normal within two minutes of renal artery interruption.[2-4] After 15 min, ATP levels decrease further to 13% of control and lactate levels rise to 11 times normal.

The cell damage that results depends on the duration of the ischemic insult. Ischemia of 25 min or less at normothermia results in mild injury, which is revers-ible.[4] Ischemia of 40 to 60 min produces more severe damage, with some recovery occurring over a period of two to three weeks. Ischemia of 40 min in experimental animals caused loss of vascular control and the production of focal segmental necrosis in muscle cells and tubular endothelium.[5] Ischemia of 60 min in the rabbit kidney has been shown to decrease fluid transport in the proximal convoluted tubule to approximately 20% of normal and to produce back-leakage in the med-ullary tubules.[6]

Cellular injury may continue to occur after restoration of systemic pressure and flow. Renal blood flow does not return to normal following resumption of circu-lation after a period of ischemia (the so-called "no reflow" phenomenon). Animal studies show that after an ischemic insult renal blood flow remains reduced by as much as 50% for many hours.[7] This interference with the resumption of normal renal blood flow distribution potentiates ischemic injury with further damage to glomerular cells and tubular epithelium.[8] Micropuncture studies have shown that a vascular abnormality persists even after restoration of normal blood pressure and flow in the intact animal and that this is caused by an increase in afferent arteriolar resistance.[9]

The cause of this lingering vasoconstriction has not been clearly proved. The most likely explanation is that an increase in proximal tubular sodium and chloride content occurs because of failure of function of tubular cells, and this increase stimulates vasoconstriction of the afferent arteriole by feedback through the jux-taglomerular apparatus[10,11] (Fig. 7-1). This vasoconstriction, plus damage to glo-merular cells causing loss of surface area for filtration,[8] results in a profound fall in glomerular filtration rate, which is perpetuated even after blood flow is restored.

Tubular obstruction by hyaline, granular, and pigmented casts is found in animal models of acute renal failure caused by ischemia. Such obstruction of the tubular lumen also contributes to the lack of excretion of filtrate in the ischemically dam-

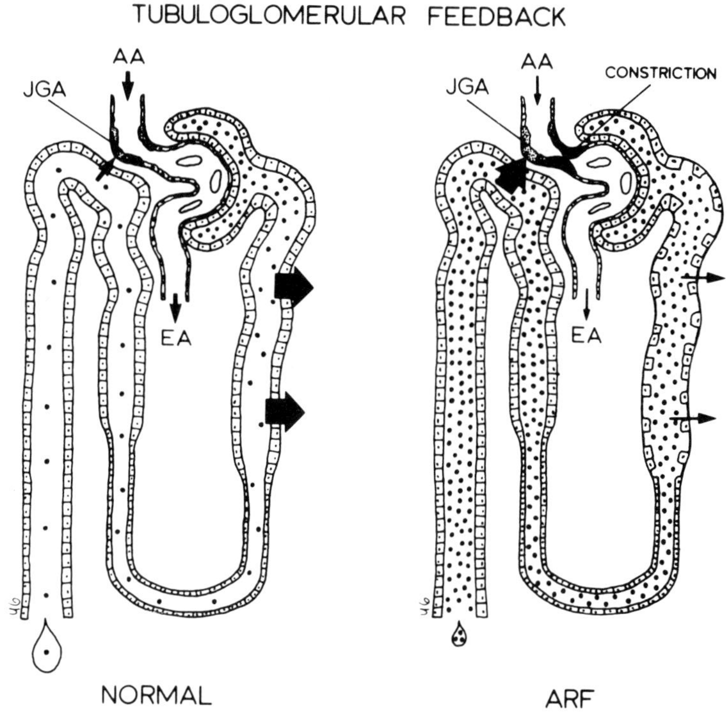

TUBULOGLOMERULAR FEEDBACK

Fig. 7-1. Tubuloglomerular feedback.

aged kidney.[12,13] Biopsies of human patients during acute renal failure have shown similar changes with collapsed glomeruli, alteration in tubular cells with necrosis and loss of the brush border, and tubular casts.[14] Ultrastructural studies of tubular cells show a profound decrease in luminal surface area caused by loss of the brush border and other alterations of the cell surface, which could lead to a decrease in sodium chloride filtration.

Other factors also potentiate ischemic injury in the kidney as in other organs. Failure of prostacyclin synthesis by glomerular endothelial cells has been suggested.[15,16] Intracellular increase in calcium concentration has also been postulated as a potentiating mechanism for cell injury both in systemic cells and in renal cells. Intracellular calcium has been shown to increase by 50% after one hour of renal ischemia.[17]

In summary it appears that renal ischemia produced by vasoconstriction, hypotension, or arterial interruption causes a progressive lesion in glomerular and tubular cells that is worsened with time. After resumption of blood flow a varying degree of circulatory insufficiency persists. Cellular injury may continue depending on local factors related to cell integrity and on tubuloglomerular feedback phenomena potentiating the abnormal blood flow state.

Toxic Injury

The effect of toxic substances on renal cells has been studied in a variety of classic models, most of which are not directly applicable to the critically ill patient.

Specific toxins such as aminoglycocides and contrast agents appear to affect renal blood flow and tubular function in a manner somewhat similar to ischemic injury. Renal failure in the critically ill patient usually occurs after the onset of sepsis and this lesion has not been well clarified in terms of renal cell functional integrity. All body cells suffer a metabolic insult in the presence of sepsis, manifested by impairment of function, cell swelling, and shift to anaerobic metabolism with production of lactic acidosis. Progressive renal damage occurs with oliguria in the presence of normal or even supranormal renal blood flow.

A fall in the cellular levels of ATP occurs rather rapidly after the administration of a variety of nephrotoxic substances,[18] but decrease in ATP levels alone may not cause renal failure without direct membrane injury. The persistence and aggravation of cell injury in toxic renal damage is thought to be caused by a tubuloglomerular feedback mechanism similar to that in renal ischemic damage, with failure of flow to cortical glomeruli.[19,20] Similarly, interference with prostaglandin synthesis may also contribute to lingering vasoconstriction or alteration in intrarenal blood flow distribution in septic states.

ACUTE RENAL FAILURE

Metabolic Effects

When patients suffering from shock or sepsis have acute renal failure it is difficult to determine precisely which metabolic alterations are caused by the underlying disease and which are caused by the onset of renal failure. Metabolic alterations in chronic renal failure in humans have been studied extensively over the past 15 years. It is thought that these alterations reflect adaptation to a chronic state and that the studies of chronic renal failure cannot be transposed directly to the patient with acute renal failure. Other information has come from experimental acute uremia produced in animals, but there may be certain species differences. Thus, although it seems quite clear that the acute onset of the uremic state in a patient already suffering from serious disease produces additional metabolic defects, the precise nature of these defects is still not completely understood.

Certain abnormalities are clearly related to the inability to excrete water and solute and the direct results of buildup of these substances in the plasma (Table 7-1). In the predialysis period the signs of uremia included overhydration and hyperkalemia as obvious results of the inability to excrete water and potassium. Such an occurrence should now be controlled or reversed by adequate dialysis. Metabolic acidosis was frequently a serious problem in the predialysis period, in part because of the inability to excrete fixed acids and in part because of a more basic metabolic disturbance. Other clinical manifestations such as malnutrition, gastrointestinal hemorrhage, and susceptibility to invasive infection clearly represent complicated responses to altered cellular metabolism. In the patient with transport shock, acute renal failure usually occurs only when the shock has been prolonged or inadequately treated for some reason. In the septic patient multiple organs and systems are usually affected in addition to the kidney. It is thus difficult to ascribe particular metabolic defects to renal failure alone.

The obvious hallmark of acute renal failure is the inability to excrete certain products of metabolism from the blood. Inadequacy of filtration function leads to overhydration, hyperkalemia, and metabolic acidosis. The cellular effect of increas-

Table 7-1.   Acute Renal Failure.

Abnormalities Produced by Filtration Failure and Tissue Catabolism with
Production of Fixed Acids

Abnormality	*Effect*
Metabolic acidosis	Intracellular acidosis
	Cerebral dysfunction
	Nausea, vomiting
Retention of nitrogen	Decreased membrane transport
compounds and toxins	Decreased cell energetics
	Insulin resistance
Overhydration	Hypotonicity
	Hyponatremia
	Cardiac overload
	Tissue edema
Hyperkalemia	Membrane instability
	Cardiac arrhythmias
Hypophosphatemia	Decreased cell energetics
Hypocalcemia	
Insulin resistance	Interference with substrate
Glucose intolerance	utilization

All abnormalities improved by nutritional support and adequate dialytic
therapy

ing levels of "uremic toxins" seems to be predominantly an interference with active membrane sodium pumping, a function which uses ATP and requires sodium/potassium ATPase. Decrease in membrane transport with fall in Na/K ATPase has been demonstrated in uremic patients.[21] Decrease in activity in membrane transport results in alteration in intra- and extracellular ion and water concentrations.[22,23] This abnormality is related to the degree of uremia, and can be demonstrated when creatinine clearance falls below 6 or 7 ml/min.[21] At this time the patients also exhibit uremic symptoms of nausea, vomiting, and anorexia.

Failure of cell reproduction and replenishment has also been shown in uremic patients. Cell division decreases in the experimental animal when plasma urea concentrations reach 100 mg/dl,[24] with similar alterations demonstrated in red blood cells,[25] fibroblasts,[26] and esophogeal epithelial cells.[27] Metabolic acidosis rapidly occurs with acute uremia caused by the hypercatabolic state. Increased metabolism of substrate releases more fixed acid, including sulphates, phosphates, and other organic anions that cannot be excreted. The potentially harmful effects of severe acidosis include insulin resistance and decrease in other intracellular enzyme activities, especially phosphofructokinase with reduction in glycolysis.[28]

One of the major alterations in general body metabolism in acutely uremic patients is a defect in carbohydrate metabolism with development of insulin resistance. The insulin response to glucose infusion in such patients is excessive, and plamsa disappearance seems prolonged, suggesting tissue insulin resistance as the basic problem.[29] However, alterations in hepatic gluconeogenesis have not been ruled out in these patients. Disorders of calcium and phosphorus metabolism occur rapidly in patients with acute renal failure. Hyperphosphatemia occurs because of inadequate excretion of phosphorus as well as leak of phosphates from intracellular locations. Hypocalcemia occurs rapidly in addition. Elevated levels of parathyroid hormone have been measured which are inversely proportional to calcium levels.[30] At the same time however, animal studies have shown deposition of calcium in tissues, including brain and muscle dependent on the elevated parathormone levels.[31] Intracellular calcium levels rise under these conditions[32] and this may aggravate cellular injury.[33] The administration of extra calcium under these circumstances may be dangerous and is not indicated unless hypocalcemic symptoms appear.

Prevention and Treatment

Renal failure occurs as the result of cellular injury from ischemia and toxic metabolites. The degree of injury appears to depend on the length of the ischemic period, and on the type, concentration, and length of exposure to toxic molecules. The metabolic effects of acute renal failure are those of interference with the basic energy mechanisms and membrane transport mechanisms of the cell, thereby contributing to total body failure. The importance of prevention of acute renal failure whenever possible is thus clear.

The primary goal of management in transport shock states is to restore optimal circulation to the kidney at the earliest possible moment. In fact, if shock or hypoperfusion is possible, pretreatment of the kidney can be accomplished to make it less vulnerable to ischemic insult. Renal cellular damage occurs more readily in states of dehydration and low blood flow, the "high-renin" states. Whether this increased susceptibility of renal cells to ischemic injury is caused by the presence of high angiotensin and renin levels within the renal substance or whether it is in fact caused by the hypertonic milieu in the renal medulla accompanying such states is not known. Suffice it to say that patients who are to undergo operative procedures with a risk of blood flow alterations should be well hydrated and producing nonconcentrated urine at the time of the operative procedure.

Resuscitation from hypovolemic shock must be precise, aggressive, and adequate. It is well known that the presence of a normal blood pressure does not mean a normal blood volume or a normal cardiac index. Mistakes continue to be made, however, by relying on the blood pressure as evidence of adequate perfusion. The use of electrolyte solutions, whole blood or packed cell transfusions, and synthetic or natural colloids must be organized, precise, and adequate in amount, monitored by evidence of adequate perfusion. Urine output itself is such evidence, and adequate cardiac preload by central venous or pulmonary artery wedge pressures, actual measurement of cardiac output when available, the presence or absence of metabolic acidosis, and the monitoring of the pulmonary venous oxygen tension are all methods that can be used to evaluate perfusion. The PvO_2, particularly, is usually available from a central line, is easily repeated at frequent intervals, and if below 30 mm Hg indicates inadequate tissue perfusion. Rapid and adequate resuscitation of the patient when shock occurs will minimize the incidence of renal failure. It is the appreciation of this fact alone that has resulted in the marked decrease in the incidence of renal failure in most major surgical centers.

Improvement in cardiac function requires the same aggressive approach but must rely on the basics of control of the cardiac rate, improvement of myocardial function by digitalis and ionotropic agents, manipulation of afterload, and the use of ventricular assist devices when indicated. Rapid restoration of adequate cardiac index by treatment of myocardial insufficiency is of obvious importance.

Reduction of the level of septic "toxic" insult to the kidney and other organs is the most serious therapeutic problem physicians face. There are few ancillary treatments available to alter or prevent the toxic effect on cells once materials liberated from infected areas or bacterial products reach the blood stream. The primary effort must be directed toward rapid and complete eradication of the septic focus. This implies aggressive diagnostic and therapeutic maneuvers using both antimicrobial agents and surgical drainage when indicated. Maintenance of optimal oxygenation and blood flow during the treatment period can clearly assist in preserving cell function but reduction in toxic injury depends upon control of infection.

Diagnosis

Attention is usually directed to the possibility of renal failure when the urine output falls below normal levels, approximately 0.5 ml/kg/hr, or when serum creatinine levels increase above the normal range. Primary attention should be directed toward the general state of the patient, especially to evaluate potential causes of prerenal failure. Thus, evidence of adequate cardiac output and circulating fluid volume must be obtained by the usual physical examination and monitoring methods. In addition, careful exclusion of causes of postrenal failure caused by urinary tract obstruction must be carried out. Most renal failure occurring in hospitalized patients is caused by intrinsic renal disease of the toxic/anoxic variety.[34]

Initial examination in a patient who is suspected of having acute toxic/anoxic renal failure should be directed toward examination of the urine. The urinary sediment in most patients with acute renal failure of this type is highly characteristic[35] and usually contains numbers of tubular epithelial cells with cellular and granular pigmented casts. Pre- and post-renal acute renal failure states usually do not show significant changes in the urinary sediment. Examination of the urine content of solute and of free water and the concentration of creatinine and urea is also valuable. In the case of prerenal acute renal failure, the oliguric patient will excrete a concentrated urine. The ratio of urine to plasma concentration of solute will be high, thus the urine to plasma ratio of osmolality will be greater than 1.1, the urine to plasma ratio of urea will be greater than 10, and the urine to plasma ratio of creatinine will be greater than 2.5. If these ratios fall below these levels in the oliguric patient, renal damage is usually present. Renal sodium excretion is also a useful measurement, since the prerenal azotemic patient will be maximally conserving sodium, and the urinary sodium level will usually be below 20 mEq/L. However, the damaged nephron will leak an increased amount of sodium into the urine, thus raising the urine sodium concentration above 20 mEq/L. The renal failure index[36] is an expression that combines these two tests, the urinary sodium content and the urine to plasma creatinine ratio, by dividing the urinary sodium concentration by the urine to plasma creatinine ratio. This index is approximately one in normal individuals. Use of the renal failure index can usually differentiate prerenal oliguric patients from those with acute renal failure.[37] The acute renal failure patients have a renal failure index greater than one. In the difficult situation in which there is a question between a prerenal oliguric patient normally conserving sodium and water and a patient suffering from acute renal failure, a careful test of volume expansion or increase in cardiac index by cardiotropic drugs can be tried while monitoring cardiac preload and function.

Therapy

Considerable differences of opinion still exist as to the precise value of the use of diuretics in the developing stages of renal failure or after acute renal failure has become established. Most investigation has concerned the use of mannitol and the use of the loop diuretics, ethacrynic acid and furosemide (Table 7-2). Animal studies have suggested that the production of a diuretic state by either type of diuretic before an anoxic or toxic insult ameliorates the renal damage.[38,39] This, however, is of little value in the patient who presents with established shock.

Diuretic therapy has been suggested in shock patients in three different situations (Table 7-3). The first is prophylactically to prevent acute renal failure. Most published studies of the early or prophylactic use of diuretics have been uncontrolled and thus are difficult to interpret. In addition, the more precise control and appropriateness of fluid therapy in such studies has raised the question as to whether better fluid support of the patient has produced the improved result. In general, it can be said that the prophylactic value of diuretics has not been proved

Table 7-2. Acute Renal Failure (ARF) and Diuretics.

	Mode of action	
Mannitol	-	Must be filtered; osmotic effects reduce tubular water resorption
Loop diuretics (ethacrynic acid) (furosemide)	-	Need not be filtered; act on tubular cells reducing sodium and water resorption

Table 7-3. ARF and Diuretics.

	EFFECTIVENESS	
Prophylactic	-	Not proved in patients with operation, trauma, hemorrhagic shock
	-	Valuable in: Patients with jaundice Contrast media Hemoglobinemia Nephrotoxic drugs (amphotericin cisplatinum) ? Hyperuricemia
Amelioration of ARF (early therapy)	-	Lower mortality if diuresis occurs (? Patient selection by drug, or real benefit)
Therapy of established ARF	-	Production of diuresis may decrease need for dialysis; no improvement in survival

in patients with surgical operations, trauma, or hemorrhagic shock. It has been proved valuable, however, in patients with severe jaundice, those with hemoglobinemia, and those to whom contrast media or other nephrotoxic drugs are to be administered.

A second use of diuretics has involved the therapy for early or developing renal failure. It seems clear that the administration of diuretics in the developing phase of renal failure can reverse oliguria in about ⅔ of patients.[40-42] It is thought that this implies an improved prognosis because of a lesser renal injury.[43,44] It may be, however, that the diuretic agents have "selected out" patients with a lesser degree of injury who thus have an improved prognosis.[45]

A third use of diuretic agents has been in the treatment of established acute renal failure. In the past, extremely high doses have been given for several days. Most studies have shown that a diuresis may be produced in some patients and the need for dialysis may be slightly reduced as a consequence, but that eventual mortality in these patients remains unchanged. The evidence at present is that diuretic therapy in the established acute renal failure patient does not change the prognosis.

The basis of therapy for acute renal failure in the post-shock period involves optimizing the general state of the patient in terms of oxygenation, hemodynamics, wound care, sepsis control, and the like; providing adequate nutrition to prevent breakdown of muscle protein and to allow the patient to rebuild tissues, heal wounds, and develop immune competence; and adequate dialytic therapy.

Optimization of the general state of the patient implies careful and frequent monitoring and adjustments of therapy to maintain vital organs in the best possible state, with special attention to the prevention and treatment of sepsis. The nutritional support of the patient presents a special problem, in that adequate calories must be supplied and yet fluid overload must be avoided. In general, caloric requirements should be calculated by established formulas or by measurement of oxygen consumption; fluid and electrolyte balance must be monitored by daily weights and calculations of intake and output, including dialytic ultrafiltration. Nutritional requirements include the need for adequate calories and nitrogen, administered by the appropriate route depending on the condition of the patient. Most guidelines for dietary therapy in acute renal failure emphasize a high percentage of glucose calories and a protein intake of approximately 40 g/day. When fluid limitations are severe, concentrated solutions of up to 50 to 70% dextrose and 8.5% amino acid solution may be required. Intravenous fat emulsions can aid in maintaining the caloric balance. Detailed discussion of surgical nutrition under these circumstances is best found in specific monographs on this topic.[46-49]

Dialytic therapy must be administered early and aggressively to prevent the syndrome of clinical uremia.[50,51] This usually means hemodialysis. Although it has been suggested since 1960 that aggressive dialysis results in better survival rates,[52,53] the acceptance of aggressive hemodialysis has come slowly over the years. Evidence has accumulated that dialysis aimed at maintaining the blood urea nitrogen (BUN) level at approximately 100 mg/dl and the creatinine level at around 10 mg/dl is beneficial.[54-56] The results of one study suggest that dialysis aimed at further reductions to a BUN level of 70 mg/dl and a creatinine concentration of 5 mg/dl may produce further improvement.[57] There have been no prospective studies published since that of Conger[57] to substantiate this claim, however. Peritoneal dialysis may be considered in situations in which hemodialysis is unavailable; however, the ability of peritoneal dialysis to ameliorate uremia is limited. For example, removal of potassium by this route rarely exceeds 12 mEq/hr, whereas exchange resins may remove up to 30 mEq/hr. Daily hemodialysis is necessary for most patients with tissue injury and renal failure.

Drug Administration

Pharmacokinetics describe the relationship between the dose of a drug given and the blood level achieved. Pharmacodynamics describe the response of the organism to a given drug concentration in the plasma. Both of these functions are altered in the patient with acute renal failure. Since intestinal absorption may be diminished, the effect of orally administered drugs cannot be predicted with certainty. Because of the basic underlying illness in most surgical situations, gastrointestinal alimentation is not available, and the intravenous route must be used for drug administration. This removes the problem of impaired absorption and gives direct access to maintenance of a serum level by dose adjustment.

The bioavailability of a drug depends on the metabolism or alteration of the drug as it circulates through various organs, especially the liver. Some drugs are inactivated rapidly, with up to 50 to 80% of the administered dose being altered by a single pass through the liver.[58] In uremia, bioavailability may be increased because of a decrease in hepatic function and reduction of the first-pass inactivation percentage.

The distribution of a drug in the body is determined by such factors as protein binding and lipid solubility. Alterations of these factors also occurs in patients with acute renal failure, changing the distribution patterns of certain drugs. The accumulation of acid metabolites may decrease protein binding of acidic drugs because of competitive displacement. Also, changes in drug-binding sites on albumin may alter its affinity for certain drug molecules. Even the net effect of decreased albumin binding is not clear. On one hand, the increased amount of free drug should enhance the pharmacologic action. But conversely, increased amounts of free drug may lead to greater and more rapid clearance from the body through residual renal function or dialysis. Reduction in the rates of drug metabolism in the kidney can clearly be related to renal cell dysfunction. The activity of liver enzymes may also be reduced, interfering with drug metabolism in the liver as well.[59-61]

A major alteration in pharmacokinetics in acute renal failure is impaired elimination of drugs by the kidney. In general, renal excretion of drugs follows first-order kinetics and the amount of drug eliminated per unit of time is proportional to the level in the plasma. As the rate of excretion declines, the half-life of the drug within the plasma increases. This in turn produces an increasing level of drug in the serum if the usual administration schedules are followed, and may produce toxic overdose. Drugs that are excreted unchanged in their active form most clearly demonstrate this phenomenon. These include aminoglycoside antibiotics, digoxin, penicillins, tetracyclines, methotrexate, and ethambutol.[58] Other drugs undergo transformation, with the production of drug metabolites, which in turn have bioactivity. These drug metabolites can also accumulate when excretory rates fall. Other untoward effects secondary to drug administration may occur in the patient with renal failure. Some patients become sensitive to central nervous

Table 7-4. Clearance of Commonly Used Drugs by Dialysis.

High clearance	Low clearance
Aminoglycosides	Cloxacillin
Penicillin G	Dicloxacillin
Carbenicillin	Cefazoline
Ticarcillin	Cefamandole
Amoxicillin	Vancomycin
Cephalothin	Clindamycin
Cephaloridine	Erythromycin
Cephaloxin	
Water-soluble vitamins	Digoxin
Lithium	Propanolol
Procainamide	Lidocaine
	Quinidine
	Phenytoin
	Insulin

system depressants and seem to react to normal dosages with an increased response. This may be caused by diminished protein binding of hypnotic drugs but also may be caused by uremic alteration of the blood-brain barrier.

Alteration of serum electrolytes can occur as the result of administration of large amounts of cation when giving antacids or antibiotics. The amount of magnesium, sodium, and potassium that can be administered by this route is significant, and overdose with cation is a distinct risk.

To further complicate the problem of drug administration in the patient with renal failure, dialysis removes many drugs along with other ions, and may thus rapidly change serum levels (Table 7-4). Commonly used drugs that are rapidly cleared by hemodialysis include aminoglycosides, cephalosporins, penicillins, and sulfonamides, as well as procainamide and cimetidine. Digoxin and propranolol, on the other hand, are little changed by dialysis,[62,63] except for slight prolongation of the maximum period of action. Dialysis has little effect on insulin levels.[64] Although clearance rates are lower with peritoneal dialysis, drugs removed by hemodialysis are also removed by peritoneal dialysis, but at a slower rate.[65]

It is clear that proper administration of needed drugs so as to achieve appropriate therapeutic levels is a complex process in the patient with diminished renal function. In patients with acute renal failure secondary to trauma and sepsis, drug administration may be one of the most vital therapeutic requirements. Reference to publications containing detailed information on each drug should be made and frequent blood levels obtained in order to treat such patients optimally.[66-70]

REFERENCES

1. Smith, H.W.: Principles of Renal Physiology. New York, Oxford University Press, 1956.
2. Hems, D.A., and Brosnan, J.T.: Effects of ischemia on content of metabolites in rat liver and kidney in vivo. Biochem. J., *120*:105, 1970.
3. Jennings, R.B., and Reiner, K.S.: Lethal myocardial ischemic injury. Am. J. Pathol., *102*:241, 1981.
4. Venkatachalam, M.A., Rennke, H.G., and Sandstrom, D.J.: The vascular basis for acute renal failure in the rat. Circ. Res., *38*:267, 1976.
5. Matthys, E., et al.: Alterations in vascular function and morphology in acute ischemic renal failure. Kidney Int., *23*:717, 1983.
6. Hanley, M.J.: Study of isolated nephron segments in a rabbit model of ischemic acute renal failure. Am. J. Physiol., *239*:F17, 1980.

7. Arendshorst, W.J., Finn, W.F., and Gottschalk, C.W.: Pathogenesis of acute renal failure following renal ischemia in the rat. Circ. Res., *37*:558, 1975.

8. Barnes, J.L., Osgood, R.W., Reineck, H.J., and Stein, J.H.: Glomerular alterations in an ischemic model of acute renal failure. Lab. Invest., *45*:378, 1981.

9. Daugharty, T.M., and Brenner, B.M.: Reversible hemodynamic defect in glomerular filtration rate after ischemic injury. Am. J. Physiol., *228*:1436, 1975.

10. Wright, F.S.: Characteristics of feedback control of glomerular filtration rate. Fed. Proc., *40*:87, 1981.

11. Wright, F.S., and Thurau, K.: Renal hemodynamics. Am. J. Med., *36*:698, 1964.

12. Finckh, E.S., Jeremy, D., and Whyte, H.M.: Structural renal damage and its relation to clinical features in acute oliguric renal failure. Q. J. Med., *31*:429, 1962.

13. Brun, C., and Munck, O.: Lesions of the kidney in acute renal failure following shock. Lancet, *1*:603, 1957.

14. Jones, D.B.: Ultrastructure of human acute renal failure. Lab. Invest., *46*:254, 1982.

15. Wardle, E.N., and Wright, N.A.: Intravascular coagulation and glycerin hemoglobinuric acute renal failure. Arch. Pathol. Lab. Med., *95*:271, 1973.

16. Dach, J.L., and Kurtzman, N.A.: A scanning electron microscopic study of the glycerol model of acute renal failure. Lab. Invest., *34*:409, 1976.

17. Trump, B.F., Strum, J.M., and Bulger, R.E.: Studies on the pathogenesis of ischemic cell injury. I, Relation between ion and water shifts and cell ultrastructure in rat kidney slices during swelling at 0–4°C. Virch. Arch. Cell. Pathol. *16*:1, 1974.

18. Trifillis, A.L., Kahng, M.W., and Trump, B.F.: Metabolic studies of $HgCl_2$-induced acute renal failure in the rat. Exp. Mol. Pathol., *35*:14, 1981.

19. Pfaller, W., Gunther, R., and Silbernagl, S.: Pathogenesis of $HgCl_2$ and maleate-induced acute renal failure. Pfluegers Arch. *379*:R18, 1979.

20. Hollenberg, N.K., et al: Acute renal failure due to nephrotoxins: Renal hemodynamic and angiographic studies in man. N. Engl. J. Med., *282*:1329, 1970.

21. Cotton, J.R., Woodard, T., Carter, N.W., and Knochel, J.P.: Resting skeletal muscle membrane potential as an index of uremic toxicity. J. Clin. Invest., *63*:501, 1979.

22. Akaike, N.: Operation of an electrogenic sodium pump in mammalian red muscle fibre. Life Sci., *14*:141, 1974.

23. Bilbrey, G.L., et al: Potassium deficiency in chronic renal failure. Kidney Int., *4*:423, 1973.

24. McDermott, F.T., Nayman, J., and DeBoer, W.G.R.M.: Effect of acute renal failure upon cell division in the jejunum: radioautographic and ultrastructural studies in the mouse. Ann. Surg., *174*:274, 1971.

25. Bozzini, C.E., Devoto, F.C.H., and Tomio, J.M.: Decreased responsiveness of hemopoietic tissue to erythropoietin in acutely uremic rats. J. Lab. Clin. Med., *68*:411, 1966.

26. McDermott, F.T., Nayman, J., and DeBoer, W.G.R.M.: Effect of acute renal failure upon wound healing: histological and autoradiographic studies in the mouse. Ann. Surg., *168*:142, 1968.

27. McDermott, F.T., Nayman, J., and DeBoer, W.G.R.M.: Epithelial cell division in acute renal failure: a radioautographic study in the oesophagus of the mouse. Br. J. Surg., *58*:52, 1971.

28. Relman, A.S.: Metabolic consequences of acid-base disorders. Kidney Int., *1*:347, 1972.

29. Kokot, F., and Kuska, J.: The endocrine system in patients with acute renal insufficiency. Kidney Int., *10*:926, 1976.

30. Massry, S.G., et al: Deralent ion metabolism in patient with acute renal failure: studies in the mechanism of hypocalcemia. Kidney Int., *5*:437, 1974.

31. Wallach, S., Bellavia, J.V., Schorr, J., and Schaffer, A.: Tissue distribution of electrolytes, ^{47}Ca and ^{28}Mg in experimental hyper and hypoparathyroidism. Endocrinology, *78*:16, 1966.

32. Guisado, R., Arieff, A.I., and Massry, S.: Muscle water and electrolytes in uremia and the effects of hemodialysis. J. Lab. Clin. Med., *89*:322, 1977.

33. Farber, J.L.: The role of calcium in cell death. Life Sci., *29*:1289, 1981.

34. Bushinsky, D.A., et al.: Hospital acquired renal insufficiency. Proc. Am. Soc. Nephrol., *12*:105A, 1979.

35. Levinsky, N.G., Alexander, E.A. and Venkatachalam, V.K.: Acute renal failure. *In* The Kidney. Vol. 1. Edited by B.M. Brenner and F.C. Rector, Jr. Philadelphia, W.B. Saunders Co., 1976.

36. Handa, S.P., and Morrins, P.A.F.: Diagnostic indices in acute renal failure. Can. Med. Assoc. J., *96*:78, 1967.

37. Espinel, C.H., and Gregory, A.W.: Differential diagnosis of acute renal failure. Clin. Nephrol., *13*:73, 1980.

38. Selkurt, E.E.: Changes in renal clearance following complete ischemia of the kidney. Am. J. Physiol., *144*:395, 1945.

39. Hanley, M.J., and Davidson, K.: Prior mannitol and furosemide infusion in a model of ischemic acute renal failure. Am. J. Physiol., *241*:F556, 1981.

40. Barry, K.G., and Malloy, J.P.: Oliguric renal failure: evaluation and therapy by the intravenous infusion of mannitol. J.A.M.A. *179*:510, 1962.
41. Kjellstrand, C.M.: Ethacrynic acid in acute tubular necrosis. Nephron, *9*:337, 1972.
42. Swartz, C., et al: Ethacrynic acid in acute renal failure. Circulation, *38*(Suppl. 6):54, 1968.
43. Baek, S.M., Brown, R.S., and Shoemaker, W.C.: Early prediction of acute renal failure and recovery. II. Renal function response to furosemide. Ann. Surg., *178*:605, 1973.
44. Kjellstrand, C.M.: Ethacrynic acid in acute renal failure. The American Society of Nephrology 2nd Annual Meeting, p. 31, 1968.
45. Levinsky, N.G., Bernard, D.B., and Johnston, P.A.: Mannitol and loop diuretics in acute renal failure. *In* Acute Renal Failure. Edited by B.M. Brenner and J.M. Lazarus. Philadelphia, W.B. Saunders Co., 1983.
46. Abel, R.M., et al: Improved survival from acute renal failure after treatment with intravenous essential L-amino acids and glucose. N. Engl. J. Med., *288*:695, 1973.
47. Baek, S.M., et al: The influence of parenteral nutrition on the course of acute renal failure. Surg. Gynecol. Obstet., *141*:405, 1975.
48. Feinstein, E.I., et al: Clinical and metabolic responses to parenteral nutrition in acute renal failure. Medicine, *6*:124, 1981.
49. Bergstrom, J., et al: Nutrition in renal failure. *In* Nutritional Aspects of Care in the Critically Ill. Edited by J.R. Richards and J.M. Kinney. New York, Churchill Livingstone, 1977.
50. Hakin, R.M., and Lazarus, J.M.: Hemodialysis in acute renal failure. *In* Acute Renal Failure. Edited by B.M. Brenner, and J.M. Lazarus. Philadelphia, W.B. Saunders Co., 1983.
51. Schrier, R.W.: Acute renal failure: pathogenesis, diagnosis and management. Hosp. Prac. *16*:93, 1981.
52. Scribner, B.H., Magid, G.J., and Burnell, J.M.: Prophylactic hemodialysis in the management of acute renal failure. Clin. Res., *8*:136, 1960.
53. Tesckan, P.E., et al: Prophylactic hemodialysis in the treatment of acute renal failure. Ann. Intern. Med., *53*:992, 1960.
54. Fischer, R.P., Griffen, W.O., Reiser, M., and Clark, D.S.: Early dialysis in the treatment of acute renal failure. Surg. Gynecol. Obstet., *123*:1019, 1966.
55. Kleinknecht, D., et al: Uremic and non-uremic complications in acute renal failure: evaluation of early and frequent dialysis on prognosis. Kidney Int., *1*:190, 1972.
56. Parsons, F.M., Hobson, S.M., Blagg, C.R. and McCracken, B.H.: Optimum time for dialysis in acute reversible renal failure. Lancet, *1*:129, 1961.
57. Conger, J.D.: A controlled evaluation of prophylactic dialysis in post-traumatic acute renal failure. J. Trauma, *15*:1056, 1975.
58. Anderson, R.J.: Drug prescribing for patients in renal failure. Hosp. Pract. *18*:145, 1983.
59. Anderson, R.J., and Schrier, R.W. (eds.): Clinical Use of Drugs in Patients with Kidney and Liver Disease. Philadelphia, W.B. Saunders Co., 1981.
60. Levy, G.: Pharmacokinetics in renal disease. Am. J. Med., *62*:461, 1977.
61. Gulyassy, P.F., and Depner, T.A.: Abnormal drug binding in uremia. Dial. Transplant., *8*:19, 1979.
62. Funkelstein, F.O., Goffinat, J.A., Hendler, E.D., and Lindenbaum, J.: Pharmacokinetics of digoxin and digitoxin in patients undergoing hemodialysis. Am. J. Med., *58*:525, 1975.
63. Lowenthal, D.T., et al: Pharmacokinetics of oral propranolol in chronic renal disease. Clin. Pharmacol. Ther., *16*:761, 1974.
64. Novalesi, R., Pilo, A., Lenzi, S., and Donato, L.: Insulin metabolism in chronic uremia and in the anephric state: effect of dialytic treatment. J. Clin. Endocrinol. Metab., *40*:70, 1975.
65. Golper, T.A.: Drugs and peritoneal dialysis. Dial. Transplant., *8*:41, 1979.
66. Bennett, W.M., et al: Drug therapy in renal failure: dosing guidelines for adults. Ann. Intern. Med., *93*:62, 1980.
67. Whelton, A., Quintiliani, R.: Antibiotic adjustments in renal failure. Infect. Surg., *3*:101, 1984.
68. Bennett, W.M.: Altering drug dosage in patients with diseases of the kidney and liver. *In* Clinical Use of Drugs in Patients with Kidney and Liver Disease. Edited by R.J. Anderson and R.W. Schreier. Philadelphia, W.B. Saunders Co., 1981.
69. Brater, D.C.: Handbook of Drugs Use in Patients with Renal Disease. Dallas, Improved Therapeutics, 1983.
70. Heel, R.C., and Avery, G.S.: Guide to drug dosage in renal failure. *In* Drug Treatment—Principles and Practice of Clinical Pharmacology and Therapeutics, 2nd ed. Edited by G.S. Avery and S. Graeme. Sidney, Austrialia, ADIS Press, 1980.

Chapter 8
LIVER IN SHOCK

Takashi Kawasaki • Seiji Marubayashi

Metabolic events in shock have been regarded as secondary effects because of decreased tissue perfusion leading to generalized cellular hypoxia, ischemia, and, finally, organ damage, although metabolic disturbance is markedly different in various organs. Increasingly successful management of renal and pulmonary problems has permitted the recognition of hepatic dysfunction in patients who survive shock.[1] Thus, the liver has been found to be especially susceptible to shock,[2,3] which causes functional and structural damage to liver cells.[4-7] Among the functional disorders, the status of energy metabolism is important in predicting viability of ischemic organs. Defective energy metabolism in the liver also has been implicated in the development of irreversible stages of shock.[8] It is valuable to study energy metabolism in the liver during hepatic ischemia and subsequent reperfusion, since experimental and clinical hemorrhagic shock are both associated with prolonged periods of low-flow state and with subsequent transfusion. Elucidating the mechanism of liver cell injury during hepatic ischemia or shock could be helpful in providing therapy for an ischemic insult or preventing ischemic cell damage. From this point of view, this chapter deals specifically with alterations in liver energy metabolism during shock, especially hepatic ischemia and subsequent reperfusion, and possible ways to prevent and correct such lesions.

ADENINE NUCLEOTIDE METABOLISM AND ITS PROTECTION

In shock, energy disturbance precedes alterations in biologic homeostasis and clinical symptoms. Studies of energy metabolism of ischemic cells as a functional unit are useful for understanding the whole metabolism of the organ. In the studies of energy metabolism during hepatic ischemia, we presented evidence that the ability of the liver to regenerate ATP and maintain adequate energy charge and total adenine nucleotide after blood reperfusion after ischemic periods could serve as a valid index of organ viability and could determine survival of the animal.[9] A similar line of evidence was presented from our laboratory in model experiments on ischemia of the rat kidney and brain.[10-13]

Ischemia drastically reduced the ATP level in the liver, and the level remained relatively steady thereafter (Fig. 8–1). Reflow of hepatic blood after various ischemic periods resulted in a recovery of the ATP level, the rate and extent of which appeared to be dependent on the length of the ischemic period. Coenzyme Q (ubiquinone) has been known to be a constituent of the mitochondrial respiratory chain and to function as an electron and proton carrier. Coenzyme Q_{10} (CoQ_{10}) is indispensable for the production of ATP in the mitochondria. As shown in Figure 8–1, CoQ_{10} administration markedly increased resynthesis of ATP during reperfusion after 90 min of ischemia. The level of total adenine nucleotide and the value

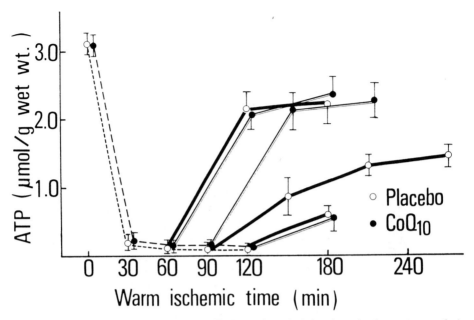

Fig. 8-1. Change in the level of hepatic ATP during hepatic ischemia and subsequent reperfusion and the effect of pretreatment with CoQ_{10}. Hepatic ischemia was induced by clamping the hepatic artery, portal vein, and bile duct. A portafemoral shunt was made by connecting a branch of the portal vein to the left femoral vein with a polyethylene tube before ischemia.[9] CoQ_{10} at a dose of 6 mg/kg of body weight was injected IV 1 hr before inducing hepatic ischemia, and in the rats receiving placebo, a solvent for CoQ_{10} preparation was injected in the same volume and same manner as CoQ_{10}. Hepatic blood flow was allowed to reperfuse at 60, 90, and 120 min after ischemia, and ATP level was determined. The solid line indicates ATP levels after reperfusion following ischemia; the dashed line indicates ATP levels after ischemia.

of energy charge were also significantly higher in the CoQ_{10}-treated group than in the placebo group. This treatment was also accompanied by a marked increase (60%) in the survival rate of ischemic rats compared to 0% in the rats receiving placebos. However, administration of CoQ_{10} did not improve a greatly decreased resynthesis of ATP after reflow following 2 hours of ischemia.

Pass, et al.[14] reported markedly reduced tissue levels of ATP in the rat during hemorrhagic shock. Schloerb, et al.[15] showed that hemorrhagic shock in rats produced a 50% mortality. Liver ATP level decreased in proportion to the volume of shed blood that had to be reinfused in order to maintain a constant level of hypotension. It was shown that deterioration in the capacity of the liver for ATP generation plays an important role in the progression to the irreversible stage of hemorrhagic shock[16] and the change in energy charge is sensitive to acute blood loss.[17] Ukikusa, et al.[17] also reported that in hemorrhagic shock hepatic energy charge level correlated significantly to mean arterial blood pressure as well as blood volume withdrawn, which in turn correlated to the various mortalities of rats. Chaudry, et al.[18] showed that a decrease in hepatic ATP in the late stage of sepsis (low-flow septic rats) is similar to that seen during early hemorrhagic shock and suggested that inadequate perfusion is the cause, since in the early stages of sepsis these rats did not show any decrease in either hepatic blood flow or tissue ATP.

Is there any possible criterion to assess tissue ATP levels? Miller, et al.[19] investigated the relationship between changes in ATP level and those in surface oxygen tension of the liver and brain during hypotension and reported that a decrease in the ATP level of the liver was correlated with a decrease in the surface partial oxygen tension during hemorrhagic shock. After reinfusion of blood, restoration of ATP level was dramatic and the surface oxygen tension of the liver returned to an essentially normal value. Pass, et al.[14] reported, however, in animals subjected to hemorrhagic shock, that arterial pH rather than arterial Po_2 may be a sensitive indicator of decreased hepatic perfusion and impaired liver ATP production. It is interesting that changes in acetoacetate/β-hydroxybutyrate ratio in arterial blood reflect a liver mitochondrial redox state and are correlated with hepatic energy charge levels in hemorrhagic shock.[2,20]

ALTERATION IN MITOCHONDRIAL FUNCTION

A decrease in ATP or hepatic energy charge after hypovolemic shock and hepatic ischemia may be explained by mitochondrial damage.[4,21−26] In studies of the role of mitochondrial damages in the pathogenesis of liver cell injury in shock or ischemia, a loss of respiratory control, a decrease in ADP:O ratio, changes in mitochodrial ultrastructure, and an increase in total cellular and mitochondrial Ca^{2+} content have been generally noted.[8,11−28]

As reported from our laboratory,[24−26] mitochondria isolated from the placebo group showed a progressive loss of respiratory control index (RCI)—a sensitive indicator of mitochondrial coupling, with a lapse in time after clamping. Although the RCI after reflow following 90 min of ischemia was recovered incompletely, CoQ_{10} administration stimulated the recovery of RCI to the normal level. However, only poor recovery of respiratory control was observed even in the CoQ_{10}-treated group after 120 min of ischemia and subsequent reperfusion.

Similar liver mitochondrial damage was observed during hemorrhagic shock in laboratory animals.[29] Mela, et al.[21] showed defective oxidative metabolism of liver mitochondria of rats in hemorrhagic and endotoxic shock. It is reported, however, that in the early stage of septic shock in animals liver mitochondrial oxidative and phosphorylative activities were somewhat enhanced, and this enhancement was depressed in the late stage.[30] These results suggest that hepatocellular damage in the early stage of sepsis may not involve liver mitochondrial damage and subsequent inadequate energy production.

There is controversy as to whether irreversible mitochondrial injury is actually a cause of irreversible damage or a secondary manifestation resulting from cellular damage. Reports from Farber's laboratory[27,28] suggest that mitochondrial alterations are not causally related to the development of irreversible cell injury on hepatic ischemia. This is based on the fact that chlorpromazine pretreatment of rats dissociates the effect of liver ischemia on mitochondrial function from the development of irreversible cell injury. Mitochondrial membranes are, however, sensitive to prolonged ischemia, and eventually permanent damage to mitochondrial membranes occurs if ischemia continues beyond a critical period.[5,23−26] Many reports, including our associates' and ours, clearly indicate that in shock or ischemia liver mitochondria cannot respond to energy needs by a normal acceleration of oxidative phosphorylation even though enough O_2 and substrate are provided [5,21−26] and that the mitochondrial phosphorylating activity of the liver plays an important role in recovery from shock[2,20] and determines mortality.[3] These results are consistent with our results, which show that the ability of liver cells to reverse ischemic mitochondrial dysfunction correlates with the ability of tissue to recover from ischemic cell injury.[24–26]

CALCIUM CONTENT OF LIVER MITOCHONDRIA

Calcium ion is well known to be an important regulator in many cellular functions, and the maintenance of calcium homeostasis is essential for cellular metabolism as well as cellular and subcellular integrity, including mitochondria.

We and our colleagues studied the effect of hepatic ischemia and subsequent reperfusion on mitochondrial Ca^{2+} content. Although the Ca^{2+} content was not altered during ischemic periods up to 120 min, 1 hour of reperfusion following 90 min of ischemia induced a twofold increase in the Ca^{2+} content, and CoQ_{10} pretreatment completely suppressed this rise. The Ca^{2+} level after 1 hour of reflow following 120 min of ischemia was not affected by CoQ_{10} pretreatment. Ca^{2+} concentration in mitochondria was also reported to increase after shock.[31] The increase in mitochondrial Ca^{2+} content is assumed to be a consequence of increased cytosolic Ca^{2+} content,[32] which probably results from damage to plasma membranes. This is supported by the fact that membrane damage caused by lipid peroxidation results in intracellular Ca^{2+} overload in ischemic myocardium.[33] A high level of Ca^{2+} is known to cause a loss of mitochondrial function.[34] The ability of biomembranes to regulate intracellular Ca^{2+} level is implicated in critical cellular functions, and this ability was found to be lost during irreversible cellular injury.[35,36] The finding[37] that increased intracellular Ca^{2+} potentiates lipid peroxidation in the erythrocyte membrane seems to support our assumption, as is described in the following section.

ROLE OF LIPID PEROXIDATION IN INDUCING CELLULAR INJURY

The precise mechanism by which shock produces liver mitochondrial damage is not known, although resultant anoxic and ischemic conditions appear to be an important factor. In addition, several factors may be responsible for alterations in mitochondrial metabolism during shock. These include 1. lipid peroxide formation in mitochondrial membrane during shock; 2. an increased mitochondrial Ca^{2+} level, as described in the preceding section; and 3. inhibition of mitochondrial functions by free fatty acids and their CoA ester derivatives.[27,28,38] Considerable evidence suggests that an elevated level of long-chain acyl-CoA esters is responsible for inhibition of adenine nucleotide translocase in ischemia and shock.[27–29,38] The tissue level of fatty acyl-CoA is usually low but increases during shock and ischemia, and most of this occurs in mitochondria[39,40] The inhibition of adenine nucleotide translocase by free fatty acids or fatty acyl-CoA esters can explain in part a loss of respiratory control of liver mitochondria during shock and ischemia.

Lipid peroxide formation has been suggested to be associated with a variety of pathologic processes, such as liver necrosis, hemolytic anemia, lung damage[41–43] ischemic heart disease,[44,45] brain ischemia,[13] and ischemic liver cell injury.[24–26,46] Lipid peroxidation is ascribed to a sequence of reactions of lipids with oxygen through formation of free radical intermediates, occurring mostly in cellular and subcellular membranes. The pathologic consequence of lipid peroxidation may reflect the alterations of membrane integrity or membrane-associated functions in subcellular organelles, such as mitochondria, microsomes, cell membranes, and lysosomes.

As shown in Figure 8–2, the level of malondialdehyde (MDA), which is an end product of lipid peroxides after they react with thiobarbituric acid, remained relatively steady during ischemic periods up to 120 min. When reflow of hepatic blood was allowed, definite changes in MDA level were observed depending on the length of ischemic periods. Ischemia for 60 min and subsequent reflow kept the level of MDA in the control range. After 90 min of ischemia and following reflow, the level increased markedly. The administration of CoQ_{10} did not affect the level of MDA during ischemic periods or that after reflow following 60 min of ischemia. However, the treatment with CoQ_{10} completely suppressed the marked elevation in the MDA level after reperfusion. Pretreatment with CoQ_{10} failed to reverse the rise in the MDA when the ischemic period was prolonged to 120 min, which suggests that irreversible hepatic cellular damages developed during the 120-min period. Changes in the MDA level of liver mitochondria and the effect of CoQ_{10} administration were quite similar to those found in the liver tissue during ischemia and after reperfusion periods. Vitamin E administration (10 mg/kg of body weight/day, i.p. for 3 days) also suppressed the marked increase in MDA level after reperfusion following 90 min of rat hepatic ischemia. The results obtained indicate that cellular damage to the livers of rats by ischemia followed

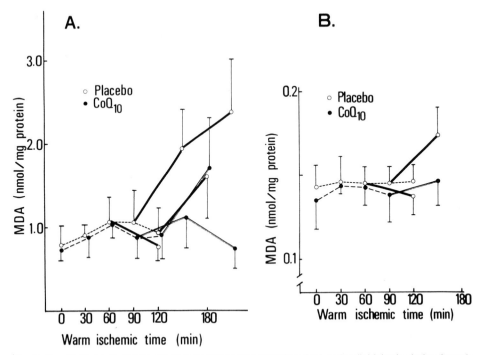

Fig. 8-2. Changes in the levels of liver tissue and mitochondrial malondialdehyde during hepatic ischemia and reperfusion and the effect of pretreatment with CoQ_{10}. Experimental conditions were identical to those given in the legend of Fig. 8–1. Lipid peroxide in liver tissue and mitochondria was measured as malondialdehyde (MDA) by a colorimetric reaction with thiobarbituric acid. (A) Liver tissue; (B) Mitochondria. Solid line indicates MDA levels after reperfusion following ischemia; dashed lines indicate MDA levels after ischemia.

by reperfusion is, in part, caused by lipid peroxidation in biomembranes. This causes mitochondrial dysfunction and perturbation of energy metabolism and cellular calcium homeostasis.

Marked lipid peroxide formation in the liver was reported in shocked animals.[47–49] Sakaguchi, et al.[47] reported the participation of lipid peroxidation in liver cell membrane damage in endotoxin-poisoned mice. They showed that the lipid peroxide level in the livers of endotoxin-poisoned mice after the administration of vitamin E or reduced glutathione (GSH) was lower than that in the controls, and these free radical scavengers prevented completely the membrane damage that arose from endotoxin challenge. A beneficial effect of free radical scavengers in traumatic shock and myocardial ischemia also was reported.[50] Ogawa, et al.[48] showed that endotoxemia gives rise to accumulation of hepatic lipid peroxides by activation of a producing system and impairment of an elimination system of superoxide radicals, since treatment of rats with allopurinol and GSH reversed an elevation of lipid peroxide and a reduction of superoxide dismutase activity induced by endotoxin. Drug-induced liver cell injury is also explained by peroxidative processes in vivo through formation of free radical intermediates, and cellular mechanisms of protection for peroxidation are proposed to be caused by actions of free radical scavengers, antioxidants, and related enzymes.[51–53]

Park, et al.[49] proposed the mechanism for oxygen radical production in ischemic organs. This involves reaction of xanthine oxidase with hypoxanthine and molecular oxygen to produce oxygen free radicals when an ischemic organ was reperfused. Their hypothesis may be supported by the fact that allopurinol, a competitive inhibitor of xanthine oxidase, substantially increased the survival rate of dogs subjected to hemorrhagic shock.[54,55] Superoxide anion undergoes further reduction to form hydrogen peroxide, the hydroxyl radical, and singlet oxygen, and the radicals derived secondarily from superoxide anion may be responsible for hepatic cellular injury.[56]

ROLE OF ENDOGENOUS ANTIOXIDANTS

Vitamin E is thought to function in vivo as a free radical scavenger as well as an antioxidant,[52,57] and the action of CoQ homologs as an antioxidant was reported in several in vitro systems.[58,59] Intracellular GSH levels in the liver are reduced after several types of shock, including hemorrhagic, traumatic, and endotoxic shock.[60–64] Jeffries, et al.[63] reported that the level of nonprotein GSH in the livers of mice declined to 60% below normal 18 hours after administration of endotoxin. It seems, therefore, to be important to determine whether or not hepatic ischemia or shock processes affect the contents of endogenous antioxidants, CoQ homologs, vitamin E, and GSH.

As shown in Tables 8–1 and 8–2, ischemia of the livers of rats for 90 min resulted in decreases of endogenous vitamin E and GSH without significant changes in the level of endogenous CoQ homologs. Restoration of the blood flow resulted in marked decreases in endogenous CoQ homologs, vitamin E, and GSH. In CoQ$_{10}$-treated animals, however, there were no changes in the levels of endogenous CoQ$_9$, vitamin E, or GSH, or in the level of enhanced CoQ$_{10}$ during the reperfusion period. A similar line of evidence was obtained with vitamin E pretreatment of the ischemic liver.[66] These results suggest that lipid soluble (CoQ

Table 8–1. CoQ Homologs and Vitamin E in Liver Mitochondria during Ischemia and Subsequent Reperfusion and the Effect of Pretreatment with CoQ$_{10}$.

Treatment				
Ischemia (min)	Reflow (min)	CoQ$_{10}$	CoQ$_9$	Vitamin E
		ng/mg protein		
Placebo				
0*		141 ± 10.2	951 ± 94.9	190 ± 12.6[c]
90	0	138 ± 18.0[a]	864 ± 99.8[b]	135 ± 20.0[c,d]
90	60	95.2 ± 5.57[a]	586 ± 94.4[b]	77.3 ± 18.8[d]
CoQ$_{10}$-treated				
0		925 ± 243	981 ± 71.0	213 ± 31.9[e]
90	0	905 ± 284	916 ± 87.2	145 ± 22.8[e]
90	60	1089 ± 122	988 ± 95.6	162 ± 26.3

Mitochondria were isolated from the ischemic liver.[24–26] Simultaneous determination of CoQ homologs and of vitamin E was carried out as previously described.[65] CoQ$_9$ and CoQ$_{10}$ represent total (oxidized and reduced) content of each CoQ homolog. Values are mean ± SD of five experiments.
*Rats received sham operation.
[a,c,d,e]$p < .001$
[b]$p < .01$

Table 8–2. Concentration of Total and Oxidized Glutathione in Liver Tissue during Hepatic Ischemia and Subsequent Reperfusion and the Effect of CoQ$_{10}$ Administration.

Treatment			
Ischemia (min)	Reflow (min)	GSH + GSSG	GSSG
		μmol/g liver	
Placebo			
0*		7.24 ± 0.53[a]	0.103 ± 0.007[b]
90	0	5.82 ± 0.58[a,c]	0.116 ± 0.006[b]
90	60	4.24 ± 0.51[c]	0.109 ± 0.011
CoQ$_{10}$-treated			
0		6.96 ± 0.44[d]	0.096 ± 0.010[e]
90	0	5.95 ± 0.53[d]	0.117 ± 0.008[e]
90	60	5.65 ± 0.68	0.099 ± 0.012

Assays of total glutathione (GSH + GSSG) and of oxidized glutathione (GSSG) are carried out as previously described.[65] Values are mean ± SD of five experiments.
*Rats received sham operation.
[a,c]$p < .001$.
[b,d,e]$p < .01$.

homologs and vitamin E) and water soluble (GSH) antioxidants function cooperatively to prevent lipid peroxidation during reperfusion.

Lipid peroxidation proceeds by a cyclic chain reaction involving free radical reactions.[57] Changes in concentrations of endogenous vitamin E, GSH, and CoQ homologs (Tables 8–1 and 8–2) suggest that free radical reactions are assumed to be initiated during the process of ischemia, and further peroxidative processes are evident after reperfusion. This is supported by the fact that a twofold increase in lipid peroxidation in liver tissue and mitochondria was observed only when oxygen, probably as oxygen free radicals, was resupplied to the liver after 90 min of ischemia (Fig. 8–2).

These results, together with those reported from our laboratory,[10−13,24−26,65,66] support the assumption that liver cell damage from ischemia or shock can be explained by free radical reaction processes. Restoration of blood flow to previously ischemic organs causes a rapid increase in tissue oxygen tension that favors the production of active oxygen species through the partial reduction of oxygen molecules, and promotes lipid peroxidative processes after the initiation of free radical reactions during ischemia.

RETICULOENDOTHELIAL FUNCTION IN SHOCK

It has been well demonstrated that the phagocytic activity of the reticuloendothelial system (RES) is depressed in various kinds of shock.[67−71] Hepatic clearance failure may become a major predisposing factor to development of pulmonary insufficiency, renal failure, septicemia, and disseminated intravascular coagulation, since liver Kupffer cells have a major role in determining the function of the RES. Animals surviving after shock manifested only transient RES depression followed by subsequent recovery, and animals that did not survive shock had a persistent and progressive depression in RES function before they died.[72]

Fibronectin is an opsonic glycoprotein that augments reticuloendothelial phagocytic clearance of nonbacterial particulates.[73] The effect of fibronectin on particle phagocytosis after augmentation of cell–cell interaction and of cell adhesion to a substratum suggests that fibronectin has opsonic as well as adhesive properties.[74] Plasma fibronectin deficiency exists in patients with serious trauma and burns[75−76] and in patients with multiple organ failure or disseminated intravascular coagulation.[77] Saba, et al.[74−76,78] showed that altered humoral opsonic activity plays an important role in changes in RES function in shock. Reversal of opsonic deficiency in injured patients in a state of septic shock was observed after infusion of fibronectin-rich plasma cryoprecipitate.

With regard to ATP content in reticuloendothelial cells and phagocytosis, a close relationship was demonstrated in in vitro systems using isolated macrophages.[79] It is suggested that a decreased ATP level and energy charge in the liver may in part contribute to a decreased phagocytic activity in animals in a state of septic shock.[68] The precise correlation between energy metabolism and phagocytic activity of RES remains to be elucidated, however.

THERAPEUTIC CONCEPT OF LIVER CELL DAMAGE

It is important to provide and maintain an adequate vascular volume during shock or after an ischemic episode. Along with this, various adjunctive agents and approaches may be used, such as buffering agents, steroids, vascular agents, vasoactive agents, and other methods of circulatory supports. Correction of specific alterations in cell function, however, may be necessary if the foregoing nonspecific therapy is not effective. From the viewpoint of energy metabolism and alteration in mitochondrial function during shock, it is necessary to enhance the cellular energy production during shock. Many experimental approaches in this regard have been studied, including the use of respiratory substrates, and other agents such as tricarboxylic acid cycle intermediates, nicotinamide, cAMP, inosine, adenosine, allopurinol, and ATP-$MgCl_2$.[3,54,55,72,80]

Studies from our laboratory have shown that CoQ_{10} and vitamin E administration proved to be beneficial in stimulating survival of animals after hepatic ischemia.[24–26,65,66] A similar line of evidence was presented from our laboratory on ischemia of the rat kidney and brain.[11–13] It is noteworthy that preservation with CoQ_{10} or vitamin E of cellular damage caused by hepatic ischemia is probably a result of protection of cellular and subcellular membranes from lipid peroxidation, so that mitochondrial functions are restored and cellular calcium homeostasis is maintained. The protective effect of GSH may be expected in liver cell injury during shock.[47,48,63]

These results suggest that administration of free radical scavengers and antioxidants such as CoQ_{10}, vitamin E, and GSH is useful for protection of liver cell injury during shock.

Figure 8–3 shows a tentative hypothesis for the sequence of events leading to liver cell injury caused by ischemia and subsequent reperfusion. Ischemia causes a loss of ATP. Oxygen supplied by reperfusion appears to react with lipids and to stimulate formation of free radical intermediates and subsequently of lipid peroxides in membranes, which results in plasma and mitochondrial membrane damages and impaired mitochondrial function. Upon reperfusion a massive influx of Ca^{2+} may occur across damaged membranes, which causes an overload of cytosolic and mitochondrial calcium. A high level of calcium in the cell is known to result in a loss of mitochondrial ATP-generating capacity. These sequential events may further elevate cytosolic Ca^{2+}, since Ca^{2+} is actively extruded from the cell

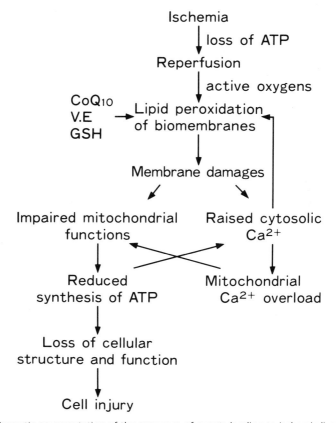

Fig. 8-3. *Schematic representation of the sequence of events leading to ischemic liver cell injury.*

by an energy-dependent process, and then the high level of cytosolic calcium further potentiates lipid peroxidation.[81] A vicious circle would be therefore established, which would result in further cellular membrane and mitochondrial damages and then finally lead to ischemic cell injury.

Preservation by CoQ_{10} or vitamin E administration of ischemic liver cell damage and survival from ischemia would therefore be the result of protection of cellular and subcellular membranes from lipid peroxidation, by which cellular calcium homeostasis is maintained and mitochondrial function is restored.

REFERENCES

1. Champion, H.R., et al.: A clinicopathological study of hepatic dysfunction following shock. Surg. Gynecol. Obstet., *142*:657, 1976.
2. Ozawa, K.: Energy metabolism. *In* Pathophysiology of Shock, Anoxia, and Ischemia. Edited by R.A. Cowley, and B.F. Trump. Baltimore, Williams & Wilkins, 1982.
3. Chaudry, I.H.: Cellular mechanisms in shock and ischemia and their correction. Am. J. Physiol., *245*:R117, 1983.
4. Chien, K.R., et al.: Accelerated phospholipid degradation and associated membrane dysfunction in irreversible, ischemic liver cell injury. J. Biol. Chem., *253*:4809, 1978.
5. Gaja, G., Ferrero, M.E., Picoletti, R., and Bernelli-Zazzera, A. Phosphorylation and redox states in ischemic liver. Exp. Mol. Pathol., *19*:248, 1973.
6. Holliday, R.L., Illner, H.P., and Shires, G.T.: Liver cell membrane alterations during hemorrhagic shock in the rats. J. Surg. Res., *31*:506, 1981.
7. Banks, J.G., Foulis, A.K., Ledingham, I.Mc.A., and Macsween, R.N.M.: Liver function in septic shock. J. Clin. Pathol., *35*:1249, 1982.
8. Delorme, E.J.: Arterial perfusion of the liver in shock. An experimental study. Lancet, *1*:259, 1951.
9. Marubayashi, S., et al.: Adenine nucleotide metabolism during hepatic ischemia and subsequent blood reflow periods and its relation to organ viability. Transplantation *30*:294, 1980.
10. Kawasaki, T., et al.: Energy metabolism in the brain of SHR after ligation of carotid arteries and reflow of circulation. Jpn. Heart J., *20*:301, 1979.
11. Tatsukawa, Y., Dohi, K., Yamada, K., and Kawasaki, T.: The role of CoQ_{10} for the preservation of the rat kidney. Life Sci., *24*:1309, 1979.
12. Takenaka, M., et al.: Protective effects of α-tocopherol and coenzyme Q_{10} on warm ischemic damages of the rat kidney. Transplantation *32*:137, 1981.
13. Yamamoto, M., et al.: A possible role of lipid peroxidation in cellular damages caused by cerebral ischemia and the protective effects of α-tocopherol administration. Stroke, *14*:977, 1983.
14. Pass, L.J., et al.: Liver adenosine triphosphate (ATP) in hypoxia and hemorrhagic shock. J. Trauma, *22*:730, 1982.
15. Shloerb, P.R., et al.: Intravenous adenosine triphosphate (ATP) in hemorrhagic shock in rats. Am. J. Physiol., *240*:R52, 1981.
16. Ozawa, K., et al.: Different response of hepatic energy charge and adenine nucleotide concentrations to hemorrhagic shock. Res. Exp. Med., *169*:145, 1976.
17. Ukikusa, M., et al.: Pathophsiology of hemorrhagic shock. II. Anoxic metabolism of the rat liver following acute blood loss in the rat. Circ. Shock, *8*:483, 1981.
18. Chaudry, I.H., Wichterman, K. A., and Baue, A.E.: Effect of sepsis on tissue adenine nucleotide levels. Surgery, *85*:205, 1979.
19. Miller, A.T., Jr., Shen, A.L., and Bonner, F.B.: Hemorrhagic shock in the rat: metabolic changes in brain and liver. Arch. Int. Physiol. *82*:69, 1974.
20. Tanaka, J., et al.: Pathophysiology of hemorrhagic shock. A role of arterial ketone body ratio as an index of anoxic metabolism of the liver in acute blood loss. Adv. Shock Res., *5*:11, 1981.
21. Mela, L., Becalzo, L.V., and Miller, L.D.: Defective oxidative metabolism of rat liver mitochondria in hemorrhagic and endotoxin shock. Am. J. Physiol., *220*:571, 1971.
22. Mela, L.: Altered mitochondrial metabolism in circulatory shock. Adv. Exp. Med. Biol., *78*:371, 1977.
23. Rhodes, R.S., Depalma, R.G., and Druet, R.L.: Reversibility of ischemically induced mitochondrial dysfunction with reperfusion. Surg. Gynecol. Obstet., *145*:719, 1977.
24. Marubayashi, S., et al.: Preservation of ischemic rat liver mitochondrial functions and liver viability with CoQ_{10}. Surgery, *91*:631, 1982.
25. Marubayashi, S., et al.: Prevention of ischemic liver cell—prevention of damage by coenzyme Q_{10}. Transplant. Proc., *15*:1297, 1983.
26. Kawasaki, T., Hayashi, K., Marubayashi, S., and Dohi, K.: Preservation of mitochondrial functions,

energy metabolism and viability of ischemic liver by coenzyme Q_{10} pretreatment. *In* Biomedical and Clinical Aspects of Coenzyme Q. Edited by K. Folkers, and Y. Yamamura. Vol. 3. Amsterdam, Elsevier North Holland, 1981.

27. Mittnacht, S., Jr., and Farber, J.L.: Reversal of ischemic mitochondrial dysfunction. J. Biol. Chem., *256*:3199, 1981.
28. Mittnacht, S., Jr., Sherman, S.C., and Farber, J.L.: Reversal of ischemic mitochondrial dysfunction. J. Biol. Chem., *254*:9871, 1979.
29. Chaudry, I.H., Ohkawa, M., Clemens, M.G., and Baue, A.E.: Alterations in electron transport and cellular metabolism with shock and trauma. Prog. Clin. Biol. Res., *111*:67, 1983.
30. Shimahara, Y., et al.: Role of mitochondrial enhancement in maintaining hepatic energy charge level in endotoxin shock. J. Surg. Res., *33*:314, 1982.
31. Mela, L.: Mitochondrial function in shock, ischemia and hypoxia. *In* Pathophysiology of Shock, Anoxia and Ischemia. Edited by R.A. Cowley and B.F. Trump. Baltimore, Williams & Wilkins, 1982.
32. Becker, G.L., Fiskum, G., and Lehninger, A.L.: Regulation of free Ca^{2+} by liver mitochondria and endoplasmic reticulum. J. Biol. Chem., *255*:9009, 1980.
33. Hess, M.L., Mahany, T.M., and Greenfield, L.J.: Calcium channel blockers in shock. Prog. Clin. Biol. Res., *111*:271, 1983.
34. Greenwalt, J.W., Rossi, C.S., and Lehninger, A.L.: Effect of active accumulation of calcium and phosphate ions on the structure of rat liver mitochondria. J. Cell Biol., *23*:21, 1964.
35. Carafoli, E., and Crompton, M.: The regulation of intracellular calcium. *In* Current Topics in Membranes and Transport. Edited by F. Bronner and A. Kleinzeller. New York, Academic Press, 1978.
36. Farber, J.L., and El-Mofty, S.K.: The biomedical pathology of liver cell necorsis. Am. J. Pathol., *81*:237, 1975.
37. Jain, S.K., and Shohet, S.B.: Calcium potentiates the peroxidation of erythrocyte membrane lipids. Biochim. Biophys. Acta, *642*:46, 1981.
38. Ohkawa, M., Clemens, M.G., and Chaudry, I.H.: Studies on the mechanism of beneficial effects of $ATP\text{-}MgCl_2$ following hepatic ischemia. Am. J. Physiol., *244*:R695, 1983.
39. Lerner, E., Shug, A.L., Elson, C., and Shrago. E.: Reversible inhibition of adenine nucleotide translocation by long chain fatty acyl coenzyme A esters in liver mitochondria of diabetic and hibernating animals. J. Biol. Chem., *247*:1513, 1972.
40. Harris, R.A., Farmer, B., and Ozawa, T.: Inhibition of the mitochondrial adenine nucleotide transport system by oleyl CoA. Arch. Biochem. Biophys., *15*:199, 1972.
41. Fridovich, I. (ed): Oxygen Free Radicals and Tissue Damages. Amsterdam, Excerpta Medica, 1979.
42. Tappel, A.L.: Lipid peroxidation damage to cell components. Fed. Proc., *32*:1870, 1973.
43. McCay, P.B.: Physiological significance of lipid peroxidation. Fed. Proc., *40*:173, 1981.
44. Hess, M.L., Okabe, E., and Kontos, H.A.: Proton and free oxygen radical interraction with the calcium transport system of cardiac sarcoplasmic reticulum. J. Mol. Cell Cardiol., *13*:767, 1981.
45. Gardner, T.J., et al.: Reduction of myocardial ischemic injury with oxygen-derived free radical scavengers. Surgery, *94*:423, 1983.
46. Parks, D.A., Bulkley, G.B., and Granger, D.N.: Role of oxygen-derived free radicals in digestive tract diseases. Surgery, *94*:415, 1983.
47. Sakaguchi, S., Kanda, N., Hsu, C.C., and Sakaguchi, O.: Lipid peroxide formation and membrane damage in endotoxin-poisoned mice. Microbiol. Immunol., *25*:229, 1981.
48. Ogawa, R., Morita, T., Kunimoto, F., and Fujita, T.: Changes in hepatic lipoperoxide concentration in endotoxemic rats. Circ. Shock, *9*:369, 1982.
49. Parks, D.A., Bulkley, G.B., and Granger, D.N.: Role of oxygen free radicals in shock, ischemia, and organ preservation. Surgery, *94*:428, 1983.
50. Lefer, A.M., Araki, H., and Okamatsu, S.: Beneficial actions of a free radical scavenger in traumatic shock and myocardial ischemia. Circ. Shock, *8*:273, 1981.
51. Tappel, A.L.: Measurement of and protection from in vivo lipid peroxidation. *In* Free Radicals in Biology. Vol. 4. Edited by W.A. Pryor. New York, Academic Press, 1980.
52. MaCay, P.B., and King, M.M.: Vitamin E: its role as a biologic free radical scavenger and its relationship to the microsomal mixed function oxidase system. *In* Vitamin E. Edited by L.J. Machlin. New York, Marcel Dekker, 1980.
53. Slater, T.F.: Mechanism of protection against the damage produced in biological systems by oxygen-derived radicals. *In* Oxygen Free Radicals and Tissue Damage. (Ciba Foundation Symposium 65). Amsterdam, Excerpta Medica, 1979.
54. Crowell, J.W., Jones, C.E., and Smith, E.E.: Effect of allopurinol on hemorrhagic shock. Am. J. Physiol., *216*:744, 1969.
55. Cunningham, S.K., and Keaveny, T.V.: Effect of a xanthine oxidase inhibitor on adenine nucleotide degradation in hemorrhagic shock. Eur. Surg. Res., *10*:305, 1978.
56. Stage, T.E., Mischke, B.S., Cox, G.W., and Daniels, K.A.: The role of free-radical inhibitors on acetaldehyde-induced increases in lipid peroxidation. Fed. Proc., *42*:513, 1983.

57. Witting, L.A.: Vitamin E and lipid antioxidants in free-radical-initiated reactions. *In* Free Radicals in Biology. Vol. 4. Edited by W.A. Pryor. New York, Academic Press, 1980.

58. Mellors, A., and Tappel, A.L.: The inhibition of mitochondrial peroxidation by ubiquinone and ubiquinol. J. Biol. Chem., *241*:4353, 1966.

59. Takayanagi, R., Takeshige, K., and Minakami, S.: NADH- and NADPH-dependent lipid peroxidation in bovine heart submitochondrial particles. Biochem. J., *192*:853, 1980.

60. Flohe, L.: Glutathione peroxidase. *In* Oxygen Free Radicals and Tissue Damage. (Ciba Foundation Symposium 65). Amsterdam, Excerpta Medica, 1979.

61. Reichard, S.M., Bailey, N.M., and Galvin, M.J., Jr.: Alterations in tissue glutathione levels following traumatic shock. Adv. Shock Res., *5*:37, 1981.

62. Yamada, H.: The protective effects of reduced glutathione (GSH) on experimental traumatic shock. Jpn. J. Anesthesiol., *26*:640, 1977.

63. Jeffries, C.D.: Liver nonprotein sulfhydryl of endotoxin-treated mice. J. Bacteriol., *86*:1358, 1963.

64. Brown, P.L., and Jeffries, C.D.: Liver glutathione and glutathione reductase response of endotoxin-treated mice. Inf. Immunity, *11*:8, 1975.

65. Marubayashi, S., Dohi, K., Yamada, K., and Kawasaki, T.: Changes in the levels of endogenous coenzyme Q homologs, α-tocopherol, and glutathione in rat liver after hepatic ischemia and reperfusion, and the effect of pretreatment with coenzyme Q_{10} Biochim. Biophys. Acta, *797*:1, 1984.

66. Marubayashi, S., et al.: Role of free radicals in ischemic liver preservation: prevention of damage by CoQ_{10} and vitamin E. Transplant. Proc., *17*:1463, 1985.

67. Kaplan, J.E., and Saba, T.M.: Humoral deficiency and reticuloendothelial depression after traumatic shock. Am. J. Physiol., *230*:7, 1976.

68. Nakatani, T., et al.: The pathophysiology of septic shock: studies of reticuloendothelial system function and liver high-energy metabolism in rats following sublethal and lethal Escherichia coli injection. Adv. Shock Res., *7*:147, 1982.

69. Carr, F.K., and Loegering, D.L.: Reticuloendothelial system function and humoral factor deficiency following acute hemorrhage. Can. J. Physiol. Pharmacol., *56*:299, 1978.

70. Cook, J.A., Dougherty, W.J., and Holt, T.M.: Enhanced sensitivity to endotoxin induced by the RE stimulant, Glucan. Circ. Shock, *7*:225, 1980.

71. Kaplan, J.E., et al.: Reticulo-endothelial phagocytic response to bacterial challenge after traumatic shock. Circ. Shock, *4*:1, 1977.

72. Altura, B.M.: Reticuloendothelial system and neuro-endocrine stimulation in shock therapy. Adv. Shock Res., *3*:3, 1980.

73. Blumenstock, F.A., et al.: Opsonic fibronectin after trauma and particle injection as determined by a peritoneal macrophage monolayer assay. J. Reticuloendothel. Soc., *30*:61, 1981.

74. Saba, T.M., and Jaffe, E.: Plasma fibronectin: its synthesis by vascular endothelial cells and role in cardiopulmonary integrity after trauma are related to reticuloendothelial function. Am. J. Med., *68*:577, 1980.

75. Lanser, M.E., Saba, T.M., and Scovill, W.A.: Opsonic glycoprotein (plasma fibronectin) levels after burn injury: relationship to extent of burn and development of sepsis. Ann. Surg., *192*:776, 1980.

76. Saba, T.M., Blumenstock, F.A., Scovill, W.A., and Bernard, H.: Cryoprecipitate reversal of opsonic α_2 surface binding glycoprotein deficiency in septic surgical and trauma patients. Science, *201*:622, 1978.

77. Mosher, D.R., and Williams, E.M.: Fibronectin concentration is decreased in plasma of severely ill patients with disseminated intravascular coagulation. J. Lab. Clin. Med., *91*:729, 1978.

78. Saba, T.M., et al.: Reversal of fibronectin and opsonic deficiency in patients. Ann. Surg., *199*:87, 1984.

79. Stossel, T.P.: Phagocytosis: recognition and injestion. Serum Hematol., *12*:83, 1975.

80. Chaudry, I.H., and Baue, A.E.: The use of substrates and energy in the treatment of shock. Adv. Shock Res., *3*:27, 1980.

81. Marubayashi, S., et al.: Preservation of ischemic rat liver cell damages by CoQ_{10} administration through restoration of cellular calcium homeostasis. Eur. Surg. Res., *14*:68, 1982.

Chapter 9
INITIAL TREATMENT OF THE PATIENT IN TRAUMATIC SHOCK

John Barrett • Lloyd Nyhus

Although the physician may be called upon to treat a patient in shock in a number of different situations and for a variety of causes, perhaps the most dramatic example of a patient requiring prompt and correct treatment is the patient with multiple trauma presenting in a state of shock with life-threatening injuries. Serious injuries to the chest, head, abdomen, and extremities are common and frequently occur in combination. The physician may therefore be called upon to make a number of judgmental decisions as to what to treat first and how best to resuscitate the patient. These decisions have to be made rapidly, since the seriously traumatized patient may have only minutes to live. In addition, these decisions are frequently made under the most adverse of conditions and often with minimal history and diagnostic information. It is important, therefore, to have a preplanned systematic approach to such patients, based on finding and treating the most life-threatening injuries first.

Our approach to the trauma patient has been divided into a number of stages (Table 9–1).[1] The initial stage consists of a quick primary survey. This survey is designed to find immediate life-threatening injuries. These are injuries that are likely to kill the patient within minutes unless discovered and managed appropriately. The management of these life-threatening injuries is the second resuscitation phase of our approach. At the conclusion of the second phase, we should have a patient in whom all of the immediate life-threatening injuries have been identified and managed. Such patients should now be in a reasonably stable condition. At this time a more leisurely secondary survey can be conducted. This consists of a head-to-toe examination of the patient to find other injuries that may have been bypassed in the primary survey, but which may be a source of later morbidity or mortality. Included in this secondary survey are various diagnostic tests, roentgenograms, ECG, laboratory investigations, CT scans, and angiograms. Such investigations are not used in the primary survey because the initial examination is focused on immediate life-threatening injuries and no time is available for such studies. At the end of the secondary survey, we should now have found all of the injuries that the patient has received. This will allow us to proceed to the fourth (and final) stage of the definitive care phase. At this stage, plans can be made for the ultimate care of the patient, various consultative services can be informed, and a coordinated plan of management formulated. It is important at all times that the patient remain under the care of a single physician, who can coordinate and orchestrate the various consultative services.

Table 9-1.   Phases of Management of Trauma Patient.*

Phase 1	Initial assessment
Phase 2	Resuscitation
Phase 3	Secondary assessment
Phase 4	Definitive care

*Advanced Trauma Life Support Course, Committee on Trauma, American College of Surgeons.

PRIMARY SURVEY

The primary survey is focused on the three conditions that are the most likely to lead to death of the patient in the initial phase. These three systems are (A)irway, (B)reathing, and (C)irculation. This sequence, which is based on the likelihood of serious fatal outcome, must be followed. The treating physician should not become distracted from the correct sequence. On many occasions, the treating physician may at least initially be alone, or with minimal support staff. In such situations, it is futile to attempt to control external bleeding as an initial step when the patient may be dying because of an obstructed upper airway. Management of the upper airway takes precedence over all other interventional modalities.

"A" IS FOR AIRWAY

There are a number of possible causes of upper airway obstruction in a multiply traumatized patient. In many instances, the obstruction may be caused by foreign material lodged in the upper airway. Vomitus, blood, mucus, fragments of tissue and broken bones, as well as broken teeth and dentures are not uncommon obstructing agents. The initial attention therefore should be to the head and face of the patient. The patient's mouth should be opened and loose foreign bodies rapidly removed by suction. It is also important at this stage to place the patient on oxygen. An assistant, if available, should hold the mask as close as possible to the mouth and nose while the upper airway is being cleaned.

Despite the fact that foreign bodies are often encountered in the upper airway, the most common cause of upper airway obstruction in the multiple trauma patient is the tongue.[2] The patient may be unconscious and because of relaxation of the jaw muscles, the tongue falls backward and obstructs the upper airway. A number of methods can be used to bring the tongue forward and relieve the obstruction. The most tempting method is to tilt the head back. This will carry the mandible forward, which because of its muscular attachments carries the tongue forward with it. In the multiple trauma patient, however, there is a grave risk of cervical spine fracture. Undue movement of the neck in such patients may result in paraplegia. Because of this fear, movement of the neck during the initial stabilization of these patients is contraindicated. Patients who are considered at risk for cervical spine injury include all patients who have head or facial trauma, and all patients who are unconscious after an automobile accident or a fall. Such patients should have cervical spine stabilization initiated immediately, preferably at the scene of the accident and before transportation. Such cervical spine stabilization must be maintained during the initial management until the possibility of injury to the cervical spine can be eliminated by diagnostic examination.

Fortunately alternative methods of moving the tongue forward without movement of the neck are available. The entire mandible can be moved forward by means of a "jaw thrust." This consists of placing the fingers behind the angle of the mandible and thrusting it forward while the head and neck are maintained in a neutral position.[2] An alternative method is to grasp the chin and lift the chin forward, the so-called "chin-lift." This offers some additional advantages in that it can be performed with one hand, leaving the other hand free to occlude the nostrils should mouth-to-mouth ventilation be required. Directly grasping the tongue and pulling it forward is difficult and places the operator at risk of having a finger bitten.

If the patient's breathing improves after the tongue has been moved forward by means of the chin-lift or jaw-thrust, airway patency can then be maintained by means of a small, curved plastic oral airway or a nasopharyngeal airway. The tongue must, however, be moved forward before insertion of such devices. To blindly push an oral airway into the mouth of an unconscious patient will serve only to push the tongue further back into the upper airway and render a bad condition even worse.

If upper airway control cannot be achieved by simple suctioning or by manual methods such as those described, it becomes necessary to intubate the trachea. There are a number of methods available to do this.

Oral Endotracheal Intubation

To successfully accomplish an endotracheal intubation, it is necessary to visualize the vocal cords. There is considerable concern that in order to do this it is necessary to move the neck by extension.[1] This is especially so for casual practitioners. Such movement is contraindicated in patients with cervical spine injuries. Oral endotracheal intubation should be used if the patient is completely apneic.[1] In this situation, we are confronted with a respiratory arrest, and the quickest airway possible should be obtained. The completely apneic patient is unlikely to be successfully intubated by the nasotracheal route.

Nasotracheal Intubation

This can be successfully carried out in most patients who have some spontaneous respiratory activity. The advantages of this approach include the fact that it can be carried out without movement of the neck, there is less cuff trauma to the trachea after insertion, and the tube is easier to fix in position.[3] In addition, it is easier for the patient since he or she does not have to "chew on the tube" and can generally swallow saliva without difficulty.

Direct Surgical Control of the Upper Airway

Should all other methods fail to gain control of the airway, direct surgical access must be obtained. This may occur when attempts at nasotracheal intubation are unsuccessful or in instances of massive facial trauma when nasotracheal intubation is contraindicated.[4] The recommended surgical approach to the airway is by a cricothyroidotomy. This procedure has now replaced the slash tracheostomy.[5-7] Advantages of the cricothyroidotomy include the speed and ease with which it can be carried out. Although it is true that the cricothyroid membrane is somewhat soft, tracheostomy tubes can be left in position through a cricothyroidotomy for several days. Should the patient still require airway control at the end of that time, the cricothyroidotomy can be easily replaced with an elective tracheostomy.

"B" IS FOR BREATHING

Once definitive airway control has been achieved, attention should then be directed toward ensuring adequate oxygenation. The upper torso should be exposed by rapidly cutting off the clothes and exposing the anterior chest. Conditions causing immediate life-threatening respiratory embarrassment should then be sought.

Tension Pneumothorax

This occurs because the accumulation of air in one hemithorax increases the pressure with subsequent movement of the mediastinum. Venous return by the great veins is reduced, and the patient dies because of inadequate venous return.[8] Life-threatening tension pneumothorax should be recognized and managed clinically. Clinical findings in such situations include tense, distended neck veins, trachea shift to the contralateral side, absent air entry with hyperresonant percussion on the involved side. Treatment consists of immediate needle decompression followed by chest tube insertion.[1,9]

Chest tube insertion in traumatized patients should be carried out in the 4th or 5th intercostal space (nipple level) at the midaxillary line. This will place the chest tube above the dome of the diaphragm and allow the tip of the tube to be directed posteriorly to drain the paravertebral gutter. All such chest tubes should be inserted by way of an open tube thoracostomy. Blind, or percutaneous, insertion of such tubes runs the risk of perforation of vital organs. This is especially true in trauma patients in whom chest tubes are frequently placed without preinsertion roentgenograms. Some patients may have diaphragmatic ruptures with herniation of liver or spleen into the chest. Blind, or percutaneous, insertion in these instances is extremely hazardous.

Sucking Chest Wounds

A sucking chest wound, or open pneumothorax, allows the equilibration of intrathoracic and atmospheric pressures. Such patients are effectively unable to breathe. The size of the defect does not have to be large; a defect approximating the size of the patient's trachea can be life-threatening. Any sucking chest wound should be considered to be serious and should be treated promptly. Treatment consists of immediate closure of the defect. This can generally be accomplished by occluding the hole with gauze packs and dressings to obtain an air-tight seal. This will convert the open pneumothorax into a closed pneumothorax. Such patients are now at risk of developing a tension pneumothorax. Because of this, all such patients should have a chest tube inserted.

Flail Chest

In flail chest, a segment of chest wall lacks continuity with the remaining chest. It occurs when a number of rib or sternal fractures allow a segment of the chest wall to become loose or "flail." Such conditions can be relatively easily recognized by the paradoxic movement of the flail segment. When the patient inhales, the flail segment will collapse, and when the patient exhales, it will expand. This paradoxic movement of the segment is characteristic and diagnostic of a flail chest.

Although it may be tempting to manage such patients by attempting to stabilize the flail segment in some manner, the initial emergency management of the flail segment in the primary survey stage of resuscitation is different. Such patients are dying because of respiratory embarrassment. Resuscitation should therefore consist of relief of the respiratory problem. Recommended treatment in this instance consists of airway intubation and volume-cycled ventilation.[10] Volume ventilation, as opposed to pressure-cycled ventilation, is recommended because the presence of the flail and the underlying pulmonary contusions will alter the compliance of the chest so that pressure-cycled ventilation will result in inadequate tidal volumes. An additional benefit from such volume-cycled ventilations is that they create an "internal pneumatic stabilization" of the flail segment.

"C" IS FOR CIRCULATION

Under this heading are considered disorders of the cardiac and circulatory system.

Cardiac Tamponade

This occurs because of the accumulation of blood between the rigid overlying pericardium and the underlying compressible cardiac chambers. Such conditions can occur after both blunt and penetrating chest trauma. The small pericardial knife wound of the stiletto type is particularly dangerous in this regard. Such injuries can create a small hole in the pericardium, allowing the blood from the underlying cardiac injury to accumulate and produce the tamponade.

As the blood accumulates in the pericardial space, the pressure begins to rise. Ultimately, the pressure will become great enough to occlude the atria and the small portions of the superior and inferior vena cava within the pericardial sac. The venous return to the heart is impaired and the patient dies because of inadequate venous return.[11] This mechanism of death is identical to that caused by the tension pneumothorax; some clinical confusion can occur when attempting to differentiate the two conditions. In tension pneumothorax, however, there should be tracheal deviation because of the mediastinal shift, and also absent breath sounds. Such findings may be difficult to elicit with certainty in a busy and noisy emergency department. Should confusion exist as to which condition is present, it is better to treat the injury as if it were a tension pneumothorax. The initial needle decompression is diagnostic and not particularly hazardous.

In the presence of a known or suspected cardiac tamponade, needle pericardiocentesis should be performed. This is best done by a subxiphoid approach, decreasing the likelihood of pneumothorax and lessening the possibility of myocardial and coronary vessel injury. The needle should be directed upward and to the left at a 45° angle to the vertical and horizontal axes. An easy method to remember is to direct the needle as if it were to strike the inferior border of the left scapula.[1] Attachment of an ECG "V" lead to the needle by an alligator clip is helpful in preventing cardiac injury. Once such a needle touches the myocardium, an injury pattern will be apparent and the needle can be withdrawn slightly. Aspiration of blood from within the pericardial sac confirms the diagnosis.

Once the diagnosis of pericardial tamponade has been confirmed in this situation, all such patients should undergo thoracotomy in the operating room. To observe such patients, awaiting the reaccumulation of the tamponade, is hazardous and results in an unacceptably high mortality.

Control of External Bleeding

External bleeding is best controlled by direct pressure. Blind clamping in the depths of actively bleeding wounds is to be condemned. It will only result in injuries to the associated structures in the neurovascular bundle. Injuries to the vein are difficult to repair, and crushing the nerve with a clamp in an attempt to control bleeding may result in serious and permanent neurologic impairment. Even if the transected arterial vessel can be identified in the wound, such vessels should not be clamped unless vascular clamps are available. Regular clamps will crush the ends of the vessels. This will frequently result in such damage that the crushed ends will ultimately require resection. Such injuries will then require interposition-reversed venous grafts instead of simple direct reanastamosis.

Venous Access

Venous access in the multiply traumatized patient has traditionally been obtained by central lines placed by subclavian or internal jugular venous access. Such lines, in general, are not placed to obtain the central venous pressure (CVP) readings. Traumatized patients who present in shock can be assumed to be in hemorrhagic shock and the CVP can be assumed to be low. Central access has been used because it affords a method of venous access in a situation in which the peripheral veins are frequently collapsed and inaccessible.

The challenge in administering fluids to such patients is to obtain a large-bore venous access. The position of the catheter is of secondary importance. It is better in these situations to have a large-bore peripheral catheter than a small-bore central one. If the physician is uncomfortable with central venous access, or unable to obtain such access (as in young children), then there should be no hesitation in resorting to direct venous cutdown. Suitable veins for cutdown include the long saphenous vein above and anterior to the medial malleolus. The long saphenous vein can also be directly approached in the groin, although care should be taken in these circumstances to prevent injury to the femoral vein. Antecubital venous access can also be obtained in the antecubital fossae of the upper extremities. Once large-bore venous access has been obtained, fluid resuscitation, as described in Chapter 2, can be carried out.

At this stage the patient should now have been returned to a relatively stable situation. Once this has occurred, the secondary survey can be conducted and additional diagnostic tests obtained to detect more subtle and occult injuries.

In a small number of instances it may prove impossible to resuscitate the patient out of the shock state. In general this will indicate a source of continued bleeding. Should such be the case, no time should be lost in obtaining appropriate surgical intervention. The patient who exhibits bleeding through a chest tube to a volume of more that 1,000 ml following initial insertion or continued bleeding at greater than 250 ml/hr will almost certainly require surgical control of the bleeding site. Similarly the patient who presents in hemorrhagic shock with blunt or penetrating abdominal trauma, and who despite adequate volume replacement cannot be resuscitated, should undergo immediate surgical exploration. In these instances surgical intervention becomes part of the resuscitative phase. Such multiply traumatized patients require immediate access to surgical services and should be managed in appropriately equipped and staffed facilities.

Trauma is now the leading cause of death of persons younger than 37 years of age. Apart from the enormous human tragedy in the loss of these lives, such deaths and disabilities are a grave socioeconomic burden to the community at large. A number of such deaths are preventable. It is particularly tragic when such preventable deaths occur after the patient has reached a hospital setting. Strict attention to the correct sequence in the management of such multiple-trauma patients is paramount. A correctly performed initial primary survey and resuscitation phase for every patient presenting with hemorrhagic shock following trauma go a long way toward reducing the enormous loss of young lives to trauma.

REFERENCES

1. Advanced Trauma Life Support Course. Committee on Trauma, American College of Surgeons, Chicago, 1981.
2. Committee on Trauma, American College of Surgeons: Early Care of the Injured Patient. Philadelphia, W.B. Saunders Co., 1982.
3. Jacoby, J.: Nasal endothracheal intubation by an external visual technique. Anesth. Analg., *49*:73, 1970.
4. Tintinalli, J.E.: Complications of nasotracheal intubation. Ann. Emerg. Med., *10*:142, 1981.
5. Brantigan, C.O.: Cricothyroidotomy elective use in respiratory problems requiring tracheotomy. J. Thorac. Cardiovasc. Surg., *71*:72, 1976.
6. Mitchell, S.A.: Cricothyroidostomy revisited. Ear Nose Throat J., *58*:214, 1979.
7. Brantigan, C.O.: Cricothyroidotomy revisted again. Ear Nose Throat J., *59*:26, 1980.
8. Ballinger, W.F., Rutherford, R.B., and Zuidema, G.D.: The Management of Trauma. Philadelphia, W.B. Saunders Co., 1968.
9. Kirsh, M.M., and Shoan, H.: Blunt Chest Trauma: General Principles of Management. Boston, Little, Brown and Co., 1977.
10. Sabiston, D.C., and Spencer, F.C.: Gibbon's Surgery of the Chest. Philadelphia, W.B. Saunders Co., 1983.
11. Symbas, P.N.: Trauma to the Heart and Great Vessels. New York, Grune & Stratton, 1978.

Chapter 10

TREATMENT OF SEPTIC SHOCK

Michael F. Adinolfi • William St. John LaCorte • Ronald Lee Nichols

Shock is a distinct clinical entity with multiple causes, including sepsis, hypovolemia, and cardiogenic, anaphylactic and neurogenic factors. It can be universally characterized by inadequate tissue perfusion, reduced blood pressure, and an increased pulse rate. This description of shock may be translated into two words that characterize physiologically its biologic state: *anaerobic metabolism,* a condition that always ensues when there is hypotension and decreased tissue perfusion.[1] Thal[2] believes that the shock state represents a survival mechanism in which blood is shunted to vital organs at the expense of anaerobic metabolism elsewhere in the body. Septic shock is a specific clinical syndrome that is characterized by systemic sepsis with evidence of circulatory insufficiency and inadequate tissue perfusion.

To the practicing clinician, septic shock may be a challenging diagnostic as well as therapeutic dilemma. Transient bacteremia in a compromised host may easily lead to septicemia, septic shock, and death. The usual originating sites for the bacteremia include skin, gastrointestinal, urinary, and respiratory infections.

Aerobic gram-negative bacilli account for 40 to 60% of all bacteremias, while anaerobes account for 8 to 12%.[3] Of the anaerobes, *Bacteroides fragilis* is the most common, accounting for 70 to 80% of all anaerobic bacteremias. The lipopolysaccharide capsule found in some bacteroides species is not, however, a biologically active endotoxin that can cause the hemodynamic changes found in the usual case of aerobic gram-negative shock. The predominant aerobic gram-negative organisms isolated from bacteremias are listed in Table 10–1.

RISK FACTORS

Many host factors can alter human resistance and render an individual susceptible to bacterial invasion. If infection occurs and becomes established, these factors play a determining role in both the outcome of the infection and in the death of the patient. Localized infections spread easily in the compromised host, causing systemic sepsis and distant infection.

Knowledge of the population at risk and a high index of suspicion are the keys to early diagnosis and treatment. Patients at increased risk for sepsis and septic shock are those whose immune system has been altered by an underlying systemic disorder such as diabetes mellitus, cirrhosis, malnutrition, and advanced age.

Another group of patients at increased risk are those with an underlying carcinoma, lymphoma, or leukemia. In addition to their predisposing underlying disorder, these patients are further compromised by medical therapy, which frequently includes radiotherapy, chemotherapy, and immunotherapy. Alone or in

Table 10-1.   Predominant Aerobic Gram-Negative Isolates in Bacteremia.

Organism	% of isolation from all instances of bacteremia
Escherichia coli	30–40
Klebsiella	15–20
Pseudomonas	10–15
Proteus	5–10
Enterobacter	5–10
Serratia	3–5
Others	5–10

combination, these factors dramatically alter host defense mechanisms and place the host at an increased risk for septic complications.

Another subset of patients at increased risk are transplant recipients or patients with prosthetic devices. Patients who undergo major thoracic or abdominal operations are at increased risk, as are those who have prolonged stays in an intensive care unit, have indwelling catheters or central lines in place for a prolonged period, or who are ventilator-dependent, requiring prolonged intubation.

PATHOPHYSIOLOGY

The pathophysiology of gram-negative sepsis and septic shock is complex and is described in more detail in other chapters. Bacterial endotoxin is the most readily identifiable microbial component responsible for septic shock. Endotoxin is the lipopolysaccharide component of the cell wall found in all aerobic gram-negative bacteria. Endotoxin exerts a variety of negative effects upon the circulatory system, including arteriolar and venular vasoconstriction in the renal, mesenteric, and pulmonic circulation. This leads to tissue hypoperfusion, hypoxia, and subsequent anaerobic metabolism with lactic acidosis. If the condition is allowed to continue untreated, there is subsequent arteriolar vasodilation but persistent venule vasoconstriction. Acidosis persists, hydrostatic pressure increases, and there is leakage of plasma into the interstitial third space. The effective circulatory volume decreases, causing further reflex vasoconstriction and further local anoxia and acidosis, with subsequent tissue damage. Further tissue damage results from venous microthrombosis.

Endotoxin also directly damages the endothelium of cells, causing release of vasoactive peptides. These peptides activate the complement and coagulation systems. Vasoactive peptides cause activation of Factor XII, which converts kallikreinogen to kallikrein, bradykinin, and other active peptides. These kinins cause further vasodilation and increased capillary permeability.

Activation of Factor XII also initiates the intrinsic system in the coagulation cascade. Fibrin thrombi become deposited in the vascular tree, causing further hypoxia, acidosis, and tissue damage. As this continues, coagulation factors are consumed, and the platelet count and fibrinogen levels in the blood decrease.

Further deposition of fibrin leads to activation of the fibrinolytic system. Fibrin split products are formed, and as the coagulation factors continue to be consumed, hemorrhage results. Laboratory analysis at this time reveals a prolonged prothrombin time, thrombocytopenia, decreased serum fibrinogen levels, and the presence of fibrin degradation products.

Endotoxin can also activate the complement system by the alternative pathway and to a lesser extent through the classic pathway. Complement consumption enhances the inflammatory process, promotes tissue damage, and increases capillary permeability.

Sepsis and the shock state affect a wide variety of organs and organ function. Both right and left ventricular performances are affected by cell membrane depolarization and dysfunction of intracellular organelles.[4] A hyperdynamic state characterized by an increased cardiac output and low systemic vascular resistance is common in septic shock.

Lefer[5] writes that in septic shock hypoxia damages lysozymal membranes in cells within the pancreas and splanchnic region, allowing release of a substance that acts as a negative inotropic agent causing myocardial depression. The issue of myocardial inhibitory factors, however, remains controversial.

DIAGNOSIS AND INTERVENTION

Septicemia with the syndrome of septic shock is an evolving dynamic process that requires aggressive medical and surgical intervention. Care of these critically ill patients calls for invasive monitoring. The diagnosis of shock is based on persistent hypotension and decreased tissue perfusion. The clinician must identify the cause of the shock state. In critically ill patients, more than one cause of circulatory failure may be present.

Regardless of the cause of the shock state, treatment should begin simultaneously with diagnostic evaluation. Early diagnosis and intervention are essential to ensure a high survival rate by treating sepsis before septic shock occurs.

History, physical examination, and the clinical setting often are helpful in identifying hypovolemic, cardiogenic, or spinal shock. Once again, as in all critically ill patients, a high index of suspicion is always helpful. Remembering the groups of patients at high risk may add further clues to the diagnosis of septic shock. Similarly, a current history of respiratory, skin, urinary, or gastrointestinal infections or recent abdominal or urologic operative intervention may guide the clinician to look for sepsis as a cause of the hypotension.

In septic shock the skin may be dry, warm, and pink. Fever, chills, and tachypnea are usually present, as are mental confusion and oliguria. Hypotension and tachycardia are common. Lactic acidosis or respiratory alkalosis secondary to tachypnea may be present.

Most patients have leukocytosis with a shift to immature forms of polymorphonuclear leukocytes. Thrombocytopenia may be seen in 50 to 60% of patients with gram-negative sepsis, although the classic findings of decreased fibrinogen level, presence of fibrin degradation products, and prolonged prothrombin time may be seen only in 5% of the instances. Appropriate Gram stains and cultures of exudates, blood, sputum, and urine may give a clue to the site or nature of the offending bacteria.

PORTALS OF ENTRY AND CAUSATIVE BACTERIA

Before an organized search for the origin of the sepsis is begun, the patient must be stabilized and treatment started. Knowledge of common portals of entry causing gram-negative bacteremia is vital. In virtually all studies, the urinary tract is the most common portal and may account for 30 to 40% of all instances of bacteremia.[6,7] The respiratory tract is the second most common portal, accounting for 15 to 20% of instances, especially in the hospitalized, intubated patient. Intra-abdominal or pelvic abscesses account for another 10 to 15%, while the surgical wound may be the causative site in 5 to 10% of instances. Burn wounds and phlebitis account for another 10%.

Ascending cholangitis may also cause septic shock. Studies[8,9] have shown that the coliforms, including most commonly Escherichia coli and Klebsiella, are the most frequent offending organisms.

As mentioned previously, the urinary tract is the most common source of bacteremia causing septic shock. The organisms usually involved in this setting are coliforms (especially E. coli), Pseudomonas, and enterococci.

Hospital-acquired pneumonia is usually secondary to invasion by the coliforms or Pseudomonas, especially in patients requiring prolonged ventilatory support.[10] Less frequently penumococci or Staphylococcus aureus may cause pneumonia and subsequent sepsis without evidence of the shock syndrome. Appropriate Gram stains or tracheal aspirations are extremely helpful in differentiating gram-positive from gram-negative pneumonia.

Female genital infections involve both aerobic and anaerobic organisms similar to those isolated from the lower gastrointestinal tract.[11,12]

Catheter sepsis is seen most commonly in patients receiving hyperalimentation. Candida albicans is a common causative yeast as are Staphylococcus, Klebsiella, Pseudomonas, and Serratia. If catheter sepsis is the suspected source, appropriate therapy initially is to remove the catheter and to culture its tip.[13] In most instances this is the only therapy necessary.

MONITORING

An aggressive, invasive approach to the monitoring of the patient in septic shock is always indicated. A Foley catheter should be placed aseptically to monitor hourly urine output. An arterial line for continuous blood pressure monitoring and access for arterial blood gas analysis is extremely useful and is recommended. Patency of the ulnar artery should be determined by the Allen test prior to radial artery cannulation for monitoring.

Thermodilution Swan-Ganz catheters are extremely helpful, both diagnostically and as a guide to therapy.[14] A characteristic finding in septic shock is a high cardiac output with a low systemic vascular resistance, the so-called "hyperdynamic state." Monitoring the pulmonary artery pressure and the wedge pressure can guide the clinician to proper management of the patient's volume status. Once the volume status has been maximized, as determined by the wedge pressure, treatment can then employ inotropic or dopaminergic agents to further stabilize the vascular status of the patient and correct any persistent hypotension.

Continuous electrocardiographic monitoring should also be used in these critically ill patients. It should allow for immediate detection and treatment of any arrhythmia that may occur secondary to electrolyte abnormalities or hypoxemia.

Progressive respiratory dysfunction may occur in these patients. If serially determined arterial blood gases reveal progressive hypercarbia and hypoxemia, intubation and mechanical ventilation may be required to correct these respiratory abnormalities.

Serial measurements of blood lactate levels may reflect improved perfusion and act as indicators of successful treatment.[15] Blood pH, electrolytes, blood urea nitrogen (BUN) level, creatinine clearances, hematocrit reading, platelet count, and coagulation profiles should also be monitored closely.

LOCALIZING THE SEPTIC SOURCE

Once the patient's condition has been stabilized cardiovascularly and treatment begun, an organized diagnostic evaluation may be undertaken. A careful history and physical examination are the most important first steps in this search. Knowledge of the common portals of entry and their frequency of occurence is also essential.

As mentioned previously, the urinary and respiratory tract account for 40 to 60% of all gram-negative septic episodes. Localizing these infections may not present much difficulty to the alert clinician. Urinalysis is a quick, reliable, and accurate test. The presence of bacteria, red and white blood cells, and casts are important diagnostic clues to urinary sepsis and possible acute pyelonephritis. The intravenous pyelogram (IVP) and computerized tomographic (CT) scan are not diagnostic or reliable in this setting, unless a perinephric abscess is considered to be the source of the sepsis. An IVP may be indicated, however, to rule out obstruction.

Gram stain and culture of sputum samples, collected either by having the patient cough or by tracheal aspiration, in conjunction with the chest roentgenogram should alert the clinician to a pulmonary source of sepsis.

An intra-abdominal or retroperitoneal abscess poses a difficult diagnostic challenge. Most abdominal abscesses result from spontaneous intra-abdominal diseases and less commonly result from abdominal trauma. In one study,[16] 71% of intra-abdominal abscesses developed spontaneously following appendicitis or diverticulitis, whereas 29% arose as a complication of various operations or procedures. The accuracy of CT scans in this series was 92%, while ultrasonography was 77% and gallium scanning 75% accurate. In a similar study,[17] ultrasonography was observed to be 75% accurate, whereas CT scans were 71% accurate. One should choose the procedure that is best done at each individual hospital. One advantage that CT scans do offer the clinician is the possibility of percutaneous drainage of the abscess. Percutaneous drainage may be a safe, reliable therapeutic tool as pointed out by several authors.[18-20] Those authors emphasize, however, several criteria that should be adhered to if percutaneous drainage is to be attempted. They are 1. a unilocular fluid collection; 2. a safe percutaneous access route; 3. joint radiologic and surgical evaluation; 4. surgical standby; 5. avoidance of penetrating sterile cavities; 6. extraperitoneal, dependent drainage; and 7. an experienced radiologist. The overall success rate in these series of percutaneous drainage was 86% with a complication rate of 8 to 15%.

Sepsis arising from a surgical wound is readily identified if the wound is inspected. The hallmarks of wound infection include local warmth, swelling, redness, and tenderness. Crepitance and bulla formation may be seen in clostridial or streptococcal infections. Immediate Gram staining will often identify the offending bacteria.

The burn wound may be a portal of entry for gram-negative bacteria in 5% of instances of gram-negative bacteremias. Bacterial invasion of the burn occurs both from the surface of the wound and from the deeper epidermal appendages. Two phases of burn-wound sepsis can occur. Early colonization of the burn wound, occurring 1 to 3 days after the injury is usually caused by gram-positive organisms such as beta-hemolytic streptococci and S. aureus.[21] Late burn-wound sepsis is usually gram-negative, with Pseudomonas aeruginosa, Proteus, Providentia stuartii, and Serratia being the major offenders. Bacteriologic monitoring of the burn wound surface is not helpful in diagnosing burn-wound sepsis. The most reliable way to make the diagnosis is with qualitative and quantitative biopsy and culture of the burn wound. More than 100,000 microorganisms per gram of tissue is diagnostic of burn-wound sepsis. It should be noted that Candida is currently being seen with increased frequency as a causative organism in burn-wound sepsis.

Phlebitis secondary to intravenous catheters should not be forgotten as a possible source of sepsis. Careful inspection of peripheral intravenous access sites may reveal erythema, a palpable cord or purulent drainage from the insertion site. Central venous catheters should be suspect when no other source is encountered. Removal of these, with Gram stain and culture of the catheter tip, may be both diagnostic and therapeutic. Rarely, excision of the involved vein may be necessary to eliminate the infection effectively.

PRINCIPLES OF TREATMENT

The mainstay of therapy in septic shock is to find and treat the underlying disorder. In all instances this includes surgical drainage of any localized collection of infection and appropriate antimicrobial therapy as well as supportive care.

No supportive regimen of antibiotics can be suggested that would be appropriate for all patients. Instead, the choice should be tailored to the clinical setting according to predicted pathogens for the suspected portal of entry (Table 10–2). Several points, however, should be adhered to. The intravenous route should be routinely employed and antibiotics should be given in sufficient dosages to achieve a therapeutic blood level. An aminoglycoside should be included in all regimens in which gram-negative sepsis is suspected. This recommendation is based on the high rates of resistance to alternative agents. Aminoglycoside agents considered adequate include gentamicin, tobramycin, netilmycin, or amikacin. The choice among these agents depends on the cost, on individual physician preference, and on the resistance profiles in each hospital. Also, in order to expand the spectrum of antibiotic coverage, two agents should be employed initially. One should use antibiotics that provide activity against anaerobes or aerobic gram-positive bacteria that may cause shock. Once culture results are available, the initial antibiotic regimen should be modified or changed according to the culture and susceptibility results. The clinician should also have knowledge of the sensitivity patterns of organisms in the individual hospital's environment.

Other supportive measures are essential for survival. Adequate tissue oxygenation must be maintained with oxygen administered either by aerosol mask or tracheal intubation and assisted ventilation if indicated. Aggressive volume replacement is the initial therapeutic modality imperative in instances of hypotension due to sepsis. The hematocrit level should be monitored and maintained at an adequate level. Crystalloids or colloids may be given to optimize the cardiac output and pulmonary artery capillary wedge pressure, thus preventing stagnant anoxia and lactic acidosis.

Table 10–2. Antibiotic Selection for Severely Ill Patients with Suspected Gram-Negative Bacteremia.

Portal of Entry	Anticipated Pathogens	Antimicrobials
Urinary tract	Coliforms Pseudomonas Enterococci	Aminoglycoside + Ampicillin
Lower respiratory tract	Coliforms, Pseudomonas Streptococcus pneumoniae Staphylococcus aureus	Aminoglycoside + Cephalosporin or Carbenicillin, Ticarcillin
Biliary tract	Coliforms Enterococci	Aminoglycoside + Ampicillin or Cephalosporin
Intra-abdominal sepsis	Coliforms Anaerobes	Aminoglycoside + Clindamycin or Cefoxitin or Chloramphenicol or Metronidazole
Female genital tract	Coliforms Anaerobes	Aminoglycoside + Clindamycin or Cefoxitin or Chloramphenicol or Metronidazole
IV catheter	Coliforms Pseudomonas S. aureus	Aminoglycoside + Cephalosporin or Oxacillin
Site unknown		Aminoglycoside + Cephalosporin or Carbenicillin, Ticarcillin or Oxacillin

The use of steroids remains controversial. Some authors have found them to be effective.[22,23] If they are used, steroids should be administered early, in sufficient dosages (methylprednisolone 30 mg/kg or dexamethasone 3 mg/kg), and for a short period of time (not exceeding a total of two doses).

Vasoactive drugs and inotropic agents are indicated only after adequate volume replacement has failed to raise the blood pressure. Two useful agents are dopamine (2 to 10 μg/min) and isoproterenol (2 to 8 μg/min). Both can cause an increased cardiac output and an increase in blood pressure. Dopamine has the added advantage of increasing renal perfusion.

Only with careful monitoring and frequent observation can the morbidity and mortality in these critically ill patients be decreased.

REFERENCES

1. McSwain, N.E.: Objective approach to the management of shock. Comp. Ther., *7(9)*:7, 1981.
2. Thal, A.P.: Shock: A Physiological Basis for Treatment. Chicago, Year Book Medical Publishers, Inc., 1971.
3. Gorbach, S.L., Bartlett, J.G., and Nichols, R.L.: Manual of Surgical Infections. Boston, Little, Brown and Co., 1984.
4. Weisul, J.P., et al.: Myocardial performance in clinical septic shock: effects of isoproterenol and glucose–potassium–insulin. J. Surg. Res., *18*:357, 1975.
5. Lefer, A.M.: Properties of cardio-inhibitory factors produced in shock. Fed. Proc. *37*:2734, 1978.
6. McCabe, W.R., and Jackson, G.C.: Gram negative bacteremia. I. Etiology and ecology. Arch. Intern. Med., *110*:847, 1962.

7. Altemeier, W.A., Todel, J.C., and Inge, W.W.: Gram negative septicemia: a growing threat. Ann. Surg., *166*:530, 1967.
8. Scott, A.J., and Khan, G.A.: Origin of bacteria in bile duct bile. Lancet, *2*:790, 1967.
9. Fukunaga, F.H.: Gallbladder bacteriology, histology, and gallstones. Arch. Surg., *106*:169, 1973.
10. Sanford, J.P., and Pierce, A.: Current infection problems—Respiratory. Proceedings of International Conference on Nosocomial Infection, Centers for Disease Control. Chicago, American Hospital Association, August 1970.
11. Thadepalli, H., Gorbach, S.L., and Keith, L.: Anaerobic infections of the female genital tract: bacteriological and therapeutic aspects. Am. J. Obstet. Gynecol., *117*:1034, 1973.
12. Rotheram, E.B., Jr, and Schick, S.F.: Nonclostridial anaerobic bacteria in septic abortion. Am. J. Med., *46*:80, 1969.
13. Bentley, D.W., and Lepper, M.H.: Septicemia related to indwelling venous catheter. J.A.M.A., *206*:1749, 1968.
14. Swan, H.J.C., and Ganz, W.: The use of balloon flotation catheters in critically ill patients, Surg. Clin. North Am., *55*:501, 1975.
15. Weil, M.H., and Afifi, A.A.: Experimental and clinical studies on lactate and pyruvate indicators of acute circulatory failure (shock). Circulation, *41*:989, 1970.
16. Saini, S., Kellum, J.M., and O'Leary, M.P.: Improved localization and survival in patients with intraabominal abscesses. Am. J. Surg., *145*:136, 1983.
17. Norton, L., Eule, J., and Burdick, D.: Accuracy of techniques to detect intraperitoneal abscess. Surgery, *84*:370, 1978.
18. van Sonnenberg, E., Ferrucci, J., Jr, and Mueller, P.R.: Percutaneous drainage of abscesses and fluid collections: technique, results, and applications. Radiology, *142*:1, 1982.
19. Johnson, W.C., et al.: Treatment of abdominal abscesses: comparative evaluation of operative drainage versus percutaneous catheter drainage guided by computed tomography or ultrasound. Ann. Surg., *194*:510, 1981.
20. Gerzof, S.: Percutaneous catheter drainage of abdominal abscesses: five-year experience. N Engl. J. Med., *305*:653, 1981.
21. Berk, J.L., et al.: Handbook of Critical Care. Boston, Little, Brown and Co., 1976.
22. Schumer, W.: Steroids in the treatment of clinical septic shock. Ann. Surg., *184*:333, 1976.
23. Hinshaw, L.B., et al.: Effectiveness of steroid/antibiotic treatment in primates administered LD_{100} Escherichia coli. Ann. Surg., *194*:51, 1981.

Chapter 11
IMMUNE RESPONSE TO SHOCK

Matti Salo

Immune defense mechanisms have become increasingly important with the progress made in the treatment of patients undergoing major operations or sustaining severe injuries or burns. Advances in recent decades in the treatment of shock have greatly improved prognosis, but now many of these patients die of multiple organ failure (MOF). Sepsis is present in the background of most instances of MOF.[1] Several factors of the immune response are depressed by major surgical procedures, severe injuries, and burns. Simultaneously, the epithelial barriers are broken, and the patients are predisposed to increased amounts of infectious material. The immune response is thus the weak link in recovery. Immunologic aspects should, therefore, be considered carefully. Modern immunology can already offer several possibilities for the treatment of patients in a state of shock.

IMMUNE DEFENSE MECHANISMS

The immune defense mechanisms beyond the epithelial barriers are phagocytosis and complement, cell-mediated and humoral immunity, which work in complicated interaction with one another and other homeostatic mechanisms.

Phagocytosis

The phagocytic system comprises polymorphonuclear leukocytes and cells of the mononuclear phagocyte system (MPS), better known as the reticuloendothelial system (RES).

POLYMORPHONUCLEAR LEUKOCYTES

More than 90% of polymorphs are neutrophils, which are important effector cells for many types of infections in the bloodstream and tissues and the first to arrive at the site of action. There are about 6×10^8 neutrophils/kg body weight in the blood circulation. About half of the intravascular pool adheres to the endothelial lining of the blood vessels (marginated pool), while the other half circulates (circulating pool). The two pools are in a dynamic equilibrium and may be enlarged at the expense of each other. The half-life of neutrophils in the circulation is 6 to 7 hr. Thereafter the neutrophils enter the tissues without reentering the circulation. In infection and injury neutrophils from the blood migrate more rapidly into the tissues in the direction of chemotactic stimuli. The bone marrow reserves of about 9×10^9 granulocytes/kg body weight may also be mobilized with an increased maturation rate.

The phagocytic process has four phases: chemotaxis, opsonization, ingestion, and bacterial killing. Chemotactic stimuli from the host or bacterial products direct the neutrophils to the site of action. The microbes are then opsonized to facilitate the uptake of the invader. This means coating of the microbe by opsonic plasma proteins which in the clearance of most bacteria is performed by antibodies and the C_{3b} and C_{5b} fragments of activated complement. The microbes are then ingested by neutrophils and killed by enzymatic and oxidative processes.

RETICULOENDOTHELIAL SYSTEM

The reticuloendothelial system is composed of blood monocytes and tissue macrophages. The monocytes are phagocytic cells and respond to chemotactic stimuli in the manner of neutrophils, but they arrive at the site of microbial invasion at a slower rate. Their half-life in the circulation is 36 to 104 hr. From the bloodstream the monocytes migrate into the tissues, where they differentiate into macrophages. These occur in the liver (Kupffer cells), spleen, lymph nodes, bone marrow, adrenal glands, brain (glial cells), skin (Langerhans cells), lungs (alveolar macrophages), and all over the body as wandering macrophages. A major portion of the RES consists of fixed macrophages lining the blood sinusoids of the liver, spleen, and bone marrow. Hepatic Kupffer cells are responsible for 80 to 85% of RES clearance capacity, while the spleen accounts for another 10 to 15%.

The primary role of the RES is the intravascular clearance of micro-organisms, endotoxins, and debris (injured cells, immune complexes, collagenous tissue debris, and intravascular coagulation products), but macrophages also have immune regulatory functions and a great variety of other important tasks. They are capable of secreting more than 50 products into their environment.

Plasma fibronectin is an important RES opsonin with its plasma concentration correlating with RES phagocytic capacity. When fibronectin concentrations decrease, RES dysfunction occurs with decreased hepatic uptake of blood-borne particulates and their increased extrahepatic localization. This may result in pulmonary insufficiency and other microvascular disturbances common in trauma and sepsis.

Complement

The complement accounts for 5% of plasma proteins. The system consists of eleven components, from C_{1q}, C_{1r}, and C_{1s} to C_9. The complement releases peptides active in inflammation, facilitates phagocytosis by opsonization, lyses invading organisms, and participates in immunoregulation. The components are normally in a dynamic inactive state. When the complement is activated, the components are sequentially involved in an event similar to the coagulation cascade. The individual components are cleaved into two or more fragments, one continuing the sequence and the others contributing to the inflammatory process and phagocytosis. The process is controlled by a balance between activator and inhibitor proteins and by the short half-lives of some activated components.

The complement may be activated by the classic or alternative pathways, both of which have the same biologic effects. The classic pathway is activated by an antibody-antigen complex, i.e., its activation requires the action of IgM, IgG_3, IgG_1, or IgG_2 against the invading organisms. By contrast, the alternative pathway may be activated by endotoxic lipopolysaccharides, teichoic acid, or other polysaccharides present in the walls of micro-organisms. The alternative pathway thus forms a defense system in a nonimmune host before generation of the antibody reponse. However, several microbes can activate the classic pathway also in the absence of antibodies. C_3 is a key component of complement combining the classic and alternative pathways. The terminal reactions are then triggered by activation of C_5 through C_6, C_7, and C_8 to C_9. Active fragments such as anaphylatoxins (C_{3a} and C_{5a}), opsonins (C_{3b} and C_{5b}), and chemotaxins (C_{3a}, C_{5a} and $\overline{C_{567}}$) are released along the activation process. These cleavage products active in the inflammatory reaction and phagocytosis may be even more important in host defenses than the final activation product $\overline{C_{56789}}$, which lyses the target cell.

Cell-Mediated Immunity

Cell-mediated immunity is the portion of the specific immune response mediated by T lymphocytes. The main subpopulations of T cells are T-helper/inducer and T-suppressor/cytotoxic cells. Contact with antigen triggers the afferent arm of the specific immune response. Macrophages take up and process the antigen and present it to T-helper lymphocytes. These activate macrophages to produce interleukin 1, a lymphocyte-activating factor. The T-helper cells, thus stimulated, release interleukin 2, which activates T- and B-effector lymphocytes. Interleukins 1 and 2 are important leukocyte transmitters, but interleukin 1 is also an inducer of the acute phase response and a factor in the release of protein catabolism in major trauma and sepsis.[2] The effector arm of cell-mediated immunity is concerned with the function of T lymphocytes on target cells (T-killer cells) and lymphokines, products of activated T lymphocytes. There are several lymphokines with nonspecific immunologic function. Chemotactic lymphokines attract macrophages to the site of antigenic stimulation, the migration inhibitory factor (MIF) retains monocytes at the site of microbial invasion, and the macrophage activating factor (MAF) activates macrophages to become potent effector cells.

Humoral Immunity

Humoral immunity is the portion of the specific immune response mediated by B lymphocytes, which together with their progeny, plasma cells, are involved in the production of specific immunoglobulins after antigenic stimulation. In the primary immune response B lymphocytes respond to antigens with or without the cooperation of T-helper cells after the antigen has been processed by macrophages. The primary immune response is provoked when a nonimmune host first encounters a foreign organism. The response consists of B-cell clonal proliferation and differentiation into immunoglobulin-producing plasma cells. In the secondary immune response, on repeat exposure to the antigen, macrophage processing is no longer necessary. The response is now more rapid and produces larger numbers of antibodies.

IMMUNE RESPONSE TO TRAUMA AND SHOCK

Profound changes occur in the immune response during operations, burns, and trauma. The changes occur progressively, their extent depending primarily on the severity of the trauma and the immune capacity of the patients. Many of the changes occurring in severe burns, trauma, and operative complications are caused partly by shock. The immune response to septic shock is well known, especially as regards complement,[3,4] but the effects of cardiogenic and hypovolemic shock as such have not been described.

Effects on Phagocytosis

POLYMORPHONUCLEAR LEUKOCYTES

Surgical trauma decreases neutrophil chemotaxis, most often measured in vitro[5,6] but also measured in vivo[7] (Fig. 11–1). The values return to normal in a few days, but may persist up to 2 to 3 months after severe injury. Although intraneutrophilic granule enzyme activities decrease even during hysterectomy,[8] ingestion and bacterial killing are decreased only in patients with severe trauma or intraabdominal infectious complications.[9,10] In burn patients random migration and chemotaxis are depressed and related to burn size in the immediately postburn phase.[11] The opsonization defect, also related to burn size, is of 2 to 3 weeks' duration.[12] In burns of more than 30% of the body surface, ingestion and bactericidal capacity are also depressed, especially in patients with septic episodes.[13,14]

A prominent feature of endotoxemia is leukopenia followed by leukocytosis. Patients with intra-abdominal sepsis show dysfunction of chemotaxis, ingestion, and intracellular killing. The abnormalities are, at least partly, caused by degranulation of neutrophils by high concentrations of chemoattractants, especially C_{5a}.[15–17] Low concentrations of chemoattractants activate neutrophils and guide them to the site of action, but high concentrations may lead to loss of all neutrophil responses and to extensive degranulation. The result is functional neutropenia and release of lysosomal enzymes necessary for the neutrophil in killing phagocytosed micro-organisms.

RETICULOENDOTHELIAL SYSTEM

Traumas of various origins decrease RES phagocytic capacity in proportion to the severity of trauma.[18] The dysfunction is reversible in a period of some hours to a few days, usually followed by a period of hyperphagocytosis. The decreased

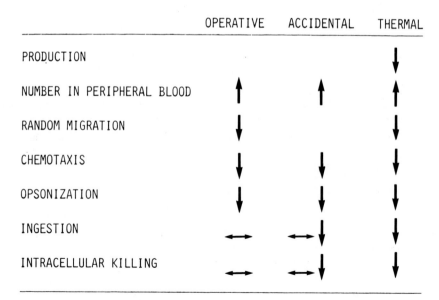

Fig. 11–1.   Effects of trauma on neutrophil leukocytes.

RES phagocytic capacity is associated with decreased plasma fibronectin concentrations.[19] Other proposed mechanisms of suppressed RES function are reduced perfusion of the main RES organs and suppression of RES by increased corticosteroid concentrations. However, no significant changes in hepatic sinusoidal blood flow have been found in animals during or after operation.[20] Low doses of corticosteroids stimulate and pharmacologic doses depress RES in animals, but in severely stressed animals administration of corticosteroids leads to RES phagocytic stimulation and enhanced resistance.[21]

Plasma fibronectin concentration is decreased after major operations, trauma, and burns, with restoration to normal or hyperopsonic values in a few hours or days.[22] In burns the decrease correlates to burn size and may be less than 10% of reference values in severe burns. Burn patients not in a septic state recover their fibronectin concentrations in 1 to 2 days but the concentrations remain low in infected and septic states.[23,24] The decrease in plasma fibronectin concentrations is greater in patients in a state of sepsis than in those not in such a state, but its predictive value for survival or death in sepsis is controversial.[25,26] Plasma fibronectin deficiency may precede the development of clinical sepsis by a few days.[23,27] The decrease may predispose the host to sepsis but it may also indicate latent sepsis.

Effects on Complement

Complement activation is observed during major surgical procedures,[28,29] but it is unclear whether it is the classic or the alternative pathway that dominates. Bacteremia during an operation may activate the complement with massive release of anaphylatoxins and lead to shock in operations such as transurethral resection of the prostate.[30] Both the classic and the alternative pathways may be activated in major trauma.[31] The alternative pathway is preferentially activated in major burns in the initial postburn phase with the extent related to the burn area. The classic pathway is activated especially in patients with septicemia developing.[32,33] The depletion is increased by the presence of nonvital tissue.[34] In patients with major trauma and burn, complement activation may be accompanied by activation of the coagulation cascade, fibrinolysis, and kallikrein-kinin systems.[35]

Sepsis and septic shock are associated with significant depletion of complement components, which is shown by decreased hemolytic complement activity and decreased serum concentrations of complement and appearance of complement activation products in the circulation. Activation of the complement in endotoxemia occurs primarily by the alternative pathway but also by the classic pathway, depending on the immune state of the patient.[3,33,36] No differences have been observed in complement activation between patients in septic shock caused by gram-positive or by gram-negative bacteria or between those who survive or those who die.[37] Complement activation is one of the earliest signs of sepsis and a significant contributor to the development of septic shock.

Effects on Cell-Mediated Immunity

The numbers of T lymphocytes, T-helper and, according to some investigators, T-suppressor cells in peripheral blood decrease in surgical, accidental, and burn trauma (Fig. 11–2). The ratio of T-helper cells to T-suppressor cells, which is more important than absolute cell numbers, is decreased[38–42] but may remain also

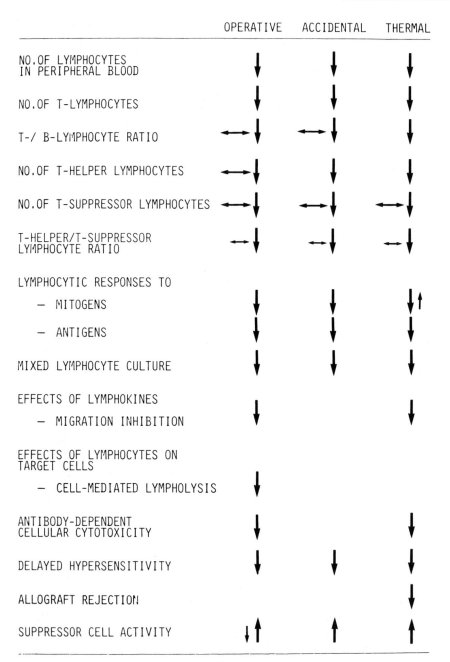

Fig. 11-2.   Effects of trauma on cell-mediated immunity.

unchanged.[43,44] Mitogen- and antigen-induced lymphocytic responses are decreased in surgical,[45] accidental,[9,46–48] and thermal trauma,[9,49,50] although increased responses have been reported in some burn patients.[51] Lymphocytic responses, decreased already during an operation, are lowest at the end of the procedure and return to normal over a period of one day to several weeks. The decreases correlate to the severity of the trauma and are lowest in patients with infectious complications.[42,46,48] A decrease in lymphocytic responses may occur when the mixed lymphocyte culture reaction, effects of lymphokines, effects of lymphocytes on target cells, and antibody-dependent cellular cytotoxicity are measured.[45] The sensitivity of lymphocytes to prostaglandin E_2 is increased post-operatively,[52] and increased suppressor cell activity has been observed in major trauma[50] and burns[39,51,53] and suspected in surgery. There may also be other types of suppressor cell populations with other characteristics.[54] The capacity of mono-nuclear cells from burned patients for producing interleukin 2 in vitro is greatly depressed for 20 to 60 days postburn, which shows failure in immune response communication. By contrast, interleukin 1 production is significantly increased early after a burn and is thereafter normal or slightly enhanced.[55] After a major operation, some patients show anergy in the delayed hypersensitivity skin test,[56,57] although anergy is uncommon in uncomplicated operations. Patients with severe trauma also have anergy.[9,58] Most patients with burns of more than 25% of the body surface and a considerable number of those with minor burns have decreased delayed hypersensitivity reactions.[59]

Effects on Humoral Immunity

The numbers of B lymphocytes are decreased in peripheral blood after trauma and operation but to a lesser degree than those of T cells (Fig. 11–3). Lymphocytic responses to pokeweed mitogen, which stimulates transformation of T and B lymphocytes, are depressed. By contrast, responses to Staphylococcus aureus Cowan I, which is mainly a B-lymphocyte mitogen, remained unchanged in open-heart operations.[60] There are decreases in serum immunoglobulin concentrations after operations and trauma, partly because of a loss of protein from intravascular spaces. The numbers of antibody-forming cells in the peripheral blood decrease, and at the same time IgG, IgM, and IgA production by artificially stimulated lymphocytes in vitro is depressed.[60] In animals the type of antigen determines if antibody response in trauma is enhanced, unaltered, or depressed.[61] Tetanus toxoid response in trauma patients is decreased,[62] but the response to polyvalent pneumococcal vaccine[63] and diphtheria toxoid[64] remains unaltered. Albumin resuscitation in shock may result in a decreased tetanus toxoid antibody response.[65]

In burn patients serum immunoglobulin concentrations are decreased, returning to normal over 1 to 2 weeks in patients without infections and to low normal in patients with infections.[9,14] Humoral immune response to new antigens is variable in burns, depressed for some and unaffected for others. Responsiveness to bacterial vaccines, tetanus toxoid, and to the infecting micro-organisms is retained in these patients.[66,67] However, no rise in agglutinin titers to infecting micro-organisms has been shown in burn patients in a state of sepsis.[33] In spite of this, there are enough opsonins in the serum for opsonization.[33]

CLINICAL IMPORTANCE

When the biologic importance of the decreased immune responses is discussed, the effects of uncomplicated operations and moderate trauma should be distinguished from the more extensive responses produced by severe trauma, sepsis, and surgical complications. The immune response is basically a physiologic reaction in which the body is trying to prevent itself from reacting against its own

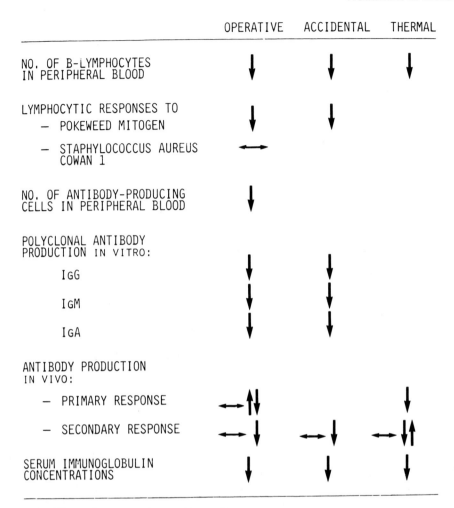

Fig. 11-3.   Effects of trauma on humoral immunity.

antigenic structures exposed and released in operations and trauma. If the decrease is prolonged and severe, it may be harmful for resistance to infections and spread of malignant disease.

By contrast, complement activation in patients with severe trauma and burns may cause the body difficulties. Complement activation is necessary in the inflammatory response and in many neutrophil functions (chemotaxis, adherence, opsonization, generation of oxygen radicals). However, massive activation together with other activated mediator systems is a major mechanism in the induction of septic shock. Excessive stimulation of neutrophils may lead to the inability of neutrophils to respond to chemotactic stimuli and to arrive at the site of microbial invasion. Excessive adhesivity and oxygen radical production and release by C_{5a} result in leukostasis and endothelial damage, contributing to pulmonary microcirculation failure. Depletion of complement may result in an ineffective complement-directed chemotaxis, opsonization, and lysis leading to bacteremia and sepsis.

RES dysfunction causes an imbalance between the amount of the material to be phagocytosed and the phagocytic capacity, which may lead to malfunction of different organs and contribute to multiple organ failure. In general, RES depression increases susceptibility to shock, while its enhancement will increase resistance.

MEASUREMENT OF THE IMMUNE RESPONSE

When the clinical status of surgical patients is evaluated, the possibility of decreased immune responses should be kept in mind, although it is not always necessary to measure the immunologic variables. High age, malnutrition, certain drugs, major trauma and operations, and several diseases are known to be associated with decreased immune responses. These factors should be taken into account in clinical decision-making even without measurement. But some patients might benefit from measurement, which may sometimes clear a problematic situation. In addition to measurement, it may also be possible to draw conclusions about the immune state indirectly. The micro-organisms cultured from the patient may provide information about the weak link, and accumulation of pus is a sign of chemotactic factor release and directed motility of neutrophils.

The delayed hypersensitivity skin test is a basic screening test[68] (Table 11–1). The test is primarily a measure of cell-mediated immunity, but the host must also be capable of maintaining an inflammatory reaction. The test is performed by injecting 0.1 ml of proper dilutions of Candida and mumps antigens, tuberculin, trichophytin, and streptokinase-streptodornase, which are most frequently used in the test, intradermally on the volar surface of the forearm. The results are read

Table 11–1.   Measurement of Immune Response in Surgical Patients.

Basic tests
    Leukocyte and differential count
    Delayed hypersensitivity skin test
Cell-mediated immunity
    T lymphocyte count
    T-helper and T-suppressor cell count
    Lymphocyte transformation by PHA, Con A, and PPD
    Mixed lymphocyte culture
    Migration inhibition test
    DNCB sensitization
Humoral immunity
    Serum immunoglobulin concentrations
    B lymphocyte count
    Lymphocyte transformation by PWM or EBV
    Immunoglobulin production in vitro
    Antibody response to diphtheria or tetanus toxoid
Phagocytosis
    Nitroblue tetrazolium dye reduction test
    Rebuck skin window
    Chemotaxis, opsonization, ingestion and bacterial killing assays
    Plasma fibronectin concentration
Complement
    Hemolytic complement
    Complement component concentrations
    Complement activation products

PHA = phytohemagglutinin; Con A = concanavalin A; PPD = purified protein derivative of turberculin; PWM = pokeweed mitogen; EBV = Epstein-Barr virus; DNCB = dinitrochlorobenzene.

at 24 and 48 hr as an induration of at least 5 mm diameter. The frequency of sepsis and mortality are higher in anergic patients with no positive reactions than in reactive patients.[69] This correlation is explained by the fact that anergy in surgical patients is associated with disturbed neutrophil and lymphocyte chemotaxis and with serum inhibitory factors.[70] The test may be valuable in guiding the treatment of surgical patients,[71,72] but contradictory opinions also exist.[73]

Leukocyte and differential counts and T and B lymphocytes and their subset numbers reflect the numbers of effector cells in peripheral blood and also have prognostic value.[74] The lymphocyte transformation test is one of the basic functional in vitro tests in clinical immunology. In the test lymphocytes are stimulated with mitogens or antigens, and their proliferative capacity is measured. The serum immunoglobulin concentration gives only a rough estimate of humoral immunity. More specific information is obtained by measuring antibody production in vitro or in vivo.

There are specific tests for measuring the various aspects of neutrophil function. Measurement of the highly peroxidase-positive neutrophils in flow cytometry, chemiluminescence techniques, and the nitroblue tetrazolium dye reduction test are rapid screening tests of neutrophil function. In testing RES function the colloid clearance techniques with isotopically labelled particles are of limited clinical value. By contrast, plasma fibronectin concentration may be measured with rapid electroimmuno- or immunoturbidometric assays.[75]

A screening test for complement is measurement of total hemolytic complement (CH_{50}). However, a decrease of individual complement components to 50% or less of reference values may have little or no effect on this test. More specific information is obtained by measuring the concentrations of different complement components and their conversion products.

SUPPORT OF IMMUNOLOGIC FUNCTIONS IN SHOCK

General Supportive Measures

Of primary importance for the immune response is the maintenance of homeostasis and treatment of the underlying disease. The body is capable of correcting even severe alterations in the immune response, if the failures in vital functions such as tissue perfusion, oxygenation and ventilation, and fluid balance can be corrected. Since many drugs have a depressing effect on the immune response, drug therapy should be based on sound indications. Even supportive measures such as mechanical ventilation with positive end expiratory pressure may decrease thoracic duct lymph flow and bacterial clearance.[76]

Immediate operation is necessary in some patients, e.g., in those with abscesses, gangrenous limbs, other nonvital tissue and toxic processes, to improve their immune responses,[34,77] but it may take weeks for some factors of the immune response, e.g., the neutrophils, to recover.[10] Treatment of malnutrition and restoration of nutritional support are important for immune responses in critically ill patients.[78] At present, the possibilities of modifying surgically induced immune responses by anesthesiologic means are not good; the importance of this modification is still doubtful. Patients with severe trauma, burns, and sepsis present a totally different problem: how to suppress exaggerated complement activation with massive mediator release while at the same time supporting other factors of the immune response.

Specific Immunotherapy

Vaccination has not proved so beneficial in severe injury and sepsis as it has in the prophylaxis of infectious diseases. The antibody response in severely injured patients is unaltered or decreased, but it takes 1 to 2 weeks before the peak of primary antibody response is achieved. Therefore, vaccination may be indicated first hand in long-term treatment. Pseudomonas vaccines have reduced mortality in moderate burns,[79] and in severe burns the frequency of Pseudomonas sepsis is decreased, but other micro-organisms may appear, resulting in death. By contrast, a booster dose of vaccine will elevate antibody levels within hours.

The use of immunoglobulin preparations in severe infections is theoretically indicated. Good results have been obtained in animals when immunoglobulins have been applied before or shortly after introducing the infective agent. Antitoxin administered to neutralize diphtheria, tetanus, botulism, and gas gangrene exotoxins has also given good results in humans when given before the toxins have irreversibly bound themselves to the tissues. Hyperimmune gammaglobulins may also be useful.[80] However, immunoglobulins obtained from nonimmunized donors lack evidence of their clinical value in severe infections in humans. Therefore, special consideration and restraint might be advisable in the use of nonspecific immunoglobulin preparations in severe infections in patients without a primary immunodeficiency disease.[81] There are, however, several types of immunoglobulin preparations for intravenous use, and differences may exist in their biologic activities depending on production methods and donor selection.[82] It is often forgotten that immunoglobulins are also given in blood transfusion and plasma administration. By contrast, plasma protein derivative (PPD) is an almost pure albumin preparation without immunoglobulins. Fresh frozen plasma is also a source of opsonizing proteins and complement factors.

The use of antisera directed to the core portion of endotoxin, which is similar in many gram-negative micro-organisms, may prove valuable in septic shock. These preparations have been shown to reduce mortality from gram-negative sepsis[83,84] and have been given prophylactically to reduce episodes of sepsis and septic shock in high-risk surgical patients.[85] A future prospect is administration of monoclonal antibodies directed against toxins and micro-organisms. Such experiments have been carried out in animals, but similar antibodies also exist in humans.[86,87]

Nonspecific Immunotherapy

Granulocyte transfusion is recommended in patients with severe infections if their blood granulocyte count is less than 0.2×10^9/L, their bone marrow failure is reversible, and they have not responded to antimicrobial treatment in 2 to 3 days. The number of neutrophils migrating into tissues already starts to decline with neutrophil blood counts of less than 1.5×10^9/L, but if there are enough monocytes, the consequences of neutropenia are less severe. To be effective, a granulocyte concentrate of 1 to 2×10^{10} granulocytes should be given once a day for several days. In general, granulocyte transfusion is considered to be effective, but studies exist that found no advantage in granulocyte transfusion over optimal antimicrobial therapy.[88,89]

RES dysfunction in patients with low plasma fibronectin concentrations may be improved by fresh frozen plasma or cryoprecipitate. Cryoprecipitate has been shown to reverse opsonic deficiency in patients with severe trauma or sepsis and improve their clinical status.[90] However, not only the amount of fibronectin but also its quality is important.[91] An imbalance between proteases and protease inhibitors may occur in major trauma and sepsis.[92,93] This may result in immune dysfunction and splitting of fibronectin.[91] The imbalance between proteases and protease inhibitors, which is probably as important as lack of fibronectin, may be corrected by administration of protease inhibitors in fresh frozen plasma or as specific concentrates (antithrombin III, alpha$_2$-macroglobulin, and alpha$_1$-antitrypsin).[91,94]

Corticosteroids, although still theoretically controversial, are widely used clinically in the treatment of septic shock. In septic shock pharmacologic doses of corticosteroids may be immunologically beneficial by suppressing responses to endotoxin and preventing nonspecific injury to cell structures[95,96] but they should be given early, preferably before the shock has fully developed.[97] In hypovolemic shock corticosteroids may not offer any such advantages and in cardiogenic shock they may be deleterious.

Use of Immunomodulators

Interleukins 1 and 2 may be used in the future therapeutically as mediators of the immune response. Interleukin 2 has already been shown to restore to normal the in vitro mixed lymphocyte culture reaction in burn patients.[98] Indomethacin, ibuprofen, and low doses of cyclophosphamide have been shown in animals to inhibit T-suppressor cells and improve immune responses.[99,100] RES stimulants such as bacille Calmette-Guérin, Corynebacterium parvum, muramyl dipeptide, and glucan have proved effective in animals. In the future such RES stimulants suitable for humans may be given to patients with burns, severe injuries, and before major operations. Abnormal neutrophil function in surgical patients may be corrected in vitro by levamisole,[101] but it has shown only marginal effects in vivo.[77] Ketoconazole, the new antimycotic with immunostimulating effects,[102] may become clinically important in mycotic infections. Complement inhibitors important in inhibiting excessive complement activation have been beneficial in sepsis in animals.[103] The use of interferon, transfer factor, and thymic factors will have to await further studies.

Plasmapheresis

Plasma exchange for the removal of immunosuppressive and other noxious agents may be used in trauma and sepsis unresponsive to conventional therapy. Clinical benefit and an immunorestorative effect of plasma exchange have been observed in burn patients but not in patients in the septic state.[104]

Different traumas have a decreasing effect on phagocytic, cell-mediated, and humoral immune responses and may also activate the complement. These reactions are primarily physiologic but if excessive they are detrimental. However, the reactions are not yet fully understood; the immunologic monitoring methods are coarse and the possibilities are limited in the regulation of immune responses and mediator systems in trauma and sepsis. The treatment of septic shock should be directed to the activated mediator systems and to the support of failing immune responses in major trauma. Improvement of antibiotic therapy, which has brought down infection rates, is no final answer to infection problems in intensive care patients. Antibiotics give the body time to respond with its own defense systems, which will ultimately clear the infection. The future treatment of choice in these patients may be a combination of antibiotics and immunoregulatory substances.

REFERENCES

1. Fry, D.E., Pearlstein, L., Fulton, R.L., and Polk, H.C.,Jr.: Multiple system organ failure. The role of uncontrolled infection. Arch. Surg., *115*:136, 1980.
2. Goldberg, A.L., et al.: Control of protein degradation in muscle by prostaglandins, Ca^{2+}, and leukocytic pyrogen (interleukin 1). Fed. Proc., *43*:1301, 1984.
3. Morrison, D.C., and Ulevitch, R.J.: The effects of bacterial endotoxins on host mediation systems. Am. J. Pathol., *93*:527, 1978.
4. Morrison, D.C., and Ryan, J.L.: Bacterial endotoxins and host immune responses. Adv. Immunol., *28*:293, 1979.
5. Bowers, T.K., O'Flaherty, J., Simmons, R.L., and Jacob, H.S.: Postsurgical granulocyte dysfunction: studies in healthy kidney donors. J. Lab. Clin. Med., *90*:720, 1977.
6. Maderazo, E.G., et al.: Polymorphonuclear leukocyte migration abnormalities and their significance in seriously traumatized patients. Ann. Surg., *198*:736, 1983.
7. Wandall, J.H.: Leucocyte mobilization and function in vitro of blood and exudative leucocytes after inguinal herniotomy. Br. J. Surg., *69*:669, 1982.
8. Davies, J.M., Sheppard, K., and Fletcher, J.: The effects of surgery on the activity of neutrophil granule proteins. Br. J. Haematol., *53*:5, 1983.
9. Alexander, J.W., et al.: A comparison of immunologic profiles and their influence on bacteremia in surgical patients with a high risk of infection. Surgery, *86*:94, 1979.
10. Solomkin, J.S., Bauman, M.P., Nelson, R.D., and Simmons, R.L.: Neutrophil dysfunction during the course of intra-abdominal infection. Ann. Surg., *194*:9, 1981.
11. Warden, G.D., Mason, A.D., Jr., and Pruitt, B.A., Jr.: Evaluation of leukocyte chemotaxis in vitro in thermally injured patients. J. Clin. Invest., *54*:1001, 1974.
12. Nathenson, G., et al.: Decreased opsonic and chemotactic activities in sera of postburn patients and partial opsonic restoration with properdin and properdin convertase. Clin. Immunol. Immunopathol., *9*:269, 1978.
13. Grogan, J.B.: Altered neutrophil phagocytic function in burn patients. J. Trauma, *16*:734, 1976.
14. Alexander, J.W., Ogle, C.K., Stinnett, J.D., and MacMillan, B.G.: A sequential, prospective analysis of immunologic abnormalities and infection following severe thermal injury. Ann. Surg., *188*:809, 1978.
15. Solomkin, J.S., et al.: Neutrophil dysfunction in sepsis. II. Evidence for the role of complement activation products in cellular deactivation. Surgery, *90*:319, 1981.
16. Solomkin, J.S., et al.: Neutrophil dysfunction in sepsis. III. Degranulation as a mechanism for nonspecific deactivation. J. Surg. Res., *36*:407, 1984.
17. Solomkin, J.S., et al.: Complement-induced expression of cryptic receptors on the neutrophil surface: A mechanism for regulation of acute inflammation in trauma. Surgery, *96*:336, 1984.
18. Schildt, B., Gertz, I., and Wide, L.: Differentiated reticuloendothelial system (RES) function in some critical surgical conditions. Acta Chir. Scand., *140*:611, 1974.
19. Saba, T.M., Lanser, M.E., and Dillon, B.C.: Opsonic fibronectin and phagocytic defense after trauma. *In* Handbook of Shock and Trauma, Vol 1: Basic Science. Edited by B.M. Altura, A.M. Lefer, and W. Schumer. New York, Raven Press, 1983.
20. Saba, T.M., and Scovill, W.A.: Effect of surgical trauma on host defense. Surg. Annu., *7*:71, 1975.
21. Altura, B.M.: Reticuloendothelial cells and host defense. Adv. Microcirc., *9*:252, 1980.
22. Richards, W.O., Scovill, W.A., and Shin, B.: Opsonic fibronectin deficiency in patients with intra-abdominal infection. Surgery, *94*:210, 1983.
23. Lanser, M.E., Saba, T.M., and Scovill, W.A.: Opsonic glycoprotein (plasma fibronectin) levels after burn injury. Relationship to extent of burn and development of sepsis. Ann. Surg., *192*:776, 1980.
24. Ekindjian, O.G., et al.: Plasma fibronectin time course in burned patients: influence of sepsis. J. Trauma, *24*:214, 1984.
25. Rubli, E., et al.: Plasma fibronectin and associated variables in surgical intensive care patients. Ann. Surg., *197*:310, 1983.
26. Brodin, B., von Schenck, H., Schildt, B., and Liljedahl, S.-O.: Low plasma fibronectin indicates septicaemia in major burns. Acta Chir. Scand., *150*:5, 1984.
27. Lanser, M.E., and Saba, T.M.: Opsonic fibronectin deficiency and sepsis. Cause or effect? Ann. Surg., *195*:340, 1982.
28. Hahn-Pedersen, J., Sørensen, H., and Kehlet, H.: Complement activation during surgical procedures. Surg. Gynecol. Obstet., *146*:66, 1978.

29. Lewis, R.E., Cruse, J.M., and Richey, J.V.: Effects of anesthesia and operation on the classical pathway of complement activation. Clin. Immunol. Immunopathol., 23:666, 1982.

30. Brandslund, I., et al.: Complement activation in shock associated with a surgically provoked bacteriaemia. Acta Pathol. Microbiol. Immunol. Scand., 91:51, 1983.

31. Bjornson, A.B., Altemeier, W.A., and Bjornson, H.S.: Host defense against opportunist microorganisms following trauma. II. Changes in complement and immunoglobulins in patients with abdominal trauma and in septic patients without trauma. Ann. Surg., 188:102, 1978.

32. Bjornson, A.B., Altemeier, W.A., and Bjornson, H.S.: The septic burned patient. A model for studying the role of complement and immunoglobulins in opsonization of opportunist microorganisms. Ann. Surg., 189:515, 1979.

33. Bjornson, A.B., Altemeier, W.A., and Bjornson, H.S.: Complement, opsonins, and the immune response to bacterial infection in burned patients. Ann. Surg., 191:323, 1980.

34. Heideman, M., Saravis, C., and Clowes, G.H.A., Jr.: Effect of nonviable tissue and abscesses on complement depletion and the development of bacteremia. J. Trauma, 22:527, 1982.

35. Zuckerman, L., Caprini, J.A., Lipp, V., and Vagher, J.P.: Disseminated intravascular multiple systems activation (DIMSA) following thermal injury. J. Trauma, 18:432, 1978.

36. Fearon, D.T., Ruddy, S., Schur, P.H., and McCabe, W.R.: Activation of the properdin pathway of complement in patients with gram-negative bacteremia. N. Engl. J. Med., 292:937, 1975.

37. León, C., et al.: Complement activation in septic shock due to gram-negative and gram-positive bacteria. Crit. Care Med., 10:308, 1982.

38. Antonacci, A.C., Good, R.A., and Gupta, S.: T-cell subpopulations following thermal injury. Surg. Gynecol. Obstet., 155:1, 1982.

39. McIrvine, A.J., O'Mahony, J.B., Saporoschetz, I., and Mannick, J.A.: Depressed immune response in burn patients. Use of monoclonal antibodies and functional assays to define the role of suppressor cells. Ann. Surg., 196:297, 1982.

40. Antonacci, A.C., et al.: Flow cytometric analysis of lymphocyte subpopulations after thermal injury in human beings. Surg. Gynecol. Obstet., 159:1, 1984.

41. Hansbrough, J.F., Bender, E.M., Zapata-Sirvent, R., and Anderson, J.: Altered helper and suppressor lymphocyte populations in surgical patients. Am. J. Surg., 148:303, 1984.

42. Levy, E.M., Alharbi, S.A., Grindlinger, G., and Black, P.H.: Changes in mitogen responsiveness lymphocyte subsets after traumatic injury: relation to development of sepsis. Clin. Immunol. Immunopathol., 32:224, 1984.

43. Grzelak, I., Olszewski, W.L., and Engeset, A.: Influence of operative trauma on circulating blood mononuclear cells: analysis using monoclonal antibodies. Eur. Surg. Res., 16:105, 1984.

44. Hole, A., and Bakke, O.: T-lymphocytes and the subpopulations of T-helper and T-suppressor cells measured by monoclonal antibodies (T11, T4, and T8) in relation to surgery under epidural and general anaesthesia. Acta Anaesthesiol. Scand., 28:296, 1984.

45. Salo, M.: Effects of anaesthesia and surgery on the immune response. *In* Trauma, Stress, and Immunity in Anaesthesia and Surgery. Edited by J. Watkins, and M. Salo. London, Butterworth, 1982.

46. Salo, M., et al.: Impaired lymphocyte transformation after accidental trauma. Acta Chir. Scand. 145:367, 1979.

47. Munster, A.M., et al.: The "in vitro skin test." A reliable and repeatable assay of immune competence in the surgical patient. Ann. Surg., 194:345, 1981.

48. Keane, R.M., et al.: Prediction of sepsis in the multitraumatic patient by assays of lymphocyte responsiveness. Surg. Gynecol. Obstet., 156:163, 1983.

49. Eskola, J., Nieminen, S., Merikanto, J., and Aho, A.J.: Impaired lymphocyte transformation after slight and moderate burns. J. Clin. Lab. Immunol., 2:143, 1979.

50. Keane, R.M., et al.: Suppressor cell activity after major injury: indirect and direct functional assays. J. Trauma, 22:770, 1982.

51. Miller, C.L., and Baker, C.C.: Changes in lymphocyte activity after thermal injury. The role of suppressor cells. J. Clin. Invest., 63:202, 1979.

52. Goodwin, J.S., et al.: Effect of physical stress on sensitivity of lymphocytes to inhibition by prostaglandin E_2. J. Immunol., 127:518, 1981.

53. Ninnemann, J.L., Stockland, A.E., and Condie, J.T.: Induction of prostaglandin synthesis-dependent suppressor cells with endotoxin: occurrence in patients with thermal injuries. J. Clin. Immunol., 3:142, 1983.

54. Salo, M., Soppi, E., Lassila, O., and Ruuskanen, O.: Suppressor lymphocytes during open heart surgery. J. Clin. Lab. Immunol., 5:159, 1981.

55. Wood, J.J., et al.: Inadequate interleukin 2 production. A fundamental immunological deficiency in patients with major burns. Ann. Surg., 200:311, 1984.

56. McLoughlin, G.A., et al.: Correlation between anergy and a circulating immunosuppressive factor following major surgical trauma. Ann. Surg., 190:297, 1979.

57. Christou, N.V., Superina, R., Broadhead, M., and Meakins, J.L.: Postoperative despression of host resistance: determinants and effect of peripheral protein-sparing therapy. Surgery, *92*:786, 1982.
58. Bradley, J.A., et al.: Cellular defense in critically ill surgical patients. Crit. Care Med., *12*:565, 1984.
59. Heggers, J.P., et al.: Skin testing. A valuable predictor in thermal injury. Arch. Surg., *119*:49, 1984.
60. Eskola, J., Salo, M., Viljanen, M.K., and Ruuskanen, O.: Impaired B lymphocyte function during open-heart surgery. Effects of anaesthesia and surgery. Br. J. Anaesth., *56*:333, 1984.
61. Kinnaert, P., et al.: Effect of surgical trauma on various aspects of the immune response in rats. Eur. Surg. Res., *16*:99, 1984.
62. Nohr, C.W., et al.: In vivo and in vitro humoral immunity in surgical patients. Ann. Surg., *200*:373, 1984.
63. Caplan, E.S., et al.: Response of traumatized splenectomized patients to immediate vaccination with polyvalent pneumococcal vaccine. J. Trauma, *23*:801, 1983.
64. Haven, W.P., Bock, D.G., and Siegel, I.: Capacity of seriously wounded patients to produce antibody. J. Clin. Invest., *33*:940, 1954.
65. Clift, D.R., et al.: The effect of albumin resuscitation for shock on the immune response to tetanus toxoid. J. Surg. Res., *32*:449, 1982.
66. Sachs, A.: Active immunoprophylaxis in burns with a new multivalent vaccine. Lancet, *2*:959, 1970.
67. Antia, N.H., et al.: The treatment of burns. Immunological studies in burns. Burns, *4*:55, 1977.
68. Salo, M.: Measurement and significance of altered immunological parameters. *In* Trauma, Stress and Immunity in Anaesthesia and Surgery. Edited by J. Watkins, and M. Salo. London, Butterworth, 1982.
69. MacLean, L.D.: Host resistance in surgical patients. J. Trauma, *19*:297, 1979.
70. Superina, R., and Meakins, J.L.: Current research review. Delayed hypersensitivity, anergy, and the surgical patient. J. Surg. Res., *37*:151, 1984.
71. Christou, N.V., et al.: The walk-in anergic patient. How best to assess the risk of sepsis following elective surgery. Ann. Surg., *199*:438, 1984.
72. Revhaug, A., and Giercksky, K.-E.: Preoperative cutaneous hypersensitivity reaction related to postoperative complications following elective surgery. Acta Chir. Scand. *150*:279, 1984.
73. Brown, R., et al.: Failure of delayed hypersensitivity skin testing to predict postoperative sepsis and mortality. Br. Med. J., *284*:851, 1982.
74. Lewis, R.T., and Klein, H.: Risk factors in postoperative sepsis: significance of preoperative lymphocytopenia. J. Surg. Res., *26*:365, 1979.
75. Saba, T.M., et al.: Evaluation of a rapid immunoturbidimetric assay for opsonic fibronectin in surgical and trauma patients. J. Lab. Clin. Med., *98*:482, 1981.
76. Last, M., Kurtz, L., Stein, T.A., and Wise, L.: Effect of PEEP on the rate of thoracic duct lymph flow and clearance of bacteria from the peritoneal cavity. Am. J. Surg., *145*:126, 1983.
77. Meakins, J.L., Christou, N.V., Shizgal, H.M., and MacLean, L.D.: Therapeutic approaches to anergy in surgical patients. Surgery and levamisole. Ann. Surg., *190*:286, 1979.
78. Renk, C.M., Long, C.L., and Blakemore, W.S.: Comparison between in vitro lymphocyte activity and metabolic changes in trauma patients. J. Trauma, *22*:134, 1982.
79. Alexander, J.W., Fisher, M.W., and MacMillan, B.G.: Immunological control of pseudomonas infection in burn patients: a clinical evaluation. Arch. Surg., *102*:31, 1971.
80. Jones, R.J., Roe, E.A., and Gupta, J.L.: Controlled trial of pseudomonas immunoglobulin and vaccine in burn patients. Lancet, *2*:1263, 1980.
81. Int. Forum: Which is the factual basis, in theory and clinical practice, for the use of intravenous gammaglobulin in the treatment of severe bacterial infections? Vox. Sang., *37*:116, 1979.
82. Hill, H.R., Augustine, N.H., and Shigeoka, A.O.: Comparative opsonic activity of intravenous gammaglobulin preparations for common bacterial pathogens. Am. J. Med., *76(3A)*:61, 1984.
83. Ziegler, E.J., et al.: Treatment of gram-negative bacteremia and shock with human antiserum to a mutant Escherichia coli. N. Engl. J. Med., *307*:1225, 1982.
84. Lachman, E., Pitsoe, S.B., and Gaffin, S.L.: Anti-lipopolysaccharide immunotherapy in management of septic shock of obstetric and gynaecological origin. Lancet, *1*:981, 1984.
85. Glauser, M.P., McCutchan, J.A., and Ziegler, E.: Immunoprophylaxis and immunotherapy of gram-negative infections in the immunocompromised host. Clin. Haematol., *13*:549, 1984.
86. Hunter, K.W., et al.: Antibacterial activity of a human monoclonal antibody to haemophilus influenzae type B capsular polysaccharide. Lancet, *2*:798, 1984.
87. McClelland, D.B.L., and Yap, P.L.: Clinical use of immunoglobulins. Clin. Haematol., *13*:39, 1984.
88. Buckner, C.D., and Clift, R.A.: Prophylaxis and treatment of infection of the immunocompromised host by granulocyte transfusions. Clin. Haematol., *13*:557, 1984.
89. Wright, D.G.: Leukocyte transfusions: thinking twice. Am. J. Med., *76*:637, 1984.

90. Saba, T.M., et al.: Reversal of fibronectin and opsonic deficiency in patients. A controlled study. Ann. Surg., *199*:87, 1984.
91. Brown, R.A.: Failure of fibronectin as an opsonin in the host defence system: a case of competitive self inhibition? Lancet, *2*:1058, 1983.
92. Witte, J., et al.: Disturbances of selected plasma proteins in hyperdynamic septic shock. Intensive Care Med., *8*:215, 1982.
93. Donnelly, P.K., et al.: The role of protease in immunoregulation. Br. J. Surg., *70*:614, 1983.
94. Sherman, L.A. New plasma components. Clin. Haematol., *13*:17, 1984.
95. Schumer, W.: Controversy in shock research. Pro: the role of steroids in septic shock. Circ. Shock, *8*:667, 1981.
96. Halevy, S., Altura, B.T., and Altura, B.M.: Pathophysiological basis for the use of steroids in the treatment of shock and trauma. Klin. Wochenschr., *60*:1021, 1982.
97. Sprung, C.L., et al.: The effects of high-dose corticosteroids in patients with septic shock. A prospective, controlled study. N. Engl. J. Med., *311*:1137, 1984.
98. Antonacci, A.C., et al.: Autologous and allogeneic mixed-lymphocyte responses following thermal injury in man: the immunomodulatory effects of interleukin 1, interleukin 2, and a prostaglandin inhibitor, WY-18251. Clin. Immunol. Immunopathol., *30*:304, 1984.
99. Hansbrough, J., Peterson, V., Zapata-Sirvent, R., and Claman, H.N.: Postburn immunosuppression in an animal model. II. Restoration of cell-mediated immunity by immunomodulating drugs. Surgery, *95*:290, 1984.
100. Maghsudi, M., and Miller, C.L.: The immunomodulating effect of TP5 and indomethacin in burn-induced hypoimmunity. J. Surg. Res., *37*:133, 1984.
101. Christou, N.V., and Meakins, J.L.: Neutrophil function in surgical patients: in vitro correction of abnormal neutrophil chemotaxis by levamisole. Surgery, *85*:543, 1979.
102. vanRensburg, C.E.J., et al.: The effects of ketoconazole on cellular and humoral immune functions. J. Antimicrob. Chemother., *11*:49, 1983.
103. Ebata, T., Kuttner, R.E., Apantaku, F.O., and Schumer, W.: Effect of a new synthetic complement inhibitor on hepatic glycolytic intermediates in septic rats. Adv. Shock Res., *9*:275, 1983.
104. Warden, G.D., Ninnemann, J., Stratta, R.J., and Saffle, J.R.: The effect of exchange therapy on postburn lymphocyte suppression. Surgery, *96*:321, 1984.

Chapter 12

PHARMACOLOGIC TREATMENT OF SHOCK

Susan J. Markowsky • Robert M. Elenbaas

Appropriate pharmacologic management of shock requires an accurate clinical assessment of its underlying cause and knowledge of the patient's initial hemodynamic status and preexisting disease states. The mainstay of therapy for most shock states is restoration of effective circulating blood volume with administration of blood, crystalloids, or colloids as indicated. Treatment goals for pharmacologic therapy are directed toward augmenting perfusion and oxygen delivery to vital organs and maintenance of coronary perfusion. In order to use pharmacologic agents effectively in the treatment of shock, an understanding of the drug's pharmacology and hemodynamic effects in different pathophysiologic states is essential.

Effective drug therapy for shock first requires repletion of intravascular blood volume, correction of acid-base abnormalities, and maintenance of adequate oxygenation and ventilation. Currently available pharmacologic agents include vasopressors to increase mean arterial pressure, inotropes to improve contractility and cardiac output, and vasodilators for afterload reduction. Pharmacologic agents may improve the hemodynamic status of cardiogenic, septic, and postcardiopulmonary bypass shock. In contrast, hypovolemic shock is best managed with intravascular volume expansion alone.

Circulatory shock states may present differently depending on the pathophysiologic stage of shock and the baseline status of the cardiovascular system. Therefore, the treatment of shock cannot be simplified to one model. Selection of vasoactive agents is based on knowledge of their pharmacologic effects, an assessment of the pathophysiologic stage of shock, determination of the patient's initial hemodynamic status, and knowledge of underlying disease states. Disease states to consider during drug selection are ischemic heart disease, recent acute myocardial infarction, congestive heart failure, and other conditions associated with compromised cardiac performance. Drug effects on myocardial oxygen demand and hemodynamic determinants of cardiac function should be considered in view of the underlying illness.

The adverse-effect profiles of the pharmacologic agents may vary based on the patient's initial hemodynamic status and underlying conditions. Adverse effects to consider when comparing agents include arrhythmogenic potential, vasoconstrictive potency, the ability to induce a "coronary steal syndrome," effect on preload, and the balance between myocardial oxygen supply and demand. Vasodilators for example may cause a "coronary steal syndrome" by decreased diastolic filling pressure of the coronary arteries. In contrast, vasopressors may raise the mean arterial pressure and increase cerebral and coronary perfusion; excessive pressor effects, however, may increase cardiac workload and sacrifice renal blood flow.

RECEPTOR PHARMACOLOGY

An understanding of drug therapy for shock is facilitated by knowledge of sympathetic receptor pharmacology. Pharmacologic activity of sympathomimetic amines depends on the receptor agonist properties that predominate at a given dose. Alpha and beta adrenergic receptors were first described by Ahlquist in 1948.[1] Beta receptors were further differentiated by Lands, et al.[2] to beta 1 and beta 2. Dopaminergic receptors were characterized by Goldberg, et al.[3] as pharmacologic receptors stimulated exclusively by dopamine.

Alpha 1 and alpha 2 receptors are located postsynaptically and presynaptically, respectively. The predominant effect of alpha 1 receptor stimulation is vasoconstriction of cutaneous, mucosal, and renal vascular beds, resulting in increased systemic vascular resistance. Stimulation of alpha 2 receptors by released norepinephrine modulates further release of adrenergic neurotransmitters, serving as a negative feedback mechanism.[4]

Beta 1 receptor stimulation results in positive inotropic and chronotropic actions on the heart. Beta 2 adrenergic agents produce bronchodilation and vasodilation of the skeletal and peripheral arteriolar beds. Beta adrenergic stimulation does not cause significant vasodilation of the renal vasculature. Dopaminergic stimulation increases blood flow to the renal and mesenteric vasculature.[5] Pharmacologic prototypes of adrenoreceptor agonists are shown in Table 12–1.

Alpha receptor blockade produces vasodilation and decreases systemic vascular resistance. Increased cutaneous and renal blood flow is seen in hypovolemic and vasoconstricted states. Effects on blood pressure are variable; however, a

Table 12–1. Pharmacologic Prototypes of Adrenoreceptor Agents.

	Agonists	Antagonists
Pure alpha	Phenylephrine	Phenoxybenzamine*
	Methoxamine	Phentolamine
Beta (nonselective)	Isoproterenol	Propranolol
		Nadolol
		Timolol
		Pindolol
B_1 Selective	Prenalterol*	Metoprolol
		Atenolol
B_2 Selective	Terbutaline	
	Albuterol (salbutamol)	
	Fenoterol*	
Mixed alpha and beta	Epinephrine	
	Dopamine**	
	Dobutamine	
	Levarterenol (norepinephrine)	
	Metaraminol	
Dopaminergic	Dopamine	Phenothiazines

* Investigational agent in the US.
** Also stimulates dopaminergic receptors.

decrease in diastolic blood pressure predominates secondary to arteriolar vaso-dilation and increased venous capacitance.[4]

SYMPATHOMIMETIC AGENTS

Sympathomimetic agents vary in their pharmacologic actions and receptor ago-nist properties (Table 12–2). Therapeutic use of these agents in shock is primarily for their inotropic effect to support cardiac pump function and improve circulatory perfusion. This may be beneficial in a variety of shock states when hemodynamic measurements indicate pump impairment since cardiac compromise may accom-pany even the noncardiogenic forms of shock. In addition, vasopressor agents may be indicated following fluid repletion to raise mean arterial pressure to 65 to 70 mm Hg and increase coronary and cerebral blood flow.

A delicate balance exists, however, between increasing perfusion of the heart and brain and compromising blood flow to the kidney and other tissues through marked peripheral vasoconstriction. Vasopressors may additionally impair cardiac function by increased systemic vascular resistance and impedance to ventricular emptying. Peripheral hypoperfusion may result in tissue anoxia and potentiate the risk of "irreversible shock." The goal of therapy is thus to raise mean arterial pres-sure, but not necessarily to normalize blood pressure. Comparison of the effects of sympathomimetic agents on regional blood flow and hemodynamic measure-ments is shown in Tables 12–3 and 12–4, respectively. Potent vasoconstrictors such as levarterenol, metaraminol, phenylephrine, and epinephrine should be reserved for severe hypotension unresponsive to other treatment modalities. An

Table 12–2. Sympathomimetic Agonist Properties.

Agonists	Alpha Vasoconstriction	Beta 1 Inotropic Activity	Beta 2 Peripheral Vasodilation	Dopaminergic Renal Vasodilation
Dopamine	↑↑↑*	↑↑	↑→	↑↑↑↑
Dobutamine	↓→↑	↑↑↑	↑↑	0
Isoproterenol	0	↑↑↑↑	↑↑↑↑	0
Epinephrine	↑↑↑*	↑↑	↑↑	0
Levarterenol	↑↓↑↑	↑	0	0
Phenylephrine	↑↑↑	0	0	0
Metaraminol	↑↑↑	↑	0	0

* Predominant receptor activity at high doses. (Key: ↑ = increase; → = no change; ↓ = decrease; 0 = lacks adrenoreceptor activity.)

Table 12–3. Comparison of Sympathomimetic Effects on Regional Blood Flow.

Agonists	Renal	Cerebral	Splanchnic	Skeletal	Cutaneous
Dopamine	↑↑↓*	↑	↑	↓	↓
Dobutamine	→	↑	↑↓*	↑↓*	→↓*
Isoproterenol	→↓	↑	↑	↑	↑
Epinephrine	↓	↑	↑↓*	↑↓*	↓
Levarterenol	↓	↑	↓	↓	↓
Phenylephrine	↓	↑	↓	↓	↓
Metaraminol	↓	↑	↓	↓	↓

*Dose-dependent effects (Key: ↑ = increase; → = no change; ↓ = decrease.)

Table 12-4. Comparison of Hemodynamic Effects of Sympathomimetic
             Agents.

Agonists	HR	SV	CO	MAP	SVR	PCWP
Dopamine	→↑↑*	↑↑	↑↑↑	→↑↑↑*	↓→↑*	→↑
Dobutamine	↑	↑↑↑	↑↑↑↑	→↑*	↓	→↓
Isoproterenol	↑↑↑↑	↑↑↑↑	↑↑↑↑	→↓↓↓	↓↓↓	↓
Epinephrine	↑↑↑	↑↑	↑↑↑	↑↑*	↓↑*	→↑
Levarterenol	→↓	↑	→↓	↑↑↑↑	↑↑↑↑	→↑

* Dose-dependent effects (Key: HR = heart rate; SV = stroke volume; CO = cardiac output; MAP = mean arterial pressure; SVR = systemic vascular resistance; PCWP = pulmonary capillary wedge pressure; ↑ = increase; → = no change; ↓ = decrease.)

advantage of dopamine as adjunctive therapy to volume repletion in hypotensive shock is its combination of inotropic, renal vasodilatory, and vasopressor effects.

Dopamine

Dopamine acts as both a direct and an indirect sympathomimetic agent. Direct and indirect stimulation of beta receptors results in positive inotropic effects,[4] while the pressor effects of dopamine are dependent upon the patient's catecholamine stores and indirect release of norepinephrine from adrenergic storage sites. Direct stimulation of renal dopaminergic receptors produces local vasodilation.

The pharmacologic effects of dopamine are dependent on the dose in μg/kg/min and the patient's initial hemodynamic status. Increased renal blood flow is typically seen at doses of 2 to 5 μg/kg/min, inotropic and chronotropic activity at 5 to 10 μg/kg/min, and alpha vasoconstrictive effects predominate at 10 to 15 μg/kg/min. The dose-response scheme depicted in Table 12–5 has evolved from studies of congestive heart failure.[6–8]

Predominant cardiovascular effects of dopamine include increased contractility, which is less than that seen with isoproterenol at equal μg/kg/min doses, and pressor effects which are less potent than levarterenol. Dopamine possesses the advantage over both of these agents of a direct action to increase renal blood flow at low doses.[5] Dopamine is also less chronotropic and arrhythmogenic than isoproterenol at equal inotropic doses.[9] Nevertheless, an increase in myocardial oxygen demand[10] may occur with increases in heart rate and contractility. While this increased demand may be offset by increased coronary blood supply secondary to increased mean arterial pressure and cardiac output, dopamine may increase infarct size in acute myocardial infarction.[11] Sodium diuresis has been demonstrated in congestive heart failure[6,12] and patients in the septic state[13] receiving dopamine.

The clinical use of dopamine is broad, including hypotension with hemody-

Table 12-5. Dose Ranges in μg/kg/min for Hemodynamic Effects of Dopamine
             and Dobutamine in Congestive Heart Failure.

	Alpha Vasoconstriction	Beta 1 Inotropic Activity	Beta 2 Peripheral Vasodilation	Dopaminergic Renal Vasodilation
Dopamine	≥ 8–10	5–10	2–7	2–5
Dobutamine	> 10–15	2–10	2–10	—

namic compromise, cardiogenic shock, cardiac support following cardiopulmonary bypass, and inotropic circulatory support in septic shock. Different pathophysiologic states of shock may respond differently to dopamine. For example, shock states associated with high systemic vascular resistance may respond unfavorably to dopamine since vasoconstrictive effects may further increase impedance to ventricular outflow, compromise renal blood flow, and exacerbate preexisting peripheral hypoperfusion. Effects on systemic vascular resistance and urine output must thus be monitored frequently when dopamine is used in this setting. In contrast, dopamine offers a beneficial hemodynamic profile in hypodynamic septic shock associated with hypotension and low systemic vascular resistance by acting to increase both coronary perfusion and cardiac output. These patients may require and tolerate higher doses of dopamine than other types of shock.[13,14]

Since the pressor effects of dopamine are dependent on the patient's catecholamine stores, prolonged infusions may result in tachyphylaxis as these stores are depleted. In such instances in which continued vasopressor administration is indicated to maintain coronary perfusion, levarterenol is a rational alternative to raise mean arterial pressure since it is a direct-acting vasoconstrictor.

Peripheral necrosis and gangrene have been reported following dopamine administration.[15,16] Patients at increased risk include those with diabetes mellitus, untreated disseminated intravascular coagulation, and pre-existing hypovolemia. In addition, peripheral necrosis is associated with high doses and peripheral vein administration of highly concentrated solutions. A central vein is thus preferred for administration. If peripheral extravasation of dopamine occurs, the intravenous site should be irrigated with normal saline solution and 5 to 10 mg of phentolamine infiltrated locally to block alpha-mediated vasoconstriction.

Dopamine has been observed to increase pulmonary artery wedge pressure in several clinical studies involving left ventricular heart failure,[7,17,18] cardiogenic shock,[19-21] septic shock,[13,22-24] and cardiopulmonary bypass patients.[25,26] This increase in pulmonary capillary pressure has been variably associated with an alpha vasoconstrictor-induced increase in pulmonary vascular resistance in animal studies.[27,28] In a study of 10 patients with pulmonary hypertension and 11 patients with normal pulmonary artery pressure,[29] dopamine raised pulmonary capillary wedge pressure significantly only in the latter group. In both groups, pulmonary artery pressure increased without a concomitant increase in pulmonary vascular resistance or right atrial pressure. Holloway, et al.[29] postulated that pulmonary pressure rose secondary to increased output from the right heart rather than pulmonary vasoconstriction. Alternatively, Regnier, et al.[22] suggested that either an increased venous return or afterload accounted for the increased pulmonary capillary wedge pressure seen in patients in septic shock. The mechanism and clinical significance of this increase in pulmonary wedge pressure are unclear. However, this effect may potentially decrease the value of this measurement for assessing preload and intravascular volume status. In addition, right atrial pressure may not be elevated in clinical states of pulmonary congestion in patients in septic shock with elevated pulmonary artery pressure following dopamine therapy, suggesting that central venous pressure is unreliable as a monitoring tool in this setting.[22]

Dobutamine

Dobutamine acts by a direct mechanism independent of catecholamine stores.[5] Dobutamine is an inotropic agent that possesses moderate beta 1 selectivity and produces less beta 2 vasodilation than isoproterenol. Dopaminergic receptors are not stimulated by dobutamine; however, increased renal blood flow may often be seen secondary to improved cardiac output. Doses of 2 to 10 μg/kg/min will primarily result in a positive inotropic effect and improved cardiac output, which may be associated with slight vasodilation and decreased systemic vascular resistance.[7,20] Alpha vasoconstrictive activity is dose-dependent and may be seen at doses of dobutamine greater than 10 to 15 μg/kg/min.

Dobutamine possesses several advantages over dopamine and isoproterenol. The decrease in systemic vascular resistance after dobutamine is given is much less than that seen with isoproterenol. Dobutamine lacks significant chronotropic effects in therapeutic doses; however, an increase in heart rate similar to that seen with dopamine has been reported in cardiopulmonary bypass studies.[25,30] At higher doses, dobutamine loses its cardioselectivity, and its arrhythmogenic potential increases.

Dobutamine is a more pure inotrope than dopamine, lacking vasoconstrictor effects in therapeutic doses. At equipotent inotropic doses, dobutamine has little effect on blood pressure in contrast to the pressor effects of dopamine and the vasodilatory effects of isoproterenol, which may actually decrease blood pressure. At doses greater than 15 μg/kg/min, the vasoconstrictor effects of dobutamine may approach those of dopamine. Dermal necrosis has been reported with high doses of dobutamine secondary to excessive vasoconstriction.[31]

In the absence of severe hypotension, dobutamine has clinical utility in states of decreased cardiac output secondary to ventricular dysfunction and may be used as an alternative to dopamine when elevated pulmonary artery wedge pressure exists. The dose range for dobutamine is 2 to 15 μg/kg/min. Central vein administration is recommended to avoid extravasation and dermal necrosis. In severe hypotension with cardiac compromise, dopamine or levarterenol is preferred to maintain coronary perfusion pressure. Once blood pressure is stabilized, dobutamine may be added for additional inotropic support.

Isoproterenol

Isoproterenol is a pure, nonselective beta-agonist with equal beta 1 and beta 2 activity. This agent possesses potent inotropic, vasodiliatory, and chronotropic actions. Isoproterenol reduces systemic vascular resistance and may induce a marked drop in blood pressure. Although peripheral perfusion is increased, vasodilation does not occur in the renal vasculature.[4]

Clinical use of isoproterenol in shock is limited by its arrhythmogenic actions, vasodilator effects on blood pressure and preload, and increased myocardial oxygen requirements. Isoproterenol may induce a "coronary steal" syndrome by a fall in diastolic blood pressure and may increase infarct size in acute myocardial infarction. Its therapeutic use should be limited to chronotropic stimulation in heart block and severe bradycardia resistant to atropine.

Inadequate experience exists with the use of isoproterenol as an inotrope in most shock states. If isoproterenol is initiated, infusions should be started at 0.5 μg/min and titrated slowly upward until the desired effect on cardiac output is achieved. This will usually require an infusion rate within 1 to 5 μg/min. Infusion rates are often limited by increased heart rate and the development of ectopic beats.

Epinephrine

Epinephrine is a mixed alpha, beta 1, and beta 2 agonist that possesses inotropic and chronotropic effects. Pressor effects are greater on systolic than on diastolic blood pressure, resulting in an increased pulse pressure. The effect on diastolic blood pressure is variable, depending on whether alpha or beta 2 effects on blood vessels predominate. A biphasic response is seen with epinephrine depending on the dose used. At low doses beta effects predominate resulting in vasodilation, while high doses are associated with alpha vasoconstriction and increased systemic vascular resistance. Blood flow to the renal and cutaneous beds is decreased.

Epinephrine may be used clinically as a vasopressor, a bronchodilator, and an inotrope after cardiopulmonary bypass. Precautions with its use include its arrhythmogenic potential, increased myocardial oxygen requirements, and excess vasoconstriction at higher doses. Because the pressor effects of epinephrine on diastolic blood pressure are variable, other agents may be preferred to increase coronary perfusion pressure. The dose of epinephrine ranges from 0.01 to 0.1 μg/kg/min.

Levarterenol

Levarterenol (norepinephrine) predominantly possesses alpha adrenergic actions and produces moderate beta 1 cardiac stimulation. Alpha vasoconstriction results in potent pressor effects on both diastolic and systolic blood pressure. Cardiac contractility may be increased by beta stimulation; however, cardiac output is often unchanged or decreased secondary to a baroceptor-mediated decrease in heart rate. Vasoconstriction occurs in renal, cutaneous, and skeletal vasculature while sparing the cerebral and coronary arteries.

Levarterenol is used in clinical shock states to restore and maintain mean arterial pressure at the critical level required for coronary perfusion. Its direct action as a catecholamine offers an advantage as a pressor agent when tachyphylaxis to dopamine is encountered in the catecholamine-depleted patient.

The dose range of levarterenol is 1 to 16 μg/min. Levarterenol has arrhythmogenic potential, especially during anesthesia with halothane or cyclopropane when the myocardium is sensitized to the effects of catecholamines. Gangrene and peripheral necrosis occur with higher frequency than they do with dopamine.

Phenylephrine

Phenylephrine is a pure alpha agonist that possesses potent vasoconstrictor properties and pressor effects. Phenylephrine is a direct-acting agent similar to norepinephrine except it lacks beta-mediated inotropic and chronotropic effects on the heart. Phenylephrine may occasionally be used as an alternative vasopressor to norepinephrine. The dose is variable, ranging from 20 to 200 μg/min.

Metaraminol

Metaraminol is a vasopressor that acts both directly and indirectly by release of norepinephrine stores. This agent is much less potent than levarterenol in its pressor effects. Dosage is initiated at 1 μg/min and titrated to effect. Since the introduction of newer vasopressors, this drug is seldom indicated.

CLINICAL EXPERIENCE WITH SYMPATHOMIMETIC AGENTS IN SHOCK

In contrast with early studies of sympathomimetic agents in shock, which consisted of heterogeneous population samples, more recent studies have investigated homogeneous models of shock including either septic, postoperative, or cardiogenic shock. Favorable and unfavorable effects of pharmacologic agents differ depending on the underlying pathophysiologic shock state.

Septic Shock

Vasoactive agents are used in septic shock to improve circulatory function and increase effective perfusion of vital organs. The effect of vasoactive agents on the morbidity and mortality of septic shock is inadequately documented.[32]

Inotropic agents are used to support the myocardium during stages of septic shock in which cardiac output is impaired. Despite adequate plasma volume expansion, ventricular function and contractility may fail to increase, an observation that has been correlated with increased mortality.[32,33]

Dopamine is the preferred inotrope in hypodynamic septic shock with severe hypotension to improve cardiac output, raise mean arterial pressure, and maintain systemic vascular resistance.[13,22–24,34] More clinical experience has accumulated with dopamine in septic shock than any other inotrope. In contrast to dopamine, isoproterenol decreases systemic vascular resistance and left ventricular filling pressure.[22]

Dopamine may increase pulmonary wedge pressure in septic shock.[22,24] In addition, both dopamine and dobutamine have been shown to increase the right to left pulmonary shunt in septic shock.[22,24,35] Nevertheless, the arterial oxygen tension in these studies was not significantly changed, indicating that dopamine and dobutamine may increase oxygen transport by improved cardiac output.

Cardiopulmonary Bypass

Epinephrine, dobutamine, and dopamine are all effective inotropes for postoperative cardiac support.[30] A dose-dependent increase in cardiac index has been demonstrated for dopamine and dobutamine in dosages from 5 to 15 μg/kg/min and 2 to 15 μg/kg/min, respectively.[30,36] Isoproterenol significantly increased heart rate to a greater extent than equipotent inotropic doses of dobutamine or dopamine.[25,37]

Dopamine and dobutamine possess similar hemodynamic profiles in postoperative cardiopulmonary bypass patients, including increased cardiac index, without a significant change in systemic vascular resistance in doses up to 10 μg/kg/min.[25] Inotropic selectivity of dobutamine has not been a consistent finding in cardiopulmonary bypass studies.[25,30] Chamberlain, et al.[25] demonstrated a significantly higher increase in heart rate for dobutamine versus dopamine at 10 μg/kg/min. Salomon, et al.[26] reported superior effects of dobutamine over dopamine in 20 patients after coronary artery bypass operations. In contrast to cardiopulmonary bypass studies demonstating dose-dependent increases in cardiac output, the maximum inotropic effect of dopamine in this study occurred at 5 μg/kg/min. Neither agent was associated with a significant increase in heart rate; however, patients were receiving therapeutic doses of beta-blocking agents, which may have altered the pharmacologic properties of the inotropic agents. Studies of inotropes in postoperative cardiopulmonary bypass patients have not consistently demonstrated advantages of dobutamine over dopamine.

Cardiogenic Shock

The ability of inotropes favorably to affect cardiac output in cardiogenic shock[10,20,21,38] and left ventricular failure[6,7,17,18] is well established. Dopamine and dobutamine possess an improved hemodynamic profile over isoproterenol in that they tend not to increase heart rate and myocardial oxygen demand or reduce mean arterial pressure as greatly.[7,10,17,18] Based upon the pharmacologic effects outlined earlier, dopamine is comparable to a combined inotrope and vasopressor (or vasodilator) depending on the dose administered, whereas dobutamine is an inotrope with minimal effects on blood pressure. Dopamine may thus significantly increase mean arterial pressure,[10,18,20,38] and therefore is the preferred agent in cardiogenic shock associated with severe hypotension. In normotensive patients with congestive heart failure and elevated peripheral vascular resistance caused by increased sympathetic tone, further increases in systemic vascular resistance may be seen with dopamine doses as low as 8 μg/kg/min.[7] This may adversely influence left ventricular performance, decrease cardiac output, and increase oxygen demand. In addition, dopamine may increase pulmonary capillary wedge pressure, an effect not seen with dobutamine.[7,17,18,20–25] In view of dopamine's potentially adverse effects on myocardial oxygen demand[10] and cardiac rhythm,[7] the optimal dose in cardiogenic shock is 5 to 7.5 μg/kg/min, although higher doses may be required to raise mean arterial pressure.

Dobutamine is the preferred inotrope in severe left ventricular failure associated with high peripheral resistance without hypotension, possessing less effect on heart rate, pulmonary capillary wedge pressure, systemic vascular resistance, and arrhythmogenicity than dopamine at equipotent inotropic doses.[7,17,20]

Combined inotropic therapy with dobutamine and dopamine resulted in a superior hemodynamic profile over either agent alone in a study of cardiogenic shock.[20] Inotropic therapy with dopamine 15 μg/kg/min, dobutamine 15 μg/kg/min, or combined therapy with both agents at 7.5 μg/kg/min were compared in eight patients. Whereas dopamine markedly increased pulmonary capillary wedge pressure, combined inotropic therapy raised mean arterial pressure and cardiac index with no effect on pulmonary wedge pressure. Dobutamine alone raised cardiac index and decreased pulmonary wedge pressure slightly, but failed to increase mean arterial pressure.

Combined inotropic and vasodilator therapy has also been used in cardiogenic shock[39] and severe left ventricular pump failure following acute myocardial infarction[40,41] with favorable hemodynamic effects. The effects of combined dopamine and nitroprusside were studied in eight patients with clinical evidence of cardiogenic shock associated with hypotension following acute myocardial infarction.[39] Once mean arterial pressure was raised to 80 to 90 mm Hg with dopamine, nitroprusside was added, resulting in decreased pulmonary capillary wedge pressure, increased cardiac index, decreased systemic vascular resistance, and an average drop in mean arterial pressure to 75 mm Hg.

VASODILATORS IN SHOCK

The use of vasodilators to increase cardiac output is well accepted in the management of congestive heart failure and left ventricular failure following acute myocardial infarction associated with increased left ventricular filling pressure and increased afterload.[42] Animal models of endotoxic and hemorrhagic shock indicate increased survival with the use of alpha blocking agents; however, these studies are difficult to extrapolate to human shock states.[43,44] While vasodilators may have a potential role in the therapy for noncardiogenic shock in patients with cardiac impairment associated with increased systemic vascular resistance or pulmonary edema, inadequate clinical experience exists to recommend their routine use at this time.

The rationale for vasodilator use has evolved from animal studies that indicate that excessive endogenous catecholamines released in shock states contribute to mortality and the development of irreversible shock. It has been proposed that the impaired cardiac function, increased systemic vascular resistance, and hypoperfusion that commonly accompany shock states would benefit from therapy aimed at increased peripheral perfusion and antagonism of the compensatory catecholamine outflow. Vasodilators are postulated to increase cardiac output by afterload reduction in addition to augmenting peripheral blood flow. However, vasodilators may decrease preload by increased venous capacitance and thus decrease cardiac output in shock states associated with decreased or normal filling pressure. In addition, therapeutic use of vasodilators may potentially decrease diastolic blood pressure and coronary perfusion, may counteract the body's natural compensation to maintain blood flow to critical organs, and is contraindicated in patients with severe hypotension.

Phenoxybenzamine

Phenoxybenzamine is an alpha receptor antagonist that predominantly blocks alpha 1 receptors.[4] The predominant hemodynamic effects following its administration are vasodilation, decreased systemic vascular resistance, and decreased diastolic blood pressure.[4] Effects on blood pressure and regional blood flow are dependent on the level of adrenergic tone present, the intravascular volume status, and the degree of alpha receptor predominance in a given vascular bed. Administration of phenoxybenzamine to hypovolemic patients will result in a precipitous drop in blood pressure, although in vasoconstricted states renal blood flow may be increased. Left ventricular filling pressure may decrease secondary to increased venous capacitance and arteriolar vasodilation.

Phenoxybenzamine was first used in the clinical treatment of shock in the early 1960s.[43] Despite the fact that it has been more than 20 years since this original report, no controlled, prospective, blinded trials have been reported. Support for the use of alpha adrenergic blocking agents in shock is limited to animal studies and clinical case reports.

Phenoxybenzamine is used investigatively in the treatment of shock, administered as a 1 mg/kg intravenous infusion over one hour.[4] Potentially adverse effects include sedation and the risk of a marked drop in blood pressure. In addition, phenoxybenzamine is not titratable and requires vigorous intravascular volume loading to prevent hypotension.

Phentolamine

Phentolamine is an alpha antagonist that blocks both alpha 1 and alpha 2 receptors.[4,45] Therapeutic doses of phentolamine result in decreased systemic vascular resistance, vasodilation, and tachycardia. Phentolamine possesses potent cardiostimulant effects and may predispose to cardiac arrhythmias.[4] Tachycardia may occur by a reflex mechanism in response to vasodilation. Additionally, presynaptic alpha 2 blockade suppresses the autoinhibitory effect of norepinephrine on neurotransmitter release, resulting in unopposed beta-mediated effects of excess norepinephrine.[45]

Phentolamine has been used in severe left ventricular failure following acute myocardial infarction with favorable effects on systemic vascular resistance and cardiac index.[46,47] This agent is less than ideal as a vasodilator, since it is not titratable and possesses potent chronotropic effects.

Nitroprusside

Nitroprusside is a titratable vasodilator that directly relaxes arteriolar smooth muscle. The vasodilatory effects of nitroprusside result in decreased preload and afterload, lowering pulmonary wedge pressure and decreasing mean arterial pressure.

Although nitroprusside has been advocated in the treatment of severe left ventricular failure following acute myocardial infarction,[48,49] few studies have specifically addressed its use in clinical states of cardiogenic shock. Nitroprusside possesses a favorable hemodynamic profile for states associated with hypertension, excessive systemic vascular resistance, and pulmonary congestion. Patients in a state of cardiogenic shock by definition have hypotension in addition to clinical signs of decreased perfusion and would not be expected to benefit from further reduction in arterial pressure. Prior stabilization of mean arterial pressure with dopamine and subsequent use of nitroprusside may combine the beneficial hemodynamic effects of nitroprusside, while maintaining an adequate arterial blood pressure.[33]

CORTICOSTEROIDS

The use of steroids in shock has been the subject of controversy for over 30 years. Steroids are thought to owe their beneficial effects in septic shock and acute respiratory distress syndrome to several mechanisms, including their ability to inhibit platelet and granulocyte aggregation, inhibit the release of vasoactive kinins and peptides, and stabilize lysosomal enzymes.[50]

An analysis of studies of steroids in shock before 1971 demonstrated a lack of prospective, double-blind, controlled trials and indicated the need for improved trial design to evaluate the effects of steroids on morbidity and mortality in septic shock.[51] Investigation of steroids in this setting is confounded by the presence of multiple disease states in patients, differences between patients in the hemodynamic stages of shock, and variation in virulence of the responsible bacterial pathogens.

A well-designed, prospective, randomized trial of 172 patients with septic shock reported a reduction in mortality from 38.4 to 10.4% in patients treated with high doses of cortocosteroids.[52] Steroids used during this eight-year study included methylprednisolone 30 mg/kg or dexamethasone 3 mg/kg. Information was appropriately specified for diagnostic criteria, severity of shock, and the underlying disease states. Although the treatment groups were generally well matched for underlying disease states and antibiotic therapy, the study samples consisted largely of patients with neoplastic diseases, immunosuppression, and concurrent chemotherapy. It has been suggested that this group of patients may receive the largest benefit from steroid therapy, and that patients with septic shock associated with peritonitis or soft tissue infections may not benefit as greatly.[53]

Lucas and Ledgerwood[53] studied 48 patients with severe sepsis and hypotension in a prospective, nonblinded, random trial of dexamethasone 2 mg/kg followed by a continuous infusion of 2 mg/kg/day for 48 hours. The patients included in this study consisted predominantly of those having peritonitis, excluding patients with neoplastic disease or concurrent chemotherapy. Steroid treatment produced no significant effects on morbidity and mortality of septic shock in this model. Statistically significant pulmonary shunting and decreased arterial oxygen tension were demonstrated in the steroid group; however, clinically significant pulmonary deterioration was not evident.

The use of steroids in hypovolemic shock has largely been limited to animal studies. Although improved survival has been demonstrated in animal models, Lucas and Ledgerwood[54] were unable to demonstrate improved survival rates in a clinical study of 114 patients with hypovolemic shock caused by blood loss and trauma. As in their investigation of septic shock, steroid use was associated with an increase in right to left pulmonary shunt and a decrease in arterial oxygen tension.

In ten patients with shock lung syndrome, therapy with 30 mg/kg methylprednisolone every six hours for 48 hours was associated with improved arterial oxygen tension and a 10% mortality.[55] While this is considerably lower than the 60 to 90% mortality historically associated with the shock lung syndrome,[55] the problems in using historical controls for this type of study are readily acknowledged.

The dosage regimens most often used in the treatment of septic shock include a single or repeated dose of methylprednisolone 30 mg/kg or dexamethasone 3 to 6 mg/kg. Complications of short-term therapy with steroids appear low in studies of septic shock. Schumer[52] reported that psychosis and gastrointestinal ulceration occurred in 1 and 2% of steroid patients, respectively, which was not significantly different from the control group. Other potential complications of steroid therapy are decreased wound healing and increased susceptibility to infection. The greatest disadvantage of steroid use in the treatment of shock may well be their high cost.

NALOXONE

Evidence has accumulated to support a role of beta-endorphins, which are endogenous opiate-like peptides, in the mediation of hypotension in shock states. Animal studies in hypovolemic and endotoxic shock models have demonstrated reversal of hypotension and increased survival rates with naloxone and outlined its dose-dependent pressor effects.[56] Naloxone is an opiate antagonist that blocks both endogenous and exogenous agonists of opiate receptors. In normal volunteers,[57] the plasma half-life of naloxone is 60 minutes.

Clinical experience with naloxone in shock is largely confined to case reports[58-61] and a few controlled clinical trials in septic shock. Although transient increases in systolic blood pressure and pulse pressure have been reported following naloxone administration, improvement in mortality has not been demonstrated.[62-64] Peters, et al.[62] reported a 45% increase in systolic blood pressure in eight of eleven patients in septic shock with prolonged hypotension. The transient increase in blood pressure lasted at least 45 min after administration of 0.4 mg to 1.2 mg naloxone. Three patients in septic shock who did not respond to naloxone had previously received corticosteroids. Peters, et al. postulated that steroid therapy interfered with the effect of naloxone by suppressing beta-endorphin release from the pituitary gland.

In a study of ten patients in a state of septic shock, a single intravenous bolus of naloxone 0.3 mg/kg produced a significant increase in blood pressure, which peaked in 15 min in 50% of patients. Two patients who responded to naloxone were receiving chronic high-dose steroid therapy. Only one out of ten patients lived.[63]

Hemodynamic effects of naloxone were studied in a double-blind, prospective, randomized trial of 29 patients in septic shock. After two successive doses of 0.8 mg and 8 mg, transient increases in mean arterial pressure occurred, which peaked at 15 min and lasted 18 min. The higher dose did not add further significant improvement in blood pressure, and neither dose affected indices of cardiac output.[64]

Further study is warranted to determine if naloxone is equally effective in reversing hypotension in both gram-positive and gram-negative septic shock, to determine the effect of naloxone on mortality in a large study sample both with and without concurrent steroid therapy, and to determine the optimal dosing range for both intravenous bolus doses and continuous infusions. Since evidence suggests that a critical dose of naloxone is required to reverse hypotension in septic shock,[56] and the pressor effects of naloxone given by bolus injection are transient, study of continuous infusions of naloxone is warranted.

NEW DIRECTIONS

Although many pharmacologic modalities have been used for the clinical treatment of cardiogenic or septic shock with favorable hemodynamic effects, a decrease in mortality has not been consistently demonstrated. Current shock research is directed toward pharmacologic modalities that counter the progression to irreversible shock. Although many agents are being studied in animal models, little is known about the interactions of complex humoral and biochemical changes that contribute to the mortality of shock. Research is being conducted to decipher the role of the prostaglandin-arachidonic acid system, humoral vasoactive substances, and catecholamines in the pathophysiology of shock.

Considerable research has been conducted on the use of antiprostaglandin agents in animal endotoxic and peritonitic septic shock models.[65] Antiprostaglandin agents have been shown to reduce mortality when administered prophylactically or soon after the induction of shock.[65] More experience has been gained with the use of indomethacin;[65,66] however, other studies have demonstrated favorable results with aspirin[67] and ibuprofen.[68] Whether or not prostaglandins play a role in the genesis of irreversible shock is unknown; the exact pharmacologic mechanism of antiprostaglandin agents in improving survival has not been clearly demonstrated. In a sublethal baboon endotoxic model, both lidocaine and indomethacin improved survival, while only indomethacin inhibited the synthesis of prostaglandin PGF-2, a potent vasoconstrictor, suggesting another mechanism of improved survival.[68]

Paradoxically, both infusions of prostaglandins and prostaglandin inhibition have been shown to increase survival rates in animal shock models. Prostaglandins are potent vasoactive agents, each possessing unique pharmacologic properties.[69] PGI2 (prostacyclin),[70] a potent vasodilator, has been studied in various experimental shock models. The rationale for its use is to counter excessive sympathetic tone and increase peripheral perfusion. PGI2 has been postulated to decrease platelet aggregation,[70] protecting the lung from injury, and may inhibit the release of vasoactive substances.[69]

Preliminary investigations of calcium channel blockers are being conducted in animal hemorrhagic shock models. Calcium channel blockers may have favorable effects on systemic vascular resistance through smooth muscle relaxant properties. It has been proposed that calcium channel blockers may inhibit transsarcolemmal calcium influx and prevent the intracellular calcium overload that occurs in ischemic reperfusion models.[71]

REFERENCES

1. Ahlquist, R.P.: A study of adrenotropic receptors. Am. J. Physiol., *153*:586, 1948.
2. Lands, A.M., et al.: Differentiation of receptor systems activated by sympathomimetic amines. Nature, *214*:597, 1967.
3. Goldberg, L.I., Talley, R.C., and McNay, J.L.: The potential role of dopamine in the treatment of shock. Prog. Cardiovasc. Dis., *12*:40, 1969.
4. Gilman, A.G., Goodman, L.S., and Gilman, A. (Eds.): The Pharmacological Basis of Therapeutics. 6th Ed. New York, Macmillan Publishing Co., 1980.
5. Goldberg, L.I.: Cardiovascular and renal actions of dopamine: potential clinical applications. Pharmacol. Rev., *24*:1, 1972.
6. Beregovich, J.: Dose-related hemodynamic and renal effects of dopamine in congestive heart failure. Am. Heart J., *87*:550, 1974.
7. Leier, C.V., et al.: Comparative systemic and regional hemodynamic effects of dopamine and dobutamine in patients with cardiomyopathic heart failure. Circulation, *58*:466, 1978.
8. Stemple, D.R., Kleinan, J.H., and Harrison, D.C.: Combined nitroprusside-dopamine therapy in severe chronic congestive heart failure: dose-related hemodynamic advantages over single dose infusions. Am. J. Cardiol., *42*:267, 1978.
9. Talley, R.C., Goldberg, L.I., Johnson, C.E., and McNay, J.L.: A hemodynamic comparison of dopamine and isoproterenol in patients in shock. Circulation, *39*:361, 1969.
10. Mueller, H.S., Evans, R., and Ayers, S.M.: Effect of dopamine in hemodynamics and myocardial metabolism in shock following acute myocardial infarction in man. Circulation, *57*:361, 1978.
11. Reid, P.R., Pitt, B., and Kelly, D.T.: Effects of dopamine on increasing infarct area in acute myocardial infarction. Circulation, *46(Suppl. II)*:210, 1972.
12. Goldberg, L.I., McDonald, R.H., and Zimmerman, A.M.: Sodium diuresis produced by dopamine in patients with congestive heart failure. N. Engl. J. Med., *268*:1060, 1963.
13. De La Cal, M.A., et al.: Dose-related hemodynamic and renal effects of dopamine in septic shock. Crit. Care Med., *12*:22, 1984.
14. Drueck, C., Welch, G.W., and Pruitt, B.A.: Hemodynamic analysis of septic shock in thermal injury: treatment with dopamine. Am. Surg., *7*:424, 1978.
15. Goibranson, F.L., Lurie, L., Vance, R., and Vandell, R.: Multiple extremity amputations in hypotensive patients treated with dopamine. JAMA, *243*:1145, 1980.
16. Winkler, M.J., and Trunkey, D.D.: Dopamine gangrene. Am. J. Surg., *142*:588, 1981.
17. Loeb, H.S., Bredakis, J., and Gunnar, R.M.: Superiority of dobutamine over dopamine for augmentation of cardiac output in patients with chronic low output cardiac failure. Circulation, *55*:375, 1977.
18. Francis, G.S., Sharma, B., and Hodges, M.: Comparative hemodynamic effects of dopamine and dobutamine in patients with acute cardiogenic circulatory collapse. Am. Heart J., *103*:995, 1982.
19. Loeb, H.S., et al.: Acute hemodynamic effects of dopamine in patients with shock. Circulation, *64*:163, 1971.
20. Richard C., et al.: Combined hemodynamic effects of dopamine and dobutamine in cardiogenic shock. Circulation, *67*:620, 1983.
21. Timmis, A.D., Fowler, M.B., and Chamberlain, D.A.: Comparison of haemodynamic responses to dopamine and salbutamol in severe cardiogenic shock complicating acute myocardial infarction. Br. Med. J. (Clin. Res.), *282*:7, 1981.

22. Regnier, B., et al.: Hemodynamic effects of dopamine in septic shock. Int. Care Med., *3*:47, 1977.
23. Regnier, B., Safran, D., Carlet, J., and Teisseire, B.: Comparative haemodynamic effects of dopamine and dobutamine in septic shock. Int. Care Med., *5*:115, 1979.
24. Jardin, F., Gurdjian, F., Desfonds, P., and Margairaz, A.: Effect of dopamine on intrapulmonary shunt fraction and oxygen transport in severe sepsis with circulatory and respiratory failure. Crit. Care Med., *7*:273, 1979.
25. Chamberlain, J.H., Pepper, J.R., and Yates, A.K.: Dobutamine, isoprenaline and dopamine in patients after open heart surgery. Int. Care Med., *7*:5, 1980.
26. Salomon, N.W., Plachetka, J.R., and Copeland, J.G.: Comparison of dopamine and dobutamine following coronary artery bypass grafting. Ann. Thorac. Surg., *33*:48, 1981.
27. Harrison, D.C., Pirages, S., Robison, S.C., and Wintroub, B.U.: The pulmonary and systemic circulatory response to dopamine infusion. Br. J. Pharmacol., *37*:618, 1969.
28. Mentzer, R.M., Alegre, C.A., and Nolan, S.P.: The effects of dopamine and isoproterenol on the pulmonary circulation. J. Thorac. Cardiovasc. Surg., *71*:807, 1976.
29. Holloway, E.L., Polumbo, R.A., and Harrison, D.C.: Acute circulatory effects of dopamine in patients with pulmonary hypertension. Br. Heart J., *37*:482, 1975.
30. Steen, P.A., et al.: Efficacy of dopamine, dobutamine, and epinephrine during emergence from cardiopulmonary bypass in man. Circulation, *57*:378, 1978.
31. Hoff, J.V., Beatty, P.A., and Wade, J.L.: Dermal necrosis from dobutamine. J.A.M.A., *243*:1145, 1980.
32. Winslow, E.J., et al.: Hemodynamic studies and results of therapy in 50 patients with bacteremic shock. Am. J. Med., *54*:421, 1973.
33. Vincent, J., Weil, M.H., Puri, V., and Carlson, R.W.: Circulatory shock associated with purulent peritonitis. Am. J. Surg., *142*:262, 1981.
34. Wilson, R.F., Sibbald, W.J., and Jaanimagi, J.L.: Hemodynamic effects of dopamine in critically ill septic patients. J. Surg. Res., *20*:163, 1976.
35. Jardin, F., et al.: Dobutamine: a hemodynamic evaluation in human septic shock. Crit. Care Med., *9*:329, 1981.
36. Sakamoto, T., and Yamada, T.: Hemodynamic effects of dobutamine in patients following open heart surgery. Circulation, *55*:525, 1977.
37. Tinker, J.H. et al.: Dobutamine for inotropic support during emergence from cardiopulmonary bypass. Anesthesiology, *44*:281, 1976.
38. Holzer, J., et al.: Effectiveness of dopamine in patients with cardiogenic shock. Am. J. Cardiol., *32*:79, 1973.
39. Keung, E.C., et al.: Effects of combined dopamine and nitroprusside therapy in patients with severe pump failure and hypotension complicating acute myocardial infarction. J. Cardiovasc. Pharmacol., *2*:113, 1980.
40. Awan, N.A., et al.: Effect of combined nitroglycerin and dobutamine infusion in left ventricular dysfunction. Am. Heart J., *106*:35, 1983.
41. Miller, R.R., et al.: Combined dopamine and nitroprusside therapy in congestive heart failure. Circulation, *55*:881, 1977.
42. Forrester, J.S., Diamond, G., Chatterjee, M.B., and Swan, H.J.C.: Medical therapy of acute myocardial infarction by application of hemodynamic subsets. N. Engl. J. Med., *295*:1404, 1976.
43. Nickerson, M.: Sympathetic blockade in the therapy of shock. Am. J. Cardiol., *12*:619, 1963.
44. Lillehei, R.C., Longerbeam, J.K., and Bloch, J.H.: Physiology and therapy of bacteremic shock: experimental and clinical observations. Am. J. Cardiol., *12*:599, 1963.
45. Saeed, M., Sommer, O., Holtz, J., and Bassenge, E.: α-Adrenergic blockade by phentolamine causes α-adrenergic vasodilation by increased catecholamine release due to presynaptic α-blockade. J. Cardiovasc. Pharmacol., *4*:44, 1982.
46. Kelly, D.T., et al.: Use of phentolamine in acute myocardial infarction associated with hypertension and left ventricular failure. Circulation, *67*:729, 1973.
47. Majid, P.A., Sharma, B., and Taylor, S.H.: Phentolamine for vasodilator treatment of severe heart failure. Lancet, *2*:719, 1971.
48. Franciosa, J.A., et al.: Improved left ventricular function during nitroprusside infusion in acute myocardial infarction. Lancet, *1*:650, 1972.
49. Chatterjee, K., et al.: Effects of vasodilator therapy for severe pump failure in acute myocardial infarction on short-term and late prognosis. Circulation, *53*:797, 1976.
50. Nicholson, D.P.: Corticosteroids in the treatment of septic shock and the adult respiratory distress syndrome. Med. Clin. North Am., *67*:717, 1983.
51. Weitzman, S., and Berger, S.: Clinical trial design in studies of corticosteroids for bacterial infections. Ann. Intern. Med., *81*:36, 1974.
52. Schumer, W.: Steroids in the treatment of clinical septic shock. Ann. Surg., *184*:333, 1976.
53. Lucas, C.E., and Ledgerwood, A.M.: The cardiopulmonary response to massive doses of steroids in patients with septic shock. Arch. Surg., *119*:537, 1984.

Table 13-1.   Etiologic Classification of Shock.

Hypovolemia
Cardiac failure
Bacteremia
Hypersensitivity
Neurogenic causes
Vascular obstructing lesion
Endocrine failure

common than hypovolemic shock. Shock can also occur as the result of massive fluid extravasation from large burns, peritonitis, or severe trauma. Hemorrhage, while an important factor, is less common in the infant and child than in the adult. Unique causes of hemorrhagic shock in the newborn include avulsion of the umbilical cord,[6] occult hemorrhage secondary to coagulation deficiencies and birth trauma,[7] transplacental hemorrhage from fetus to mother,[8] and twin-to-twin transfusion syndrome.[9] In addition, gradual fluid loss of 10% of body weight or greater often leads to symptoms of shock.

Cardiogenic shock is uncommon in pediatric patients, but may occur in children with acute arrhythmias or congestive heart failure, or in surgical patients after open heart surgery. The underlying defect is poor myocardial function despite adequate venous return, resulting in diminished cardiac output. A useful manual for managing patients with cardiac dysfunction, including the latest inotropic and chronotropic drug regimens, was written and is periodically updated by Behrendt and Austen.[10]

Sepsis is common in newborn infants, particularly premature and small-for-gestation infants, and shock should be suspected whenever sepsis is present. Bacteremic shock is caused by toxins released into the blood stream by microbial agents, most commonly endotoxins shed by gram-negative bacteria. Although the mechanism is not completely understood, it is known that endotoxin has a direct effect on the heart and blood vessels, increases vascular permeability, activates the coagulation system, severely deranges intermediary metabolism, and releases endogenous vasoactive substances including kinins,[11] endorphins,[12] and prostaglandins.[13]

Hypersensitivity shock is an extreme form of allergy leading to sudden vascular collapse and is often associated with asthma-like symptoms and severe bronchial constriction. It may be seen after injection of a drug or, less commonly, after an insect bite. The mechanism is a direct toxin effect plus loss of intravascular volume through tissue edema, leading to a hypovolemic type of shock.[1,7]

Neurogenic shock is the result of severe impairment of the central nervous system caused by trauma or by the administration of certain CNS-blocking or depressant drugs. The mechanism is a loss of vasomotor tone leading to circulatory failure because of a disproportion between vascular volume and vascular capacity. The intravascular volume is normal, but the capacity of the vascular system, especially on the venous side, is greatly expanded. This leads to a rapid fall in intravenous pressure and a diminished cardiac output. Remarkable improvement follows expansion of vascular volume.[1,7]

Vascular obstruction leading to shock is rare in pediatric patients, and includes pulmonary emboli,[14] spontaneous thrombosis of the inferior vena cava, renal veins, or distal aorta, and disseminated microvascular obstruction associated with consumption coagulopathy.[7] The common denominator is a major impediment to venous return resulting in decreased cardiac output.

Endocrine failure can result in shock, especially in adrenal, thyroid, and pituitary disorders. The common basic mechanism is a failure of cellular metabolism, with specific manifestations depending on the endocrine organ involved. An example is shock associated with pheochromocytoma, which is caused by excessive vasoconstriction and cardiac failure.

PHASES OF SHOCK

Although diverse in its causes, shock is progressive with common characteristics that lead to a useful division into three clinical phases: compensated, uncompensated, and irreversible. In the first phase, an insult has occurred, but compensatory mechanisms maintain an adequate blood pressure even though ominous shifts in tissue perfusion are apparent. The classic clinical manifestations of this stage include pallor, clammy skin with cool extremities, apprehension, and tachycardia—all a result of increased sympathetic activity. If the insult continues, or if compensatory mechanisms fail, the second phase ensues. In the second or uncompensated phase, blood is diverted to vital organs at the expense of reduced perfusion elsewhere, leading to regional ischemia, anaerobic metabolism, acidosis, and cellular injury. The patient becomes progressively obtunded as the circulation fails, poor skin turgor and dry mucous membranes signal fluid loss, and oliguria reflects diminished renal perfusion. Jaundice, petechiae, and peripheral or local edema may be part of the general appearance. Although major organs may be damaged at this phase, the deteriorating clinical situation is still amenable to corrective therapy. If this phase is left untreated, there is continued decompensation to the third or final phase of shock. i.e., irreversible tissue damage and death despite therapy that may temporarily return cardiovascular measurements to normal levels. "The skilled clinician recognizes Phase 1, reverses Phase 2, and prevents Phase 3."[1]

CLINICAL MANIFESTATIONS

The classic clinical manifestations of a patient in shock have already been alluded to in discussion of the phases of shock. Several special considerations are important for effective diagnosis and treatment of infants and children.

First, the infant with inadequate tissue perfusion may exhibit a unique syndrome called "sclerema neonatorum"—a diffuse, rapidly spreading, nonedematous, tallowlike hardening of the subcutaneous tissue during the first few weeks of life.[15] Until the mid-1960s, sclerema was looked upon as a rare disease of unknown cause with an almost uniformly fatal prognosis. Because of isolated reports of therapeutic success with steroids, antibiotics, and transfusions, steroid therapy was regarded as possibly specific for this unusual disorder. It now appears more likely that sclerema represents a state of poor perfusion in shock that may have a number of underlying causes.[16] The infant's subcutaneous tissues undergo a unique pathologic change, but otherwise the basic pathophysiology appears similar to shock syndromes in older patients.

Second, the pulse rate of a patient in shock is generally thought of as being elevated, although this is not always true, and has perhaps been overemphasized in adults as well as in children. Weil and Shubin[5] analyzed the heart rate of 25 patients with shock caused by myocardial infarction and found that the average rate was essentially the same as the rate in 125 patients in whom myocardial infarction was not complicated by shock. Evaluation of heart rate as an indicator of cardiovascular decompensation is even more complicated in infants, in whom the normal range is much more variable than in adults. Therefore, it is unreliable to use isolated determinations of an infant's heart rate as an index of impending circulatory collapse. Instances of sudden cardiovascular collapse have been reported without the warning of a noticeable elevation in heart rate, and brady-cardia usually develops in newborn infants during the early phase of shock.[17]

Third, reduced blood pressure is also generally regarded as an important com-ponent of the shock syndrome, although it is possible to have serious forms of shock with elevated blood pressure and associated increased vascular resistance. The infant or small child in a state of shock is difficult to evaluate inasmuch as blood pressure is technically difficult to measure accurately under conditions of circulatory decompensation. Moreover, the range of normal blood pressure changes considerably over the first two weeks of life, and mean pressures that would be considered shock levels for an adult can be normal pressures for an infant. Moss, et al. reported normal values obtained by umbilical artery catheter-ization that range from 44/24 to 84/54 mm Hg in premature infants, and 53/33 to 91/61 mm Hg in full-term infants.[18,19] This wide variability in normal values underscores the importance of following trends with serial pressure measure-ments because individual determinations may appear to be alarmingly low. The difficulties in clinical evaluation of such basic measurements as pulse and blood pressure emphasize the importance of precise methods of clinical monitoring.

MONITORING

Monitoring the pediatric patient in shock has the following four broad goals: 1. find the etiologic factors and cardiorespiratory pattern helpful in diagnosis, prog-nosis, and treatment; 2. permit continuous assessment of vital organ function; 3. provide a means of assessing the response to therapy; and 4. minimize the fre-quency of complications by detecting correctable problems early, thereby facili-tating rapid resolution.

Measurements for monitoring shock in infants and children are listed in Table 13–2. In general, these are the same measurements that are monitored in adults, but the technical aspects of measurement are frequently more difficult and exact-ing in the pediatric age group.

Standard blood pressure techniques with a cuff are unreliable in vasoconstricted infants. Because of the large range of extremity size in the pediatric age group, cuffs are frequently either too large or too small relative to the circumference of the extremity, and mechanical errors frequently occur.[20] In addition, intravascular arterial pressure measured directly by strain-gauge transducers may be consider-ably higher than cuff pressure obtained by auscultation or palpation due to the initially higher vascular resistance in some patients with shock, which dampens or eliminates the Korotkoff sounds or radial pulses.[21] Failure to recognize that low cuff pressure does not necessarily indicate arterial hypotension may lead to dan-gerous errors in therapy. Therefore, for a sick, unstable child with a need for fre-quent or continuous blood pressure monitoring, we insert a radial or umbilical arterial line and measure the pulse and mean arterial pressure directly.[22] The line

Table 13-2. Monitoring Infants and Children in Shock.

Essential		Desirable
Arterial pressure	Hematocrit	Pulmonary arterial pressure
Central venous pressure	WBC	Pulmonary wedge
Heart rate	Differential count	pressure
Continuous EKG	Platelets	Cardiac output
Respiratory rate	Clotting time	Lactic acid
Rectal temperature	Fibrinogen	Urine osmolality
Surface temperature	Partial thromboplastin time	Liver function tests
Abdomen	Sodium	Bilirubin
Extremities	Potassium	SGOT
Inspired O_2 concentration	Chloride	SGPT
Arterial Po_2	BUN	LDH
Arterial O_2 saturation	Creatinine	Amylase
Arterial Pco_2	Glucose	Transcutaneous O_2, CO_2
Arterial pH	Urine sugar	
Base excess	Bacterial cultures	
Fluid input	Blood	
Urine output	Urine	
Serial roentgenograms—chest	Sputum or tracheal	
and disease-specific	aspirate	
Daily weight	Specific local infections	

is also used for obtaining arterial blood gas tensions, pH, and other important blood chemistries with minimal discomfort to the patient.

Although central venous pressure (CVP) is technically more difficult to obtain in the infant than it is in the adult, it has the same clinical usefulness and probably the same physiologic significance in infants as it does in older children and adults. As has been emphasized by many authors, changes in central venous pressure can be used as an index of the heart's ability to pump the volume of fluid presented to it, and changes in CVP are not an index of the circulating blood volume, the cardiac output, or the size of the venous reservoir.[7,23,24] The subclavian approach is the usual route we use for central venous access. In newborn infants, subclavian cannulation is much more difficult and hazardous than in older children, and the external jugular vein or internal jugular vein is preferred for cannulation. It is rarely feasible to thread a catheter from the antecubital space up the basilic vein and into the superior vena cava in a newborn infant, although a proximal saphenous vein cutdown can be used for access to the inferior vena cava. Subclavian catheterization in an infant requires experience and careful attention to technical details if serious complications are to be avoided. A closed syringe and needle system must be used to avoid pneumothorax and air embolism. The insertion maneuver must not incorporate any change of needle direction once the skin has been penetrated, and the needle must be completely withdrawn before changing direction in order to avoid tearing vessels.

Although usually not required for management of shock except in pediatric cardiac patients or patients with cardiogenic shock from malignant sepsis, a pulmonary artery catheter (pediatric Swan-Ganz) can be placed to measure pulmonary arterial pressure and pulmonary wedge pressure (PWP). Since many patients with septic cardiogenic shock or cardiac dysfunction on the basis of congenital heart disease show poor correlation between pressure on the right side of the heart (CVP) and pressure on the left side of the heart (PWP), both measurements are needed to manage successfully volume replacement and inotropic and chronotropic drug administration.[25] In addition, these catheters are available with an incorporated thermister, which can be used for measuring cardiac output by use of the principle of thermodilution. The thermodilution technique compares favorably with more traditional methods for estimating cardiac output. Determinations can be made frequently and rapidly by injecting a room-termperature physiologic saline solution as the indicator.[26] No blood need be withdrawn from the patient, and small volumes of indicator cause no siginficant blood temperature changes even in patients of less than 10 kg body weight. These catheters are inserted percutaneously using the Seldinger technique with the femoral vein being the favored venous entry site. A portable fluoroscopic image intensifier facilitates placement, although measuring the pulmonary artery pressure and noting the difference after the catheter balloon tip is inflated and "floated" into the pulmonary wedge position is generally sufficient.[25]

Continuous monitoring of heart rate with an oscilloscope to display rhythm patterns and a cardiotachometer for ease of recording is essential for all shock patients. Reliable miniaturized adhesive leads are available and convenient even for premature infants.

Temperature monitoring is extremely important in infants and small children. Protection against thermal stress is often overlooked in the urgency of performing a variety of procedures and therapeutic maneuvers for a patient in shock. In addition to underdeveloped thermoregulatory mechanisms, premature infants have a much higher ratio of body surface area to total body mass than older children or adults, resulting in greater heat loss. Negative thermal balance can increase oxygen consumption and energy expenditure several times over and prove highly detrimental, defeating other therapeutic attempts to counter shock in an infant.[27] In addition to core temperature, surface temperature monitoring is important in that peripheral surface temperature is related to the state of perfusion. An infant well perfused has a small temperature gradient between the central portions of his or her body and the periphery.[7]

As with adults, frequent measurement of urine volume in infants and children is a useful index of renal perfusion and function. Infants and children are less likely than adults to retain urine on the basis of immobility or mechanical problems, and they void much more frequently (up to 20 times a day for a newborn infant). The more delicate and short urethera in the infant and small child makes complications of uretheral instrumentation and induced infection more likely. For these reasons, urine should be collected by external appliances when feasible. If this is unsatisfactory, however, catheter drainage must be used so that urine output can guide appropriate therapy.

Laboratory measurements should always include serial hematocrit readings, white blood cell counts, and differentials. Trends in the hematocrit reading are useful if one takes into account the time lag necessary for dilutional changes. Serum sodium, potassium, and chloride levels must be monitored for adequate fluid management. Blood urea nitrogen and serum creatinine levels are followed as part of the renal evaluation, and osmolarity, of both serum and urine, is desirable if available. Serial blood glucose determinations are particularly important in newborn infants in a state of shock because of the increased frequency of hypoglycemia and its complications. Arterial blood pH and gas partial pressure measurements are important to adjust respiratory settings and to provide measurements for correcting respiratory and metabolic acidosis. Blood lactate levels are also desirable as a measure of metabolic acidosis and as an index of the severity of shock. Ongoing evaluation of the coagulation system is important because of the known changes in coagulability with certain types of shock, and because heparin anticoagulant therapy may be essential in shock associated with disseminated intravascular coagulation.[28] Newborn infants, however, are rarely heparinized because of their increased risk of intracranial bleeding under conditions of physiologic stress. Serial cultures of blood, urine, and any other focus of infection must be followed carefully to guide antibacterial therapy. Serial chest roentgenograms and other appropriate roentgenologic imaging relevant to the clinical problem are always a part of shock management. Serial enzyme studies, including liver function tests, are a useful measurement of organ function and the severity of shock injury. In that infants and children have unique metabolic requirements because of their need for body growth and central nervous system development, we have started to measure resting energy expenditure by means of indirect calorimetry. This allows for provision of more appropriate calorie levels on a daily basis, and is particularly important during the patient's weaning from a respirator and during recovery from shock.[29]

TREATMENT

The usual approach of diagnosis first and treatment later may not be appropriate in shock. Rather, physicians must initiate orderly treatment immediately and gain insight into the cause of the patient's illness as the treatment proceeds. The child's own compensatory mechanism and defenses are generally inadequate to protect those organs with little margin for interruption of oxygen and nutrients. Cells deprived of oxygen and energy rapidly reach an irreversible state of injury, and cell death may proceed even if circulation is later restored. Therefore, a plan directed at the pathology common to all types of shock allows prompt treatment in this life-threatening condition. The plan includes first correcting hypoxia by appropriate airway management, stopping massive hemorrhage, gaining vascular access, splinting unstable fractures, administering fluids and appropriate drugs, identifying sepsis and starting antibiotics, considering early administration of steroids, and monitoring the patient as described in the previous section. Outlines for managing the most commonly encountered forms of shock, hypovolemic (including hemorrhagic) and septic, are provided in Figures 13–1 and 13–2.

Airway

The patient's airway and oxygen status should receive first and immediate attention. A low threshold should be maintained for early intubation. Early and frequent monitoring of arterial blood gases and pH is important. Abnormalities in oxygenation, ventilation, and acid-base balance can adversely affect cardiovascular performance and systemic oxygen transport, and should be corrected early and reassessed frequently.

The lung is one of the most sensitive organs in shock; respiratory failure can develop rapidly, and if support is delayed until respiratory failure is obvious, mortality is greatly increased.[30,31] The use of paralytic or sedative drugs will further reduce the oxygen cost of breathing as well as enhance positive pressure ventilation.[32]

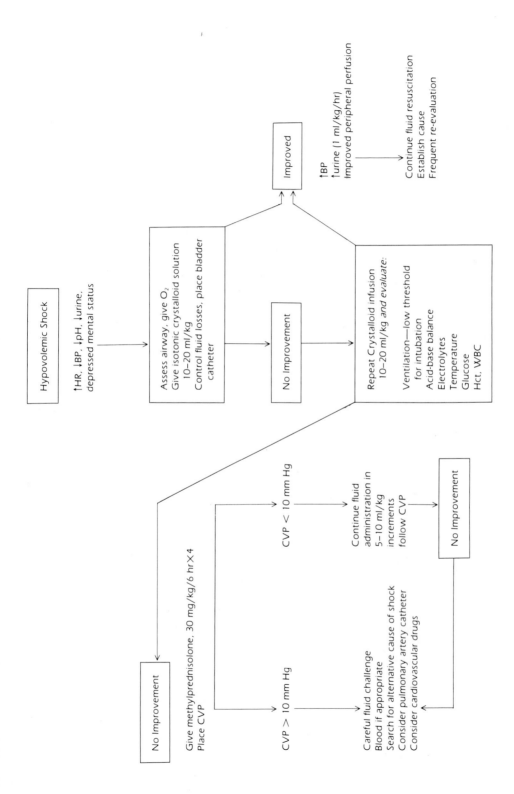

Fig. 13-1. Algorithm for the treatment of hypovolemic and hemorrhagic shock.

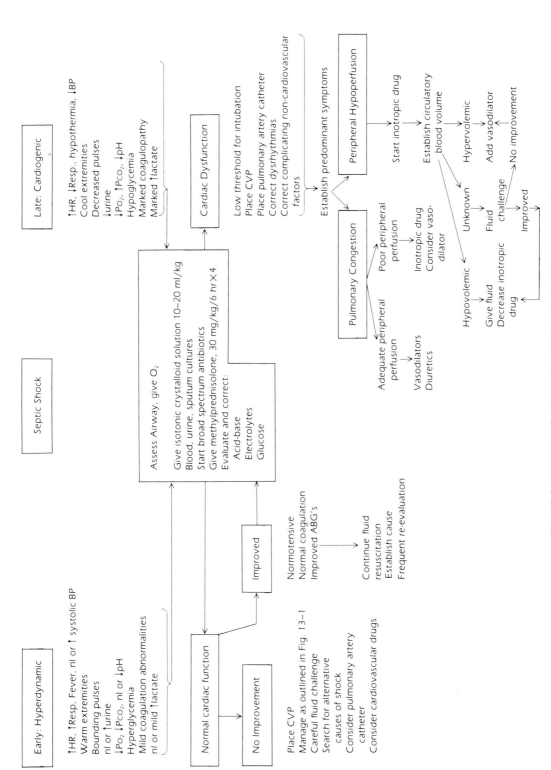

Early: Hyperdynamic

↑HR, ↑Resp. Fever, nl or ↑ systolic BP
Warm extremities
Bounding pulses
nl or ↑urine
↓Po₂, ↓Pco₂, nl or ↓pH
Hyperglycemia
Mild coagulation abnormalities
nl or mild ↑lactate

Septic Shock

Late: Cardiogenic

↑HR, ↓Resp. hypothermia, ↓BP
Cool extremities
Decreased pulses
↓urine
↓Po₂, ↑Pco₂, ↓pH
Hypoglycemia
Marked coagulopathy
Marked ↑lactate

Assess Airway, give O₂

Give isotonic crystalloid solution 10–20 ml/kg
Blood, urine, sputum cultures
Start broad spectrum antibiotics
Give methylprednisolone, 30 mg/kg/6 hr × 4
Evaluate and correct:
    Acid-base
    Electrolytes
    Glucose

Cardiac Dysfunction

Low threshold for intubation
Place CVP
Place pulmonary artery catheter
Correct dysrhythmias
Correct complicating non-cardiovascular
    factors
Establish predominant symptoms

Normal cardiac function

Improved

Normotensive
Normal coagulation
Improved ABG's

Continue fluid
resuscitation
Establish cause
Frequent re-evaluation

No Improvement

Place CVP
Manage as outlined in Fig. 13–1
Careful fluid challenge
Search for alternative
    causes of shock
Consider pulmonary artery
    catheter
Consider cardiovascular drugs

Pulmonary Congestion

Adequate peripheral
    perfusion

Vasodilators
Diuretics

Poor peripheral
    perfusion

Inotropic drug
Consider vaso-
    dilator

Hypovolemic

Give fluid
Decrease inotropic
    drug

Peripheral Hypoperfusion

Start inotropic drug

Establish circulatory
    blood volume

Unknown

Fluid
challenge

Hypervolemic

Add vasodilator

No improvement

Improved

Fig. 13–2. Algorithm for the treatment of septic shock.

Vascular Access

Simultaneously with airway management, adequate vascular access must be established. The traditional saphenous vein percutaneous insertion or cutdown in infants and small children is rapidly performed in experienced hands, and is reliable for the administration of blood and crystalloid at rapid rates. However, a central venous line is also desirable for ready measurement of central venous pressure (CVP), which is a helpful variable to follow during fluid resuscitation in a sick infant. Serial CVP measurements together with pulmonary wedge pressures obtained from a balloon-tipped pulmonary artery catheter are necessary for successful treatment of patients in the later phases of shock. As has already been described, the variability and potential unreliability of cuff blood pressures make it advisable to maintain a low threshold for inserting a radial or umbilical arterial line to follow mean arterial pressure accurately, and to have ready access for arterial blood gas and pH measurements.

Fluid Administration

Once dependable venous access has been established, a fluid challenge of 10 to 20 ml/kg is administered rapidly, and systemic arterial pressure response to the fluid challenge is assessed. If shock is on the basis of hemorrhage, a blood sample is sent immediately for typing and cross-matching, and blood is administered as soon as available. If systemic arterial pressure does not return to and remain at normal levels for the patient's age following the fluid challenge, additional volumes are infused and titrated against central venous pressure as outlined in Figures 13–1 and 13–2. Initially CVP levels are followed because of the greater ease in obtaining these measurements. If circulatory instability persists after achieving adequate CVP levels (10 to 15 mm Hg), however, a balloon-tipped, flow-directed pulmonary artery catheter should be placed to obtain pulmonary wedge pressure, which more accurately reflects filling pressure of the left heart and allows measurement of cardiac efficiency by thermodilution cardiac output.

As has been demonstrated by several investigators, one of the most important therapeutic maneuvers in shock is to restore an adequate circulatory volume with a physiologic salt solution that has some oncotic pressure and yet is readily reabsorbed from the extravascular "third space" once the integrity of leaky capillary beds has been restored.[33,34] Lactated Ringer's solution or lactated Ringer's solution with 5% albumin has the best therapeutic record as the initial fluid choice both clinically and experimentally.[17,33,35,36] However, subsequent fluid resuscitation must take into account what type of fluid has been lost, the specific underlying physiologic problems, the need for maintaining an adequate oxygen-carrying capacity for the patient, and the physiologic actions of each fluid type.[34]

Fluid replacement programs should include an allowance for extracellular deficit as well as extra free water in the form of glucose solution to enhance renal tubular flow and urinary output. This usually starts out as a calculated fluid infusion of 110 to 125% of the estimated losses, but may require a threefold or greater increase before changes in CVP are observed. While a CVP of 10 mm Hg is generally regarded as a safe upper limit before inotropic cardiotonic drugs are initiated, it is most important to look for a change in CVP in response to the fluid infusion rather than look for an absolute value.

Corticosteroids

If septic shock has been diagnosed or is highly suspected, then a large pharmacologic dose of short-acting steroids should be administered. Steroids act to stabilize cellular and subcellular (lysosomal) membranes, and block complement (C_{3A}, C_{5A}) as well as the synthesis of certain prostaglandins and endorphins recently found to be important mediators in shock.[37-40] An appropriate short-acting steroid dose is 30 mg/kg of methylprednisolone sodium succinate (Solumedrol).[41,42] This should be infused over 30 min and continued every 6 hr for no longer than 12 to 18 hr in order to avoid the deleterious tissue anti-inflammatory effects of steroids administered for longer periods. Broad-spectrum antibiotics, including an aminoglycoside, should be started at the same time. The same inflammatory systems responsible for defending against bacterial invasion into tissues can produce septic shock when activated intravascularly by bacterial endotoxins, and hence early steroid treatment is essential in order to be predictably effective.[43,44] Since there is no reliable biochemical marker for early septic shock, clinical findings are important and include extremes of body temperature, altered mental status, unexplained edema, leukopenia, thrombocytopenia, and tachypenea or hypoxemia with development of a metabolic acidosis. In the neonate thrombocytopenia is often the first evidence of impending septic shock.[45]

Other Drugs

The clinical history and physical examination will usually lead the physician to administer cardiac drugs if myocardial failure is the primary cause of shock. If the CVP is elevated in the presence of inadequate peripheral perfusion, specific measures must be directed toward improving myocardial efficiency. Any of the following may be indicated, depending on the clinical situation: increased inspired oxygen, drugs to correct an abnormal rhythm or rate, digitalis preparations,[10] isoproterenol,[7] or dopamine.[46] The latter two drugs stimulate cardiac and peripheral beta receptors that have positive inotropic and selective vasodilator effects, depending on the dose, which must be carefully regulated.[47] Dopamine is particularly useful in low doses (less than 10 μg/kg/min) to dilate renal and mesenteric vascular beds and in conjunction with appropriate volume therapy is effective in helping to restore renal and gastrointestinal circulation.[47,48] As has been alluded to previously, bicarbonate infusion in appropriately calculated doses is temporary, and immediate therapy is needed to acutely correct low pH so that myocardial contractility and systemic enzyme function can be optimized.[25] Bicarbonate rarely maintains arterial pH unless perfusion and oxygenation are simultaneously corrected.

Other promising drugs that have been shown to be effective for the treatment of shock in experimental or clinical situations are: naloxone (an endorphin antagonist),[49-52] antiserum to endotoxin,[53] indomethacin (a prostaglandin inhibitor),[54] ibuprofen (a prostaglandin inhibitor),[7,55,56] and prostacyclin.[57] The latter is a prostaglandin that, in contrast to a number of prostaglandins with deleterious inflammatory effects, exerts a number of beneficial effects in endotoxin shock in animals, including vasodilatation, stabilization of lysosomal membranes, reduction of platelet aggregation, and suppression of thromboxane formation.[57] Many of these new and experimental drugs have not yet been tried in immature experimental animals or in pediatric patients. As we learn more about the pathophysiology of the several types of shock in the pediatric age group, drugs with increasingly more specificity can be administered to block, reduce, or reverse the shock syndrome.

NEW DIRECTIONS

Continued progress in experimental shock research and clinical application in the pediatric age group will require increasingly more sophisticated monitoring devices and a means of identifying patients at risk for hypovolemic or septic shock at an earlier time, when they can be treated with a greater expectation of success. One of the new monitoring devices on the horizon for clinical application is the micro pH probe.[58] This probe allows constant read-out of tissue pH by a microprobe inserted percutaneously—a good indicator of tissue perfusion.

More sophisticated use of drugs to alleviate the shock syndrome is already happening, and as the role of specific mediators—certain prostaglandins, endorphins, complement factors, and endotoxins—become better understood, blocking agents will be developed to counteract their effects. For example, although no effective parenteral antiprostaglandin drugs are available for clinical use at present, they are being developed with the goal of maximizing the intravascular anti-inflammatory effect in the second phase of shock—especially septic shock—without impairing the host's tissue-based anti-inflammatory and immune mechanisms.[38] On the basis of experimental shock research, there is little question that large doses of short-acting steroids are effective in the first and early second phases of shock because they inhibit the synthesis and occupy the receptor sites of a number of deleterious prostaglandins, endorphins, and complement factors. The problem with the use of corticosteroids is that they are only effective early and briefly, and interfere with important host defenses, especially those against microbial invasion.[13]

When the usual medical means of treating shock in the newborn with severe respiratory distress have failed, we have placed the infant's lungs at complete rest by means of extracorporeal membrane oxygenation (ECMO), and have been encouraged by its success in carefully selected patients.[59]

An easily detectable marker of the shock syndrome is needed to help identify patients in the early phases. Serum assays for complement (C_{5A}) as an early marker have not lived up to expectations. However, another mediator, vasopressin, is currently being evaluated as a marker, since it has recently been shown to be elaborated in increased amounts by the central nervous system of dogs in early shock, (J. Cronenett and J.N. Sheagren, personal communication).

Thus, the most important new direction of shock therapy in all age groups is earlier identification of the patient who is in the process of having the shock syndrome develop, since the primary cause of a poor outcome is usually failure to institute therapy early enough. The identification of an early marker and the administration of specific antimediator drugs to infants and children in shock also holds the promise for greater success in the treatment of shock in the future.

REFERENCES

1. Stiehm, R., and Rich, K.: Recognition and management of shock in pediatric patients. Curr. Probl. Pediatr. *3(4)*:3, 1973.
2. Segar, W: The critically ill child: Salicylate intoxication. Pediatrics, *44*:444, 1969.

3. Schafir, M.: The management of acute poisoning by ferrous sulfate. Pediatrics, *27*:83, 1961.

4. Perkin, R., and Levin, D.: Shock in the pediatric patient, Part 1. J. Pediatr., *101*:163, 1982.

5. Weil, M.H., and Shubin H.: Diagnosis and Treatment of Shock. Baltimore, Williams & Wilkins, 1967.

6. Sheldon, R.: Management of perinatal asphyxia and shock. Pediatr. Ann., *6*:227, 1977.

7. Johnson, D.G.: Shock and its management. Ped. Clin. North Am., *16*:621, 1969.

8. Shiller, J: Shock in the newborn caused by transplacental hemorrhage from fetus to mother. Pediatrics, *20*:7, 1957.

9. Becker, A., and Glass, J.: Twin-to-twin transfusion syndrome. Am. J. Dis. Child., *106*:624, 1963.

10. Behrendt, D., and Austen, W.: Patient Care in Cardiac Surgery. 3rd Ed. Boston, Little, Brown and Co., 1980.

11. Hodes, H.L.: Care of the critically ill child: endotoxin shock. Pediatrics, *44*:248, 1969.

12. Carr, D.B., et al.: Endotoxin-stimulated opioid peptide secretion: Two secretory pools and feedback control in vivo. Science, *217*:845, 1982.

13. Sheagren, J.N.: Septic shock and corticosteroids. N. Engl. J. Med., *305*:456, 1981.

14. Buck, J.R., et al.: Pulmonary embolism in children. J. Pediatr. Surg., *16*:385, 1981.

15. Hughes, W.E., and Hammond, M.L.: Sclerema neonatorum. J. Pediatr., *32*:676, 1948.

16. Warwick, W.J., Ruttenberg, H.D., and Quie, P.G.: Sclerema neonatorum—a sign, not a disease. J.A.M.A., *1984*:680, 1963.

17. Strodel, W., et al.: The effect of various resuscitative regimens on hemorrhagic shock in puppies. J. Pediatr. Surg., *12*:809, 1977.

18. Moss, A.J., Liebling, W., and Adams, F.H.: The flush method for determining blood pressures in infants. II. Normal values during the first year of life. Pediatrics, *21*:950, 1958.

19. Moss, A.J., and Adams, F.H.: Problems of Blood Pressure in Childhood. Springfield, Ill., Charles C Thomas, 1962.

20. Steier, M.,: Neonatal and pediatric cardiovascular crisis. J.A.M.A., *235*:1105, 1976.

21. Cohn, J.: Blood pressure measurement in shock. J.A.M.A. *199*:118, 1967.

22. Coran, A.G.: Mechanical support and monitoring procedures in the pediatric surgery patient. *In* Manual of Preoperative and Postoperative Care, 3rd Ed. Edited by S.J. Dudrick, et al., Philadelphia, W.B. Saunders Co., 1983.

23. Weil, M.H., Shubin, H., and Rosoff, L.: Fluid repletion in circulatory shock. Central venous pressure and other practical guides. J.A.M.A. *192*:668, 1965.

24. Wilson, J.N., et al.: Central venous pressure in optimal blood volume maintenance. Arch. Surg., *85*:578, 1962.

25. Raphaely, R.C.: Shock. *In* Textbook of Pediatric Emergency Medicine. Edited by G.R. Fleisher, and S. Ludwig. Baltimore, Williams & Wilkins, 1983.

26. Callaghan, M.L., Weintraub, W.H., and Coran, A.G.: Assessment of thermodilution cardiac output in small subjects. J. Pediatr. Surg., *11*:629, 1976.

27. Adamsons, K., Jr., Gandy, G.M., and James, L.S.: The influence of thermal factors upon oxygen consumption of the newborn human infant. J. Pediatr. *66*:508, 1965.

28. Sonnenschein, H.: Endotoxin shock in infants and children. Med. Trial. Tech. Q., *19*:134, 1973.

29. Dechert, R., et al.: Measurement of resting energy expenditure in premature infants. J.P.E.N., *8*:100, 1984.

30. Aubier, M., Trippenbach, T., and Roussos, C.: Respiratory muscle fatigue during cardiogenic shock. J. Appl. Physiol., *51*:499, 1984.

31. Bone, R.: Treatment of severe hypoxemia due to the adult respiratory distress syndrome. Arch. Intern. Med., *140*:85, 1980.

32. Macklem, P.T.: Respiratory muscles: The vital pump. Chest, *78*:753, 1980.

33. Rowe, M., and Arango, A.: The choice of intravenous fluid in shock resuscitation. Pediatr. Clin. North Am., *22*:269, 1975.

34. Shoemaker, W.C., and Hauser, C.J.: Critique of crystalloid versus colloid therapy in shock and shock lung. Crit. Care Med. *7*:117, 1979.

35. Moss, G., et al.: Colloid or crystalloid in the resuscitation of hemorrhagic shock: A controlled clinical trial. Surgery, *89*:434, 1981.

36. Benner, J., et al.: Fluid resuscitation in live escherichia coli shock in puppies. J. Pediatr. Surg., *15*:527, 1980.

37. Sheagren, J.N.: Glucocorticoid therapy in the management of severe sepsis. *In* Septic Shock: New Concepts of Pathophysiology and Treatment. Edited by M.A. Sande, and R.K. Rott. New York, Churchill Livingstone, 1985.

38. Russo-Marie, F., Seillan, C., and Duval, D.L.: Glucocorticoids as inhibitors of prostaglandin systhesis. Bull. Europ. Pathophys. Resp., *17*:587, 1981.

39. Carr, D.B., et al.: Endotoxin-stimulated opioid peptide secretion: two secretory pools and feedback control in vivo. Science, *217*:845, 1982.

40. Greisman, S.E.: Experimental gram-negative bacterial sepsis: optimal methylprednisolone requirements for prevention of mortality not prevented by antibiotics. Proc. Soc. Exp. Biol. Med., *170*:436, 1982.

41. Hinshaw, L.B., et al.: Survival of primates in LD-100 septic shock following steroid/antibiotic therapy. J. Surg. Res., *2;8*:151, 1980.

42. Schumer, W.: Steroids in the treatment of clinical septic shock. Ann. Surg., *184*:333, 1976.

43. Connors, R., et al.: Combined fluid and corticosteroid therapy in septic shock in puppies. World J. Surg., *7*:661, 1983.

44. Hoffman, S.L., et al.: Reduction of mortality in chloramphenicol-treated severe typhoid fever by high-dose dexamethasone. N. Engl. J. Med., *310*:82, 1984.

45. Rowe, M.I., Buckner, D.M., and Newmark, S.: The early diagnosis of gram negative septicemia in the pediatric surgical patient. Ann. Surg, *182*:280, 1975.

46. Goldberg, L.: Drug therapy: Dopamine-clinical uses of an endogenous cathecholamine. N. Engl. J. Med., *291*:707, 1974.

47. Perkin, R., and Levin D.: Shock in the pediatric patient, part 2. J. Pediatr., *101*:319, 1982.

48. Driscoll, D., Gillette, P., and McNamara, D.: The use of dopamine in children. J. Pediatr., *92*:309, 1978.

49. Albert, S.A., et al.: Effects of naloxone in hemorrhagic shock. Surg. Gynecol. Obstet. *155*:325, 1982.

50. Faden, A.I., and Holaday, J.W.: Experimental endotoxic shock: the pathophysiologic function of endorphin and treatment with opiate antagonists. J. Infect. Dis., *142*:229, 1980.

51. Peters, W.P. et al.: Pressor effect of naloxone in septic shock. Lancet, *1*:529, 1981.

52. Brandt, N.J., et al.: Hyper-endorphin syndrome in a child with necrotizing encephalomyelopathy. N. Engl. J. Med., *303*:914, 1980.

53. Ziegler, E., et al.: Treatment of gram-negative bacteremia and shock with human antiserum to a mutant escherichia coli. N. Engl. J. Med., *307*:1225, 1982.

54. Fletcher, J.R., and Ramwell, P.W.: Indomethacin treatment following baboon endotoxin shock improves survival. Adv. Shock Res., *4*:103, 1980.

55. Jacobs, E.R., et al.: Ibuprofen in canine endotoxic shock. J. Clin. Invest., *70*:536, 1982.

56. Wise, W.C., et al.: Ibuprofen improves survival from endotoxic shock in the rat. J. Pharmacol. Exp. Ther., *215*:160, 1980.

57. Lefer, A.M., Tabas, J., and Smith, E.F.: Salutary effects of prostacyclin in endotoxic shock. Pharmacology, *21*:206, 1980.

58. Das, J.B., Indira, J.D., and Philippart, A.I.: End-tidal CO_2 and tissue pH in the monitoring of acid-base changes: A composite technique for continuous, minimally-invasive monitoring. J. Pediatr. Surg. *19*:758, 1984.

59. Bartlett, R.H., et al.: Extracorporeal circulation in neonatal respiratory failure: A prospective randomized study. Pediatrics (in press).

INDEX

Page numbers in *italics* indicate figures; page numbers followed by "t" indicate tables.